HLA and Disease

EDITED BY

Jean Dausset
Institut de recherches sur les maladies du sang,
Hôpital Saint-Louis, 2 Paris Xe

Arne Svejgaard
Tissue-Typing Laboratory of the Blood-Grouping Department,
State University Hospital of Copenhagen

Munksgaard
Copenhagen

North and South America:
Williams & Wilkins Co.
Baltimore

HLA AND DISEASE
1st edition

Cover by Poul Breuning

ISBN 87-16-02287-4

Published simultaneously in the USA by
Williams & Wilkins Co., Baltimore

Contents

Introduction

J. Dausset & A. Svejgaard

This book has been written following the First International Symposium on HLA and Disease held in Paris in June 1976, under the auspices of INSERM (Institut National de la Santé et de la Recherche Médicale, Paris, France) and supported by the EEC (European Economic Community). This was the first meeting in which both physicians and biologists interested in this matter were brought together. Rather than constituting the proceedings of this scientific meeting, this is the first book to deal comprehensively with this new and important chapter in human genetics and medicine in general.

The aim of the book has been to present to clinicians and biologists a general view of both the theoretical possibilities involved and the practical consequences which may be drawn from the associations of various markers of the main histocompatibility system in man, the HLA system, with susceptibility to many diseases.

Numerous, and mostly negative, investigations have been conducted in the past, using other genetic markers, particularly those of the ABO blood-group system. Arthur Mourant, the world specialist in this field of research, describes in his chapter the progress that has been made so far.

As regards the HLA system, the field is completely new and the harvest has already proved immensely rich.

Readers should not be afraid of the genetic terms which are often used in this volume. The basic knowledge of immunogenetics necessary for a fruitful reading is given in Rose Payne's chapter and is relatively simple. This chapter explains the details of the highly polymorphous HLA system which controls a great number of various transplantation antigens, some components of the complement cascade, and most likely a variety of immune responses.

Each vertebrate species studied so far has a genetic system very similar to HLA. These systems play a fundamental role in transplantation and are usually referred to as Major Histocompatibility Complexes (MHC). The MHC of mice, the H-2 complex, has been studied in most detail and is described by D. Shreffler. It appears that the H-2 and HLA systems control similar functions in mouse and man respectively and, as much more is known of the fine genetic structure of the H-2 complex, this system provides a model for the human HLA system. In particular, the existence of immune-response (Ir) determinants within the H-2 system is of relevance for understanding many of the associations between HLA and disease.

One of the most important aspects of

the relationship between HLA and disease concerns the heredity of the disorders in question. In fact, almost all of the diseases which have so far been found associated with HLA have previously had an unknown mode of inheritance. As discussed by Kidd, Ceppellini, and co-workers, the fact that there are now dominant genetic markers which are associated with these diseases enables investigators to dissect their genetics into more detail. Both population and family studies are relevant in this respect, and Kidd and Ceppellini have developed a formula which can provide estimates of the frequencies of HLA-linked genes controlling disease susceptibility. Thomson & Bodmer have done so independently and give examples as to how the classical sib-pair method of Penrose, recently extended by Day & Simons, can also be used in this context.

The following chapter is a general discussion on the association concept with notes on the value of analyzing detailed HLA-phenotype data, and on diagnostic use of HLA typing. In addition, this chapter contains the results of combined calculations of almost all available data on HLA and disease associations. The statistical limits used have been set rather conservatively in order to avoid too many 'false' (chance) associations. However, doubtful associations may also be important and they are discussed in the following ten chapters dealing with the various disease groups.

These chapters also describe the pathology and signs of the various diseases and have been written by expert clinicians within their respective fields: D. A. Brewerton, W. C. Lobitz, T. Fog, J. Nerup, W. Strober, I. R. Mackay, A. L. de Weck, M. J. Simons, B. Dupont, and P. J. Morris.

Probably the most fruitful consequence of the relationship between HLA and diseases relates to the fact that they can give important information on the etiologies and pathogenetic pathways of the diseases in question. Examples of these are given in the above surveys, and the chapters of Zinkernagel & Doherty and of Amos & Ward are devoted to thorough discussions of various mechanisms which can explain the associations described in the earlier chapters.

Bodmer & Thomson give a detailed review of the evolutionary aspects of the HLA system with special emphasis on the linkage-disequilibrium phenomenon which is of special relevance for the understanding of the associations.

The chapter by Dausset is a general discussion of how the relationship between HLA and disease can be used in terms of nosology, diagnosis, prognosis, and preventive medicine.

McDevitt ends the book with a status of the present situation and outlines the fascinating perspectives of future studies.

It is the editor's hope that this book may give inspiration to many of the clinicians, biologists, geneticists, and other scientists who are working in one or more of the many fields discussed herein. If all of the important information inherent in the relationship between HLA and disease is to be utilized to the maximum benefit of patients, it is vital that there is a cross-fertilization between many different areas of research. The symposium in Paris was the first attempt in this direction and this book is the second. If this objective is accomplished, it will mainly have been due to the authors of the various chapters of this book and to the many other active participants in the symposium.

HLA-A- and -B-antigen frequencies (per cent)

HLA	Europeans	Middle Easterns	Indians	Mongoloids	American Indians	African Blacks
A1	31	24	23	4	2	8
A2	48	36	28	33	73	34
A3	28	19	14	2	2	15
A9	17	34	26	65	44	24
A10	12	10	14	14	0	15
A11	12	12	33	24	2	2
A28	8	12	12	4	17	17
A29	8	2	2	2	0	10
AW23	4	12	4	4	0	15
AW24	14	24	23	63	44	10
AW25	4	2	2	4	0	2
AW26	8	8	12	10	0	14
AW30	4	8	2	4	2	29
AW31	2	4	2	–	17	4
AW32	8	8	6	–	–	8
AW33	4	10	14	14	8	14
B5	12	28	34	17	19	15
B7	24	6	10	4	2	23
B8	21	6	15	2	–	8
B12	29	17	19	6	2	23
B13	4	6	4	8	–	2
B14	8	8	–	–	2	6
B18	10	10	4	6	2	6
B27	8	4	4	6	6	2
BW15	12	2	15	29	26	8
BW16	8	12	2	8	23	2
BW17	8	10	15	4	2	38
BW21	4	17	2	–	8	2
BW22	6	6	6	24	–	2
BW35	19	24	23	12	4	12
BW40	12	8	12	4	8	14

The frequencies are those obtained during the Fifth International Histocompatibility Workshop *(Histocompatibility Testing 1972,* eds. Dausset, J. & Colombani, J., Munksgaard, Copenhagen, 1972.)

NOTE: Unless otherwise stated, those papers quoted in the References were presented at the 1st Int. HLA & Disease Symposium, Paris, June 1976, sponsored by INSERM.

Disease Associations with Polymorphisms other than HLA

A. E. Mourant

Introduction

The chapter originally submitted at the Paris Colloquium on HLA and disease was too long for the space allowed. Having listened to the discussions at the Colloquium, the author concluded that his tables were more important than the text, and the latter has therefore been drastically reduced. The data presented in the table and discussed in the text are drawn from a more comprehensive work (1) by the present author and his colleagues (by kind permission of the publishers, Oxford University Press). The larger work reproduces the complete observational data, with full bibliographic references (totalling about 1,000), and discusses the results at length.

TABLE I

Associations of ABO groups and other polymorphisms with disease

Disease	Number tested	Relative incidence A/O	χ^2	Relative incidence B/O	χ^2	Other significant associations and additional remarks
Malignant neoplasms						
Tongue, gum, buccal mucosa & cheek	1202	1.22	5.84	1.12	1.86	
Oesophagus	2705	1.10	4.65	1.29	16.11	
Stomach	63439	1.21	402.76	1.04	8.76	
Large Intestine	10270	1.08	11.77	0.99	0.04	
Pancreas	1394	1.16	6.11	1.28	6.90	
Larynx	1611	0.99	0.06	0.94	0.58	
Lung & Bronchus	16414	1.06	7.37	1.004	0.02	
Breast	12190	1.07	11.34	1.02	0.59	PTC tasting
Cervix uteri	23255	1.09	28.68	1.02	0.68	
Corpus uteri	4656	1.06	3.31	0.99	0.08	PTC tasting
Ovary	3175	1.23	25.21	1.09	1.90	PTC tasting
Prostate	1467	1.18	7.87	1.01	0.01	
Glial tumors	3959	1.15	16.09	1.03	0.30	
Meningiomas	1380	1.07	1.03	1.31	7.44	
Hodgkin's disease	1651	0.90	3.32	0.95	0.52	Rh-negatives
Myeloid Leukaemias	1784	1.05	0.78	1.12	5.10	Hp 2
Lymphatic Leukaemias	960	0.97	0.12	0.97	0.11	Hp 2

Serological Population Genetics Laboratory, St. Bartholomew's Hospital, West Smithfield, London.

Benign neoplasms

Salivary glands	891	1.56	33.29	1.06	0.20
Uterus	5472	1.17	20.02	1.07	2.21
Ovary	1071	1.24	8.19	1.27	8.19
Chromophobe adenoma of pituitary	1269	0.96	0.49	1.08	0.59

Infectious diseases

Typhoid fever	956	0.87	3.21	0.94	0.39	Rh-negatives
Shigella flexneri dysentery	1050	1.02	0.12	0.94	0.40	
Escherichia coli enteritis	999	0.93	0.89	1.24	5.03	
Enteritis, infants, no evidence of E. coli	1316	1.11	2.91	0.99	0.005	
Pulmonary Tuberculosis	24966	0.93	15.05	0.98	1.10	Rh-negatives Hp 1
Tuberculosis of bones and joints	886	0.97	0.07	1.23	3.52	
Leprosy	18724	1.04	4.70	1.02	0.43	Rh-positives PTC tasting
Syphilis, all	18141	1.06	10.32	1.09	10.69	
Syphilis treated Wr+	1701	1.49	32.11	1.56	27.42	
Wr–	3197	0.97	0.38	0.96	0.48	
Poliomyelitis paralytic/abortive	1838/ 1681	0.82	3.80	0.70	5.60	All cases, Hp 1
Smallpox	3083	1.22	9.91	0.91	2.41	Highly hetero- geneous
Chickenpox	1290	1.08	1.43	0.95	0.29	
Measles	2030	0.88	4.50	0.93	1.01	Rh-negatives
Infectious hepatitis	3168	1.01	0.03	1.03	0.20	
Malaria	3643	1.31	19.30	1.01	0.06	

Diseases of the circulatory system

Rheumatic fever	3144	1.14	9.04	1.10	2.33	ABH non- secretion
Rheumatic heart disease	5103	1.23	36.53	1.28	24.65	
Hypertension	4710	1.00	0.00	1.03	0.40	M
Malignant hypertension	180	0.60	6.60	0.61	4.02	
Angina pectoris and coronary occlusion with- out (mention of) thrombosis	1631	1.05	0.91	1.01	0.02	
Coronary thrombosis	7124	1.29	76.26	1.19	18.00	Rh-positives
Thrombosis in pregnant or puerperal women	931	1.51	32.18	1.38	8.00	
Thrombosis in women on oral contraceptives	236	2.96	40.47	3.07	24.44	
Other thromboses	2691	1.23	22.08	1.14	3.16	
Various haemorrhages	2478	0.75	31.81	0.80	10.70	
Arteriosclerosis	3282	1.21	20.74	1.13	4.31	ABH non- secretion

Metabolic diseases

Diabetes mellitus (all)	23735	1.07	18.83	1.05	4.13	ABH secretion PTC non-tasting Heterogeneous for ABO & non-tasting
under 20	826	0.88	2.67	0.80	2.95	
over 20	11372	1.08	11.00	1.12	9.95	
Thyrotoxicosis	1950	0.89	4.43	0.95	0.38	
Goitre	3923	0.99	0.03	0.89	3.87	tox. PTC tasting non-tox. PTC non-tasting
Coeliac disease	209	1.05	0.09	1.08	0.07	

Diseases of the digestive system

Gastric ulcers (all)	30391	0.87	107.46	0.87	49.64	ABH non-secretion
Bleeding	600	0.74	10.75	0.54	12.98	ABH non-secretion
not bleeding	890	1.02	0.07	0.96	0.14	
Duodenal ulcers (all)	37160	0.73	624.04	0.80	161.46	ABH non-secretion Rh-positives
Bleeding	2648	0.70	66.75	0.64	37.65	ABH non-secretion
not bleeding	4348	0.86	16.65	0.83	10.37	ABH non-secretion
Appendicitis	4025	0.99	0.12	0.97	0.28	
Cirrhosis of liver	2837	1.24	24.88	1.18	6.66	
Cholelithiasis	14660	1.15	43.80	1.01	0.07	
Cholecystitis	1582	1.34	20.88	1.09	1.11	

Diseases of the genito-urinary system

Urinary Calculi	4270	1.07	2.47	0.99	0.06	
Hyperplasia of prostate	3701	1.05	1.41	1.06	0.89	Rh-negatives

Perinatal disorders

Mothers of abortions	4559	0.87	13.34	0.78	17.35	
Premature infants	1634	1.16	4.92	1.30	7.38	

Diseases of skin

Psoriasis	2102	0.91	2.66	0.90	1.48	M
Vitiligo	1247	0.95	0.40	1.12	2.32	

Mental disorders

Schizophrenia	12608	1.02	0.49	1.17	20.74	Low M
Manic depressive	1856	0.89	4.53	1.05	0.35	
Alcoholism	1392	1.03	0.23	0.97	0.67	ABH non-secretion
Mental retardation	2281	0.97	0.45	1.08	1.04	

Diseases of the nervous system and sense organs

Multiple sclerosis	2242	0.89	5.01	0.89	2.03	
Epilepsy	3072	1.02	0.28	1.22	10.45	

Diseases of the musculo-skeletal system and connective tissues					
Rheumatoid arthritis	2960	0.73	51.12	0.80	17.66 Heterogeneous
Ankylosing spondylitis	352	1.07	0.32	1.18	1.18
Bone fractures	2649	1.12	6.25	1.12	2.59
Congenital anomalies					
Pyloric stenosis	756	0.77	8.22	1.12	0.74
Down's syndrome	3457	1.05	1.58	1.01	0.02
Diseases of the blood					
Pernicious anaemia	3446	1.25	32.31	1.19	7.89
Allergies					
Eczema	883	1.03	0.13	0.97	0.07
Asthma	1684	1.13	3.72	1.47	20.30
Hay fever	320	0.94	0.22	1.26	1.49

Table I gives the results of computations on all diseases, and homogeneous groups of closely related diseases, for which data for the ABO system on more than 1,000 patients are available. Some large but obviously heterogeneous collections of diseases, such as unlocated cancers, have been excluded, and a few series of less than 1,000 have been included somewhat arbitrarily. The main reason for including all series exceeding 1,000 is to show that there is a fairly well-defined dichotomy between diseases where the difference of the combined incidence (or relative risk) A/O from unity is quite non-significant, and those where it is highly significant.

In the Table, the combined relative incidences A/O and B/O, computed by Woolf's (2) method, are listed, together with the values of χ^2 for difference from unity. Values of χ^2 for homogeneity have been omitted but can be found in the work of Mourant *et al.* (1). Woolf's method has been applied without Haldane's (3) correction, but in view of the large numbers involved the latter would have made hardly any difference. In the last column, significant associa-

tions with phenotypes of the MN, Rhesus, secretor, taster, and haptoglobin systems are shown, together with indications of any marked heterogeneity of the ABO data. Since nearly all series of patients who were tested at all were tested for the ABO system, and since the A/O and B/O relative incidences are tabulated in every case, the conventional limiting value of χ^2, 3.841, for one degree of freedom and a probability of 1 in 20, is applicable. For the other systems the same value of χ^2 has been used to qualify for mention in the last column, though it is realised that in some cases a higher limiting value would have been appropriate in view of the multiplicity of tests carried out.

Since the Table is to be allowed to speak for itself, the main purpose of this accompanying text will be to mention those associations not included, to draw attention to relations between associations with HLA and those with other polymorphisms, and to appeal for new data in fields where they might throw important light on the aetiology of particular diseases.

15

Perinatal disorders

Since Dienst (4) in 1905 first drew attention to pregnancy iso-immunisation and tried to relate it to the aetiology of eclampsia, an enormous amount of research has been carried out and thousands of papers have been written on the immunogenetics of pregnancy. Now that Jenkins *et al.* (5) have suggested a failure of the mother to respond to the HLA antigens of her foetus as a cause of eclampsia, further studies on the blood group, HLA, and other antigens of affected women, their husbands, and their children are needed.

Extensive family studies strongly suggest that there are two distinct main causes of spontaneous abortion, cytological abnormality, and ABO incompatibility between mother and foetus. However, there are very few data indeed on the blood groups of aborted foetuses themselves, and it is desirable that anyone who has access to the chemically untreated products of spontaneous abortions, even in small numbers, should carry out ABO tests and as many other immunological tests as possible, both on the foetuses and on the families from which they come.

Neoplastic diseases

A large proportion of the marked associations between blood groups and diseases concern cancers of various organs, and that between carcinoma of the stomach and group A (based on observations on 63,000 patients) remains the most firmly established of all. Nearly all carcinomas are in some degree associated with group A, and in most cases the association is statistically significant. Most are also associated with group B (in contrast to group O) but the relative incidences mostly depart much less from unity than the values for A/O, and only in a few cases are they statistically significant.

Some of the closest associations are those for organs which secrete blood-group substances. It might therefore have been expected that those neoplasms associated with secreting cells would show some association with the secretor factor, but there are, unfortunately, very few data on the secretor types in malignant disease. Carcinoma of the stomach appears to be weakly associated with the secretor type.

Infectious diseases

There is a close biochemical and immunological relationship between the antigens of the ABO blood groups and those of some micro-organisms. It might therefore have been expected that some infectious diseases would show associations with the ABO groups. Only a few infectious diseases, however, show strong associations, and indeed the smallness of the departures from unity of the combined relative incidences A/O and B/O serve as a sort of control to emphasize the consistent manner in which these values exceed unity for the malignant diseases.

One of the most striking features of the infectious diseases is the strong association with groups A and B in cases of syphilis with a persistent Wassermann reaction after treatment.

The apparent strong association of smallpox with group A must remain in some doubt because of extreme disagreement between the results of different groups of workers.

Malaria, probably still the most widespread of all the infectious diseases, shows a highly significant association with group A. However, a variety of epidemiological and parasitological

16

studies suggests that susceptibility is affected by the phenotypes of a very wide range of polymorphisms.

Peptic ulcers

Among the most striking associations with the ABO groups are those of gastric and duodenal ulcers with group O (6, 7). It has however been suggested (8) that these associations are not with the ulceration process itself, but with the bleeding which brings the patients into hospital and causes them to be included in surveys. The total data suggest that this may be the complete explanation for gastric ulcers but, though bleeding cases of duodenal ulcers show higher frequencies of O than non-bleeding ones, the latter still have significantly raised O frequencies. Ulcers of both organs show enhanced frequencies of non-secretors, but these, unlike O frequencies, are not significantly affected by the subdivision into bleeders and non-bleeders.

Rheumatic diseases

Rheumatic fever, which is a special form of reaction to infection with the α haemolytic streptococcus, and its sequel, rheumatic heart disease, both show a marked excess of A and B groups, and a deficiency of ABH secretors. Other infections with the same organism, on very small numbers, show similar characteristics except for a quite non-significant deficiency of B.

Rheumatoid arthritis, however, shows a marked deficiency of A and B, and an excess of group O, though the data are highly heterogeneous. Ankylosing spondylitis, with its unique association with HLA-B27, shows only a non-significant excess of A and B.

Thrombosis and haemorrhage

Coronary thrombosis, on over 7,000 cases, shows a strong association with group A and a slightly weaker one with group B. It also shows a particularly strong and significant, though rather heterogeneous, association with the Rh-positive phenotype.

A collection of nearly 2,800 other cases of thrombosis shows a closely similar association with A and B, but thrombosis of various kinds in pregnant and puerperal women, and in women on oral contraceptives, as well as coronary thrombosis in young men, are much more strongly associated still with groups A and B. Unfortunately, the contraceptive cases recorded are few, but this finding is so important in advising women on contraception that efforts should be made, by organising prospective surveys at advisory clinics, to collect larger numbers of records.

Haemorrhage, on the other hand, is strongly associated with group O. This is shown not only by a series of nearly 2,500 cases presenting primarily as haemorrhage but, as mentioned above, by haemorrhagic as compared with non-haemorrhagic cases of gastric and duodenal ulcer, as well as of pulmonary tuberculosis. This may, at least in part, be related to the higher average level of anti-haemophilic globulin in the serum of A than of O (8, 9).

Other vascular conditions

In a study of coronary thrombosis (10), it became clear that while this condition was strongly associated with blood groups A and B, coronary occlusion and angina pectoris without thrombosis were not. This may have a bearing on the prognosis in coronary disease. Hypertension also is not associated with the ABO blood groups, though, on a small sample, malignant hypertension appears to be associated with groups A and B to a slightly lesser extent than coronary thrombosis.

Diabetes mellitus

A total of over 23,000 patients with diabetes shows small, but (because of the large numbers tested) significant, excesses of both A and B. There is, however, a highly significant heterogeneity between the results published by different workers. This heterogeneity has been partly resolved as a result of the finding that diabetes of juvenile onset (but not that of adult onset) is associated with HLA antigens. Using the detailed observations of Andersen & Lauritzen (11), supplemented by others, it is clear that juvenile diabetes may be associated, but only weakly if at all, with group O, while the adult type is strongly associated with group A. Schernthaner et al. (12) have recently distinguished between an association with HLA-B8 only in diabetes of childhood onset and one with HLA-B8, HLA-BW15 and HLA-CW3 in disease of later juvenile onset. This is consistent with the progressive, rather than sudden, increase with age of the association with group A.

Diabetes mellitus is also very significantly associated with ABH secretion and with PTC non-tasting, but the data are insufficient to determine whether this is related to age of onset, and further age-based data are needed on these associations.

Goitre

Toxic and non-toxic goitres are associated respectively with ability and inability to taste phenylthiocarbamide and other related thyroid-inhibiting substances (some of which occur in food plants). The precise classification of associated and non-associated goitre types is discussed elsewhere (1), as is the possibility that the taster polymorphism is a balanced one, related to the amounts of iodine and thyroid inhibitors in the diet. Thyrotoxicosis is associated also with group A. It is associated with HLA-B8 in Europeans, and with HLA-BW35 in Japanese. Like thyrotoxicosis, thyroid carcinoma is associated with the taster type.

HLA and other associations

A few diseases merit special mention here because they are associated with HLA antigens as well as being associated (or failing to be so) with other hereditary polymorphic factors. Mention has already been made of ankylosing spondylitis, diabetes mellitus, and thyrotoxicosis. In addition, Hodgkin's disease, multiple sclerosis, and psoriasis, all of which have marked HLA associations, are also associated with group O.

It is desirable that HLA investigations should be carried out on patients suffering from a number of diseases shown to have blood-group associations, but not hitherto investigated for HLA. This applies particularly to various forms of cancer, which in general show strong group-A associations. Most of the types of cancer so far investigated have failed to show significant HLA associations.

As mentioned above, most forms of cancer are associated with blood-group A and some also with group B. On the other hand, there are indications of a tendency for auto-immune diseases to be associated with group O. Following lines thought initiated by Burnet (13), this suggests a very tentative hypothesis that many human tissues, both normal and neoplastic, may contain a blood-group A-like antigen at levels which are usually inaccessible to immune processes. However, in the course of an autoimmune process, or the immune response to a growing neoplasm, the antigen may become accessible. Then an A organism, which cannot make anti-A, will be more likely to tolerate the neoplasm than an O one, but less likely to attack its own tissues than an O one. If this is true for A, then it is also possibly true of other genetically determined antigens.

References

1. Mourant, A. E., Kopeč, A. C. & Domaniewska-Sobczak, K. (1977) *Blood groups and diseases.* Oxford University Press, Oxford, N. York, Toronto.
2. Woolf, B. (1954–5) On estimating the relation between blood group and disease. *Ann. hum. Genetics* **19**, 251.
3. Haldane, J. B. S. (1955-6) The estimation and significance of the logarithm of a ratio of frequencies. *Ann. hum. Genetics* **20**, 309.
4. Dienst, A. (1905) Das Eklampsiegift. *Zbl. Gynäk.* **29**, 353.
5. Jenkins, D. M., Need, J. A., Scott, J. S. & Rajah, S. M. (1976) HLA and severe pre-eclampsia. *Proc. HLA and Disease,* Abstracts, p. 250 Institut National de la Santé et de la Recherche Médicale, Paris.
6. Aird, I., Bentall, H. H., Mehigan, J. A. & Roberts, J. A. F. (1954) The blood groups in relation to peptic ulceration and carcinoma of colon, rectum, breast, and bronchus: an association between ABO groups and peptic ulceration. *Brit. med. J.* **2**, 315.
7. Clarke, C. A., Cowan, W. K., Edwards, J. W., Howel-Evans, A. W., McConnell, R. B., Woodrow, J. C. & Sheppard, P. M. (1955) The relationship of the ABO blood groups to duodenal and gastric ulceration. *Brit. med. J.* **2**, 643.
8. Langman, M. J. S. & Doll, R. (1965) ABO blood group and secretor status in relation to clinical characteristics of peptic ulcer. *Gut* **6**, 270.
9. Preston, A. E. & Barr, A. (1964) The plasma concentration of factor viii in the normal population. ii. The effects of age, sex and blood group. *Brit. J. Haematol.* **10**, 238.
10. Mourant, A. E., Kopeč, A. C. & Domaniewska-Sobczak, K. (1971) Blood-groups and blood-clotting. *Lancet* **i**, 223.
11. Andersen, J. & Lauritzen, E. (1960) Blood groups and diabetes mellitus. *Diabetes* **9**, 20.
12. Schernthaner, G., Ludwig, H. & Mayr, W. R. (1976) Juvenile diabetes mellitus: HLA-antigen frequencies dependent on the age of onset of the disease. *J. Immunogenetics* **3**, 117.
13. Burnet, F. M. (1968) A modern basis for pathologi. *Lancet,* **i**, 1383.

The HLA Complex: Genetics and Implications in the Immune Response

R. Payne

The major histocompatibility systems of man and mouse share many attributes in common, but these also differ in curious, perhaps basic manifestations. Their independent study has provided and will continue to provide unique insights with respect to disease susceptibility and to the evolutionary process, (subjects included in other sections of this volume). The study of these two species, man (an outbred population) and laboratory mice (in the main consisting of inbred populations), have each contributed distinctly different sorts of data which on comparison and synthesis enrich each field of investigation. Recent reviews of interest on the MHS of mice and man and on Ia provide a more extensive discussion of this area than is possible here (1, 2, 3, 4, 5).

A brief recapitulation of genetic terms employed in the text follows:

A locus (plural loci) indicates the position of a gene on a chromosome. *A gene* is a segment of DNA that directs the synthesis of a given polypeptide chain or protein. Each locus of the HLA region possesses multiple alleles. *An allele* represents an alternative form of the same gene which has arisen by mutation or duplication. When two or more alleles occur at one locus with appreciable frequency in the same population, this is referred to as a polymorphism. Identifiable characteristics in an individual are referred to as the phenotype. The genetic basis of the phenotype is deduced from the inheritance pattern among the offspring of a family, and is called the *genotype*. Differing genotypes may have identical phenotypes. The *haplotype* is that combination of closely linked HLA genes on the same chromosome, which are transmitted by one of the parents. Two haplotypes, one from each parent, make up the genotype. Thus in the HLA system, the haplotypes consist of components from each locus. These are transmitted as dominant characters from parent to child in a block, which is a reflection of the close linkage between the loci. *Linkage* is defined as the tendency of genes on the same chromosome to segregate together.

The HLA region has been called the Major Histocompatibility System of man. This term refers to a genetic region on a chromosome which plays a dominant role in the survival of grafted tissue. The letter H in HLA designates human and L designates leukocytes, as these were the first cells shown to carry the antigens of this complex. The ca-

Department of Medicine, Stanford University School of Medicine, Stanford, California 94305.

pital letter A was originally a locus designation. In 1967, when the nomenclature was agreed upon, after considerable discussion on a logical form, HL-A was written with a hyphen between HL and the locus symbol A. Investigators introduced a shorthand style of referring to the entire system as HLA. Subsequently, genes controlling other functions were also identified in the HLA region and on this basis, in 1975, the International Nomenclature Committee assigned HLA without the hyphen as the official term for the entire region. A hyphen still separates the region designation from a series of letters denoting loci. At first only two loci were recognized; by 1970 a third was proposed, and by 1975 four loci for the leukocyte specificities were agreed upon with designations A, B, C and D (6).

Then in a cascading series of observations, other characteristics such as specific red-cell groups, as well as complement factors, were found to be closely linked to HLA.

The polymorphic character of the HLA loci A, B, C and D is illustrated in Table I. There are 18 antigenic determinants at the A and 22 at the B locus. The brackets indicate that what at one time appeared to be a single specificity has now been subdivided into several. A well-accepted specificity is identified by its locus and a number. A W in front of a number indicates that the specificity was studied in an International Workshop but still requires further definition. A summary statement of the number of loci, the number of alleles, and how these are identified is shown in Table II. The two more recently recognized loci, C and D, have fewer alleles, but on further study this number will undoubtedly increase. The A, B and C loci are detected serologically making use of antisera which lyse a test lymphocyte preparation if the antigen is present. Several sera are routinely employed to ascertain the presence of any specificity. This guarantees accuracy of definition inasmuch as sera in use may not all be monospecific. Further, one or more sera may be anticomplementary thus giving occasional false

TABLE I
HLA antigens of the A, B, C and D loci

A1	B5	CW1	DW1
A2	B7	CW2	DW2
A3	B8	CW3	DW3
AW23 ⎤	B12	CW4	DW4
AW24 ⎬ A9	B13	CW5	DW5
9.3 ⎦	B14		DW6
AW25 ⎤	B18		
AW26 ⎬ A10	B27		
AW34 ⎦	BW15		
A11	BW38 ⎤ BW16		
A28	BW39 ⎦		
A29 ⎤	BW17		
AW30 ⎮	BW21		
AW31 ⎬ AW19	BW22		
AW32 ⎮	BW35		
AW33 ⎦	BW37		
AW36	BW40		
AW43	BW41		
	BW42		

BHs in Orientals, BW22J in Japanese and BTT in Caucasians and Blacks are antigens more recently identified. There is current evidence to suggest that BW21 and BW22 may be further subdivided.

TABLE II
HLA antigens

Highly polymorphic system
Four closely linked loci – A, B, C, D
Number of alleles at four loci

A	B	C	D
18	22	5	6

Definition
A, B, C – serologic –
D – cell-cell interaction
(one-way MLC test with homozygous-typing cells)

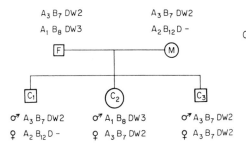

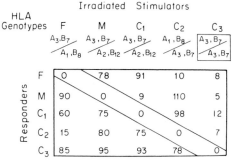

Figure 1. Identification of an HLA-D homozygote.

F = father   M = mother   C = child

If the two pairs, M with C_1 and F with C_2 are mutually nonstimulatory, this indicates A3B7 haplotypes of M and F share same MLC type.

Then, C_3 will not stimulate any family member and is therefore MLC homozygous.

TABLE III

Identification of a D-locus homozygote in a family study

Numbers express relative responses (RR) calculated as:

$$RR = \frac{A\,Bx - A}{\text{Median response} - A} \times 100$$

Where Abx = cpm of responder A to stimulator B; A = cpm of responder alone; median A response = median response of responder A to all frozen "valid" stimulators

Nonstimulation – all values < 20 %

F = father   M = mother   C = child

negative results. Because of the strong linkage disequilibrium between the B and C loci, antisera defining specificities at the C locus are still not readily distinguishable. The D-locus antigens are identified in a one-way mixed-lymphocyte culture using nonresponding lymphocytes which are homozygous for a D specificity as the typing tool. Homozygous typing cells (HTCs) have been detected by two approaches. In the first, families were sought in which a member was homozygous at the A and B loci, thus indicating the parents shared a haplotype (see Figure 1). The assumption made was that in a proportion of such members, the D-locus specificity would also be homozygous. The chance for this to occur would be greater in inbred populations and therefore, in the early investigations, families in which cousin marriages had occurred were tested (7). An example of one-way mixed-lymphocyte reactions between family members (not inbred) is shown in Table III. In this test, the lymphocyte of each family member (previously irradiated or mitomycin treated) are tested for their ability to stimulate all other members to synthesize DNA. The treat-

ed cells can stimulate but do not proliferate (thus a one-way test). Degree of stimulation, measured by the uptake of tritiated thymidine is expressed in terms of relative response (RR). Nonstimulation of the parents by the offspring (homozygous for A and B antigens) indicated that 1) the parent shared the same D-locus specificity, and 2) the child was homozygous not only for the A and B, but also for the D loci. In the second approach to detection of HTCs, lymphocytes from a restricted population are tested against each other until mutually nonstimulating cells are found. Stastny (8) succesfully employed this technique in a study of rheumatoid arthritis patients, and Sasazuki *et al.* (9) similarly tested random healthy Japanese persons against each other. Both groups of investigators identified frequently occurring D-locus specificities in their respective populations. Having identified a series of HTCs, one can then proceed to test for the D-locus specificities of other individuals. Thus, lymphocytes (homozygous for a D allele) take the place of an antiserum. If the lymphocytes being tested are stimulated by the homozygous typing cell to proliferate, the two have differing D-locus alleles (or types). If proliferation does not take place, they are presumed to share the D type. The procedure is slow and laborious, requiring days, and hopefully will soon be replaced by a serologic method. Encouraging data to support this view are already evident (5, 10).

Recording of the HLA type of an individual would be as follows:

Phenotype: A1, A3, B7, B8, CW1, CW2, D-

Genotype: A1, B8, CW1, D-/A3, B7, CW2, D-

Haplotype: A1, B8, CW1, D-

Each of the four loci is listed. A minus sign after the loci C and D in a phenotype indicates either a presumed antigen exists but cannot be identified with the reagents used, or that the individual is homozygous. The genotype and haplotype were deduced from a family study. Inheritance patterns in pedigrees have demonstrated that each individual carries two alleles for each of the A and B loci. The picture is not as clear for the number of loci that may be included in the C and D regions. It is assumed that two alleles exist for each of these with the reservation, however, that additional loci may be defined by the sera being employed (11).

When one considers all the known HLA alleles, an enormous number of phenotypes could result from all the possible combinations. Theory predicts there could be as many as 20 million phenotypes. So far, a small fraction of these have been observed; the numbers found in Caucasians show that each phenotype occurs at a low frequency.

From this vast number, it is obvious that each individual is exquisitely distinct. As is well recognized, a marked deviation from normal of any frequency for a given allele or haplotype, as in certain disease states, opens the door to enquire into their etiology and mechanism.

General characteristics of the HLA-A and -B loci antibodies and antigens are provided in Table IV. The antibodies which identify the antigenic determinants of the three loci A, B and C are not naturally occurring but are found after exposure to foreign HLA antigens, as for example in the serum of previously gravid women, of multi-transfused patients, and of transplant recipients. These antibodies are ordinarily IgG in nature and, with the usual techniques employed, either cytotoxicity or agglutination, are customarily of low titer. Antisera monospecific for an HLA specificity are not rare, but multispecific examples are more common.

TABLE IV

Characteristics of HLA-A and B

ANTIBODIES

A response to foreign antigens
Usually IgG (7S)
Sera frequently multispecific, some monospecific, often crossreactive within A locus
  e.g. B7, B27, BW22, BW42, most are of low titer
Activity may be cytotoxic and/or agglutinating

ANTIGENS

Occur on membrane surface
Shed into plasma and body fluids
Develop early in fetal life ∞ 6 weeks
Persist throughout life
On all nucleated cells examined
1–2 % of membrane proteins
Consist of two polypeptide chains
  Heavy chain – glycoprotein mol. wt.
  ∞ 44,00 daltons
  Light chain – $\beta 2$ microglobulin
  ∞ 12,000 daltons

Many antisera exhibit crossreactivity with several other HLA-antigenic determinants, usually within the same locus. For example, if an individual is immunized with the B7 antigen, a monospecific B7 serum may be produced. Another individual immunized with this same B7 could produce a serum with activity for B7, BW22, and B27 lymphocytes. The controlling mechanism, which determines whether or not a crossreacting serum is produced, is not understood. When the biochemistry of these HLA antigens and their arrangements on the cell surface have been worked out more thoroughly, the phenomenon of crossreactivity may be better understood.

The HLA-antigenic determinants occur within the surface membranes of a cell and are present on leukocytes, both T and B lymphocytes, on platelets and on all nucleated cells that have been examined. Metabolic processes induce shedding of these antigens or components thereof into the plasma and other body fluids after which regeneration occurs. These membrane constituents develop early in fetal life and persist through the life span. The precise biologic functions of these membrane constituents have not been disentangled but they are most likely related to cell recognition and immunologic response (12). One additional function of HLA, not preordained by nature, has been an investigator's bonus. The enormously polymorphic HLA system is incomparable for providing genetic markers for the study of linkage and of human populations.

The HLA antigens comprise 1–2 % of the cell-membrane and consist of two polypeptide chains, a heavy glycoprotein chain and a lighter chain made up of $\beta2$ microglobulin (13). The genes controlling the heavy chain are on Chromosome # 6 and those controlling the lighter chain are on Chromosome # 15 (14). The molecular weight of the heavy chain is approximately 44,000 daltons; the light chain has a weight of 12,000. $\beta2$ microglobulin has not been shown to be polymorphic. Sequencing analyses of the amino acid structure of the heavy chain suggest that different antigenic specificities of HLA are determined by variations in the amino acid sequences (15).

A special feature of the HLA-antigen complex is that the frequency of a particular antigen will vary widely among the different ethnic groups. A comparison of the B-locus antigens in American Blacks, African Blacks and American Caucasians clearly illustrates

TABLE V

Antigen frequencies

	Amer. Bl. N= 356	Afr. Bl. 411	Amer. Cau. 503
B5	12	4	11
B7	20	18	23
B8	6	7	20
B12	13	16	24
B13	3	4	6
B14	5	9	11
BW15	4	6	7
BW16	3	4	12
BW17	26	33	7
B18	4	10	9
BW21	10	2	4
BW22	3	1	.5
B27	2	1	8
BW35	32	14	17
BW37	2	0	5
BW40	4	2	12
BW41	1	0	1
BW42	6	16	0
HR*	3	1	1
TT	5	7	1
1AG**	34	31	12

(16) Payne *et al.* (1976)
*A possible antigen in the B5-BW35 complex
**One antigen only at the B locus

24

this point (Table V) (16). The boxed values, expressed as a percentage, outline those antigens that have a markedly higher frequency in Blacks. These differences demonstrate the importance of taking ethnic background into consideration when evaluating data on HLA and disease association. Another aspect relating to differing populations has been the observation that some HLA antigens and/or variants of them seem to be restricted to a particular set of populations. As seen in this table, BW42 was not observed in Caucasians of the United States. A total lack or very infrequent presence of an antigen has been seen not only for the B locus but for the other loci as well. For example, in very recent work on the D-locus antigens among Japanese, DW3 was not detected among 70 persons tested (9).

Is it invariably the case that each parent transmits one of his or her haplotypes to each offspring? In the HLA system this is true about 99 % of the time. Family studies however, indicate that exceptions, known as recombinants, do occur about 1 % of the time. These exceptions are the consequence of crossing over, which occurs at meiosis. An example is shown in Figure 2. In the central portion, the point of crossover is illustrated. The actual pedigree is given in Figure 3. The symbols A/B and C/D represent the abbreviated expressions for the hyplotype combinations of the two parents. Six out of seven children inherited the parental haplotypes as expected. The first child received B from father and D from mother, the child labeled C4 received B from father and C from mother. The last child inherited the crossover haplotype. She received from the mother A2 from the C haplotype and B12, C blank, D blank from the D haplotype. Such a crossing over occurring between the A and C loci explains why these loci are ordered A, C, B and D on the chromosome. Crossover between the loci have permitted mapping of the different loci in the HLA system.

Another important aspect of the genetics of HLA is referred to as linkage disequilibrium. It is defined as nonrandom association of antigens in a population; or expressed in another way, it is the situation in which two specific alleles of two linked genes occur together on the same chromosome significantly more frequent than expected from random matings. In the HLA system, the association of two antigens can be characteristic of a particular ethnic group. For example, the A1, B8 haplotype is in strong disequilibrium in Caucasians; A2, BHs is so in Chinese and AW26, BW17 is found in Blacks.

Further evidence for ethnic variation is illustrated in Table VI. The blocked areas illustrate that the African Black population and the American Caucasian population each have disequilibrium unique unto themselves. All underlined values are highly significant. The haplo-

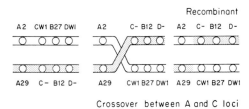

Figure 2. Illustration of crossover in the HLA region between A and C loci during meiosis.

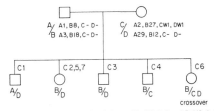

Figure 3. Recombinant family.

25

TABLE VI

Linkage disequilibrium
Selected delta values (x10⁴) – A and B series

	Amer. Bl.	Afr. Bl.	Amer. Cau.
A1, B8	*180* ***	−3	*615* ***
AW25, B18	*75* ***	−13	*156* ***
A3, B7	66	−6	*230* ***
AW26, BW39	22	7	*69* ***
AW32, B14	6	−16	*81* ***
AW33, B14	−16	5	*30* ***
AW30, BW42	113*	*210* ***	— — —
AW23, B14	30	*114* ***	−11
AW25, B12	4	*64* ***	−26
AW26, B17	−20	*209* ***	−7
A29, BW42	−13	*142* ***.	— — —
A29, B12	33	*115* **	212

* $p < 0.05$,
** $p < 0.01$,
*** $p < 0.001$.

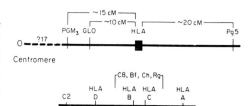

Figure 4. The lower half represents an enlargement of the HLA region on Chromosome 6.

types A1, B8 and AW25, B18 are in linkage disequilibria in both American Blacks and Caucasians. The admixture of Caucasian genes in United States Blacks is estimated roughly as 10–20 %. Neither of these two haplotypes is in disequilibrium in the Africans. What is curious is that the haplotype disequilibria seen in Africans are not found in American Blacks. The relation of linkage disequilibrium to disease is discussed in another section of this volume.

How was the location of HLA on Chromosome # 6 established? First, it was shown by family studies that the locus for PGM3, an intracellular enzyme, was linked to the HLA region (17). Then studies of interspecific somatic-cell hybrids revealed that the locus for PGM3 was on Chromosome # 6 of man (18). This established a chromosomal assignment for the HLA region. Confirmatory data for this was obtained from a family with a pericentric inversion on # 6 (19): It was noted that a specific HLA haplotype was seen in each person with the inversion.

Closely linked to the four HLA loci A, B, C and D are genes for two red-cell groups, Chido and Rogers, which are reminiscent of the G region in mice. Several complement functions Bf or properdin, C2, C4 and C8 are also located here (20). By analogy with the mouse it is probable that genes controlling immune responses affecting disease susceptibility and "Ia" antigens occur in this region. Also on Chromosome #6 but *not* closely linked are genes controlling the enzymes glyoxalase, phosphoglucomutase-3 and other factors.

A current map of Chromosome # 6 is given in Figure 4. It is unknown on which arm HLA occurs. The enlarged version of the HLA region from this map provides some indication of the close linkage of these loci.

Currently, the most exciting facet under investigation in this field is the genes controlling immune responsiveness and the Ia antigens. These are now under intensive study in man, and much more will be heard about them in the next few years. Immune-response genes, Ir, are defined as histocompatibility-linked genes determining specific recognition of foreign antigens. When one tests for Ir one measures a function, for example, an antibody level in response to a specific antigen.

The Ia genes of the mouse, as discussed in another section of this volume, occur in the I region of Chromosome 17 between the H2-K and -D regions. It is thought that in man, Ia antigens may be determined by genes at the D locus and at other, as yet, undefined but closely linked loci. In the mouse these genes determine the structure of a series of lymphocyte cell-surface allo-antigens which appear to have a central role in regulating the immune response. These Ia alloantigens which can be detected serologically have a restricted tissue distribution in both mice and man. In the murine species these are found, for example, on B lymphocytes, sperm, macrophages, to a lesser degree on T cells, but are absent from platelets (21). The distribution is similar in man. The antigens are glycoprotein with a two-chain structure. It is thought these may be T-lymphocyte receptors and may be intimately involved in antigen recognition by both helper and suppressor cells. Less is known about these antigens and functions in man. The molecular weights of Ia antigens in the mouse are 25,000 and 30,000 daltons and in man 28,000 and 33,000 (5). Ir and Ia map in the same area as the locus for the mixed-lymphocyte reaction. What is required now is resolution of the questions: are the loci for Ia and MLC the same? and are the Ia antigens the gene product of Ir?

What is the evidence for Ir in man? It is of interest in this regard that in primates Ir genes appear to map along with antigens eliciting the MLC reaction (22). One line of evidence for the location of Ir in the HLA region in man is based on the observations that immune responsiveness to streptococcal antigens, to live influenza vaccine, and to ragweed antigen Ra5, is associated with the HLA antigens B5, B14 and B7 respectively (23, 24, 25). The second line of evidence comes from family studies.

One group of workers observed a relation between response to ragweed allergen E and an HLA haplotype in families (26); this study was not confirmed by a second group of investegators (27). Another report showed concordance of antibody titer for measles in HLA identical twins (28). Definitive demonstration of Ir genes in humans will probably require deliberate immunizations with protein antigens. So far, difficulties have been encountered in performing precise family studies to define the Ir genes. For instance, studies after deliberate immunization of random individuals with the synthetic peptide GLT* (which is under Ir-gene control in guinea pigs) demonstrated no association with HLA (29). Here family studies are needed. Studies using diphtheria toxoid in families showed high and low T-cell responsiveness but these were not linked to HLA (30).

Another category of evidence for Ir genes in man, which is less convincing, is findings in autoimmune diseases. In Addison's disease, autoantibodies to the adrenal are reported to correlate with the presence of B8 and CW3 (31). In contrast, there is disagreement as to whether a similar correlation exists in Graves' disease (32, 33), also associated with B8 and DW3 in Caucasians.

What is known about Ia in man? Based on mouse data, a lively search has gone on in the last few years for antisera which detect antigens on human B lymphocytes. Specific antisera have been obtained from various sources, namely, from previously gravid women immunized by fetal cells, from patients who have received multiple transfusions or rejected a renal transplant, and from donors selected for HLA-A and -B identity who were deliberately immu-

* A random terpolymer of glutamic acid, lysine, and turosene.

nized against each other. As B lymphocytes make up only 10–30 % of the lymphocytes of peripheral blood from normal healthy individuals, enrichment procedures are employed to increase the proportion of B cells in the test preparation. Other approaches have been to use the blood of patients with chronic lymphocytic leukemia (CLL) as a test cell because of its high concentration of B lymphocytes or cultured lymphoid-cell lines derived from B lymphocytes. Many of the anti-Ia sera are contaminated with HLA-A and -B antibodies. These can be removed by absorption with platelets which lack B antigens. An alternative method has been developed by van Rood et al. for recognition of B-cell determinants of normal peripheral blood using two-color fluorescence (34). If widely applicable, this approach will eliminate the need for B-cell enrichment procedures which are tedious and time consuming.

The usual assay for serum activity is the complement-dependent cytotoxic assay; less often, cell binding and MLC inhibition assays have been utilized. The cytotoxic assay is similar to the routine one employed in HLA serology, with the exception that incubation time is often longer and the complement is carefully screened to eliminate nonspecific cytotoxic activity against the test B lymphocyte. B cells, for a variety of reasons, are often more sensitive to complement than the lymphocytes used in routine HLA typing. The various methods are in the development stage as yet and will become more standardized in the future.

Most of the data regarding these presumed Ia antigens in man come from the serologic work. In Table VII illustrative data are presented (from a few selected laboratories) on the number of Ia specificities found, a list of the D-locus specificities which seem to be identified by these sera and the type of cells tested in the cytotoxic assay. Each laboratory has used its own nomenclature, e.g. OX1 refers to antigen 1 at Oxford. Some of the B-lymphocyte serologic specificities include one for the DW locus and others are roughly equivalent to one or more. The group working at Oxford has found clusters of sera which identify five different B-cell spe-

TABLE VII

Ia antigens recognized in representative laboratories

LABORATORY	SPECIFICITIES		SOURCE OF B CELLS
	B CELL	D LOCUS	
BODMER (5)	OX 1—5	W1, 3, 4,5	HTC, PB
		LD107	CELL LINES
VAN ROOD (35)	5	W1, 2, 3	HTC, PB
	(incl. Ag-non-	LD107	
	HLA)		
WALFORD (37)	MERRIT 1–19	W1, 2, 3	CLL
			CELL LINES
DAUSSET (36)	LY-LI		CELL LINES
	(non-HLA)		
TERASAKI (38)	11		CLL, P.B.
AMOS (40)	DIg 1–7		PB

HTC-D locus homozygous-typing cell; PB – peripheral blood B lymphocytes, CLL – B cells from chronic lymphocytic leukemia.

cificities (5), the group at Leyden also has five different specificities, one of which, called Ag (35), is not linked to HLA. In Paris, investigators have independently found what they have designated the Ly-Li antigen of the Ly system also not linked to HLA (36). In Los Angeles, in Walford's laboratory, 19 antigenic determinants were identified on CLL cells (37), and in Terasaki's laboratory 11 were detected on peripheral blood B cells from healthy individuals (38). The last workers noted that their Group 2 antigen was completely lacking in patients with CLL. Mann et al. (39) found a B-cell specificity associated with gluten-sensitive enteropathy. Other disease associations with B-cell specificities are rapidly accumulating with evidence that these are more closely associated to the disease than antigens of other loci in the HLA region.

Research on B-lymphocyte antigens, although in its early stages, is progressing at a rapid pace. In 1977 at Oxford, another International Histocompatibility workshop will be held with major emphasis on this subject. Investigators will jointly work out the relation of the B-lymphocyte antigens identified in the various laboratories to each other and establish a standard nomenclature. A large series of antisera will be contributed to be tested on selected cells to sort out the number of loci and their chromosomal location; in addition, some diseases will be studied for association with Ia antigens.

In conclusion, the genetics of the HLA region have been briefly summarized. Current research is oriented toward understanding the functions of the Ia antigens and other products determined by genes in this region. Hope-

fully, this information will contribute an understanding to the mechanisms of disease susceptibility.

References

1. Svejgaard, A., Hauge, M., Jersild, C., Platz, P., Ryder, L. P., Staub Nielsen, L. & Thompson, M. (1975) The HLA System – An introductory survey. *Monogr. Human Genet.* **7**, 1.
2. McDevitt, H. O., Delovitch, T. L., Press, J. L. & Murphy, D. B. (1976) Genetic and functional analysis of the Ia antigens: Their possible role in regulating the immune response. *Transplant. Rev.* **30**, 197.
3. McDevitt, H. O. (1975) Genetic considerations in atopic and other dermatologic conditions. *Proc. Brook Lodge Conference on Immune Mechanisms in Cutaneous Disorders*, p. 1.
4. Klein, J. (1975) Biology of the mouse Histocompatibility-2 complex, Springer-Verlag, N.Y.
5. Barnstable, C. J., Jones, E. A., Bodmer, W. F., Bodmer, J., Arce-Gomez, B., Snary, D. & Crumpton, M. (1976) Genetics and serology of HLA linked human Ia antigens. *Cold Spring Harbor Symp.*, (in press).
6. WHO-IUIS Terminology Committee, Nomenclature for factors of the HLA system (1975) *Histocompatibility Testing*, p. 5.
7. van den Tweel, J., van Oud, A. B., Keuning, J. J., Goulmy, E., Termijtelen, A., Bach, M. L. & van Rood, J. J. (1973) Typing for MLC (LD): I. Lymphocytes from cousin-marriage offspring as typing cells. *Transplant. Proc.* **5**, 1535.
8. Stastny, P. (1974) Mixed lymphocyte culture typing cells from patients with Rheumatoid Arthritis. *Tissue Antigens* **4**, 571.
9. Sasazuki, T., McMichael, A., Payne, R. & McDevitt, H. O. (19766) HLA haplotype differences between Japanese and Caucasians. (Submitted for Publication.)
10. van Rood, J. J., van Leeuwen, A., Keuning, J. J. & van Oud Alblas, A. B. (1975) The serological recognition of the human MLC determinants using a modified cytotoxicity technique. *Tissue Antigens* **5**, 73.
11. Payne, R., Radvany, R., Grumet, F. C., Feldman, M. & Cann, H. (1975) Two third series antigens transmitted together.

This work was supported by NIH grant HL 03365.

29

A possible fourth SD locus. *Histocompatibility Testing,* p. 343. Munksgaard, Copenhagen.

12. Bodmer, W. F. (1972) Evolutionary significance of the HL-A system. *Nature (Lond.)* **237**, 139.

13. Strominger, J. L., Chess, L., Herrmann, H. C., Humphreys, R. E., Malenka, D., Mann, D., McCune, J. M., Parham, P., Robb, R., Springer, T. A. & Terhorst, C. (1975) Isolation of histocompatibility antigens and of several B cell specific proteins from cultured human lymphocytes. *Histocompatibility Testing,* p. 719. Munksgaard, Copenhagen.

14. Goodfellow, P., Jones, E., van Heyningen, V., Solomon, E., Brobrow, M., Miggiano, V. & Bodmer, W. F. (1976) The β2 microglobulin gene is on chromosome # 15 and not in the HL-A region. *Nature (Lond.)* **254**, 267.

15. Bridgen, J., Snary, D., Crumpton, M. J., Barnstable, C., Goodfellow, P. & Bodmer, W. F. (1976) Isolation and N-terminal amino acid sequence of membrane-bound human HLA-A and HLA-B antigens. *Nature (Lond.)* **261**, 200.

16. Payne, R., Feldman, M., Cann, H. & Bodmer, J. G. (1976) A comparison of HLA data of the North American Black with African Black and North American Caucasoid populations. *Tissue Antigens,* (in press).

17. Lamm, L. U., Kissmeyer-Nielsen, F. & Henningsen, K. (1970) Linkage and association studies of two Phosphoglucomutase loci (PGM$_1$ and PGM$_3$) to eighteen other markers. *Human Hered.* **20**, 305.

18. von Someren, H., Westerveld, A., Hagemeijer, A., Mess, J. R., Meera Khan, P. & Zaalberg, O. B. (1974) Human antigen and enzyme markers in man – Chinese hamster somatic cell hybrids. Evidence for synteny between the HL-A, PGM$_3$, ME$_1$ and IPO-B loci. *Proc. nat. Acad. Sci. (Wash.)* **71**, 962.

19. Lamm, L. U., Friedrich, U., Petersen, G. B., Jorgensen, J., Nielsen, J., Therkelsen, A. J. & Kissmeyer-Nielsen, F. (1974) Assignment of the major histocompatibility complex to chromosome no. 6 in a family with a pericentric inversion. *Human Hered.* **24**, 273.

20. Bodmer, W. F. (1976) Report on Chromosome 6. In: *Proc. of Third Human Gene Mapping Conference.* Cytogenics and Cell Genetics, (in press).

21. Shreffler, D. C. The H-2 model: Genetic control of immune functions. HLA and Disease Symposium, Paris 1976. Munksgaard, Copenhagen, p. 32.

22. van Vreeswijk, W., Roger, J. H. & Balner, H. (1975) *Genetics of "Ia-like" Antigens of Rhesus Monkeys: Provisional Mapping of Two Loci in the RhL-A Complex.* Annual report, Radiobiological Institute TNO, Netherlands, p. 151, see also Balner, H., van Vreeswijk, W. & Roger, J. H. *Transplant. Rev.* **30**, (in press).

23. Greenberg, L. J., Gray, E. D. & Yunis, E. J. (1975) Association of HLA-5 and immune responsiveness in vitro to streptococcal antigens. *J. exp. Med.* **141**, 935.

24. Speneer, M. J., Cherry, J. D. & Terasaki, P. I. (1976) HL-A antigens and antibody response after influenza A vaccination. *New Eng. J. Med.* **294**, 13.

25. Marsh, D. G., Bias, W. B. & Hsu, S. H. (1973) Association of the HL-A7 crossreacting group with a specific reaginic antibody response in allergic man. *Science,* Feb., p. 691.

26. Levine, B. B., Stember, R. H. & Fotino, M. (1972) Ragweed Hayfever: Genetic control and linkage to HL-A haplotypes. *Science* **178**, 1201.

27. Bias, W. B. & Marsh, D. B. (1975) HL-A linked antigen E immune response genes: An unproved hypothesis. *Science* **188**, 375.

28. Haverkorn, M. J., Hofman, B., Masurel, N. & van Rood, J. J. (1975) HL-A linked genetic control of immune response in man. *Transplant. Rev.* **22**, 120.

29. Green, I. (1974) Genetic control of immune responses. *Immunogenetics* **1**, 4.

30. McMichael, A., Sasazuki, T. & McDevitt, H. O. (1976) The immune response to Diphtheria toxoid in humans. *Transplant. Proc.,* (in press).

31. Thomsen, M., Platz, P., Andersen, O. 0., Christy, M., Lyngsøe, J., Nerup, J., Rasmussen, K., Ryder, L. P., Nielsen, L. S. & Svejgaard, A (1975) MLC typing in juvenile Diabetes Mellitus and idiopathic Addison's disease. *Transplant. Rev.* **22**, 125.

32. Thorsby, E., Seegaard, E., Solem, J. H. & Kornstad, L. (1975) The frequency of major histocompatibility antigens (SD and LD) in Thyrotoxicosis. *Tissue Antigens* **6**, 54.

33. Grumet, C. G., Payne, R., Konishi, J. & Kriss, J. (1974) HL-A antigens markers for disease susceptibility and autoimmunity in Graves' disease. *J. Clin. Endocrin. & Metab.* **39**, 1115.

34. van Rood, J. J., van Leeuwen, A. &

Ploem, J. S. (1976) A method to detect simultaneously two cell populations by two colour fluorescence. *Nature (Lond.),* (in press).

35. van Rood, J. J., van Leeuwen, A., Jonker, M., Termijtelen, A. & Bradley, B. (1976) Polymorphic B Cell determinants in man. *Cold Spring Harbor Symp.* Series V41, (in press).

36. Legrand, L. & Dausset, J. (1975) A second lymphocyte system (Ly-Li). *Histocompatibility Testing,* p. 665, Munksgaard, Copenhagen.

37. Walford, Roy L., Ferrara, G. B., Gatti, R. M., Liebold, W., Thompson, J. S., Mercuriali, F., Gossett, T. & Naeim, F. (1976) New groups and segregant series among B-cell alloantigens of the Merrit system: A study of leukemia cells, peripheral B-cells and lymphoblastoid cell lines. *J. exp. Med.* Supplement, (in press).

38. Ting, A., Mickey, M. R. & Terasaki, P. I. (1976) B-lymphocyte alloantigens in Caucasians. *J. exp. Med.* **143**, 981.

39. Mann, D. L., Nelson, D. L., Katz, S. I., Abelson, L. D. & Strober, W. (1976) Specific B-cell antigens associated with gluten sensitive enteropathy and Dermatitis Herpetiformis. *Lancet,* **i**, 110.

40. Johnson, A. H., Pool, P. A., McKeown, P. T., Bigelow, R. A., Kovarsky, D. B., Ward, F. E. & Amos, D. B. (1976) Analysis of sera specific for human B cells. *Transplant. Proc.,* (in press).

The *H-2* Model: Genetic Control of Immune Functions

Donald C. Shreffler

The purpose of this chapter is to introduce the major histocompatibility complex (MHC) and its role in the genetic control of a variety of immune functions that influence disease resistance. In the past five years, it has become obvious that the MHCs of a number of species play a critical role in these phenomena. The most thoroughly investigated of the MHCs with respect to immune function is the mouse histocompatibility-2 *(H-2)* gene complex. Of course, the unique value of the mouse model is its susceptibility to genetic manipulation. It has proven to be a particularly useful model because the *H-2* system is remarkably similar (homologous) to the human MHC, the HLA system. In fact, all of the currently defined MHCs show very close homologies. Many species have been studied and to date, ten species have relatively well-defined MHCs, all initially defined in the transplantation context as the species' major transplantation barriers. Three transplantation features have been found to be common to all defined MHCs: 1) acute graft rejection; 2) induction of antibodies against serologically defined MHC products; and 3) stimulation of the mixed leukocyte reaction (MLR).

Supported by U.S.P.H.S. Research Grant AI-12734.

Washington University, School of Medicine, Department of Genetics, St. Louis, Missouri 63110.

The ten species with well-defined MHCs (cf. 1) are shown in Figure 1. Most of these are mammals. However, it is particularly noteworthy that a well-defined MHC has been described in a higher amphibian, *Xenopus laevis,* and another in an avian species, the chicken. This implies that the MHC had a relatively early origin in evolution and suggests that it probably occurs in some form in most, if not all, higher vertebrates.

In addition to the common transplantation features, most of these MHCs also have certain genetic features and associated traits in common. Basic genetic features of the MHC include: 1) the existence of multiple tightly linked genes in a cluster in a short segment of

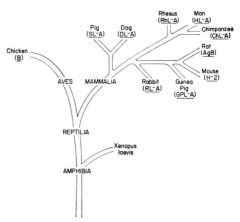

Figure 1. Species having defined major histocompatibility complexes. Note in particular the amphibian and avian species.

a single chromosome; 2) diverse, but functionally interrelated, traits and gene products; and 3) extensive genetic polymorphism, meaning the occurrence, with some appreciable frequency in a population, of multiple alleles at a single locus. Polymorphism is a feature of many loci in the MHC.

The MHCs, as typified by the *H-2* complex, determine three broad sets of traits (cf. 1, 2, 3). These traits are shown in Figure 2 for the *H-2* complex. They are controlled by four discrete genetic regions of the complex, called K, I, S, and D. The K and D regions determine the classical transplantation antigens, which are the principal antigenic targets for cell-mediated cytotoxicity in graft rejections and were the first MHC products to be detected serologically. As noted later, these products also appear to play a role in immune surveillance. The *S* region determines one or more components of the serum complement system – probably several components. The *I* (immune-response) region determines the principal factors that stimulate the mixed-leukocyte reaction (MLR), and a variety of functions relating to immune responses, particularly functions that involve specificity of antigen recognition and restrictions on interactions between lymphoid cells.

As noted above, the mouse model offers particular advantages for genetic analysis and this genetic map of the *H-2* complex was derived by extensive analyses of intra-*H-2* genetic recombination (2, 3). Three intra-*H-2* recombi-

nants are represented in Figure 3. All originated from similar or identical *H-2*-heterozygous parental combinations. In the first case, *H-2*[tl] was the result of a crossover between the *H-2*[al] chromosome and the *H-2*[s] chromosome. This crossover separated the *H-2K* locus, the marker for the *K* region, from the *Ir-1* locus, the marker for the *I* region, and for the remainder of the *H-2* complex. In the second case, the crossover occurred between the *Ir-1* and *Ss* loci, thus separating the *I* and *S* regions. In the third case, the crossover occurred between the *Ss* and *H-2D* loci, thus separating the *S* from the *D* region. More than 50 such intra-*H-2* recombinants have been detected and most have been extensively analyzed. The results of these analyses have yielded a much more detailed map of the *H-2* complex, including more loci than are shown in Figure 3.

The current detailed genetic map of the *H-2* complex is shown in Figure 4 (2, 3, 4, 5, 6). Nine discrete genetic loci have been defined. Each locus determines a distinct trait or product and each has been separated from the rest by one or more intra-*H-2* crossovers. In addition to the *K, I, S,* and *D* regions, a new region, *G*, defined by a locus determining an erythrocyte antigen, has

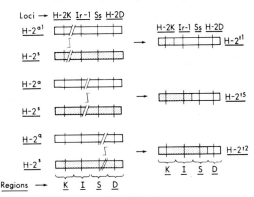

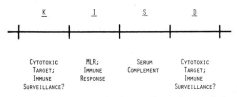

Figure 2. The principal genetic regions of the mouse *H-2*-gene complex and the general classes of traits controlled by them.

Figure 3. An example of the intra-*H-2* crossovers which have contributed to the recombination mapping of the *H-2*-gene complex.

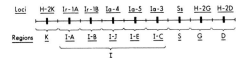

Loci	H-2K	Ir-1A	Ir-1B	Ia-4	Ia-5	Ia-3	Ss	H-2G	H-2D

Regions	K	I-A	I-B	I-J	I-E	I-C	S	G	D

Figure 4. The current detailed genetic map of the *H-2*-gene complex.

also been defined (6). In addition, the *I* region has been divided into five sub-regions, called *I-A, I-B, I-J, I-E,* and *I-C* (2, 4, 5). It should be emphasized that the genetic *loci* of the complex are single genetic units defined in terms of specific traits or products, while the genetic *regions* of the complex are segments of chromosome defined by the crossovers that have separated the various marker loci (2). The important distinction is that a genetic region might very possibly include many genes, in addition to the specific marker gene shown. In the following sections the various traits of immunologic significance that have been associated with each of the four principal regions of the *H-2* complex will be considered. Some key *H-2* alloantigenic specificities that

TABLE I

Principal specificities of some key H-2 haplotypes

Haplotype	H-2K specificity	H-2D specificity
H-2b	33	2
H-2d	31	4
H-2f	26	9
H-2k	23	32
H-2q	17	30
H-2s	19	12

define the gene products of specific *H-2K* and *H-2D* alleles are shown in Table I. Each specificity is defined by a different alloantiserum. As with the *HLA* complex, the antisera defining these specificities have proven to be very useful reagents for the identification and classification of the products of discrete *H-2* genes and alleles and for the purification and characterization of the products.

Extensive biochemical analyses have been conducted on the products of the *H-2K* and *H-2D* loci (7, 8). A schematic diagram of these molecules is pre-

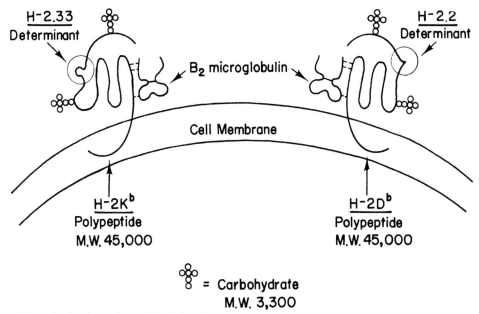

Figure 5. A schematic model of the glycoprotein products of the *H-2K* and *H-2D* genes.

sented in Figure 5. The products of the *H-2K* and *H-2D* loci are single polypeptides, each of molecular weight about 45,000 daltons. The *H-2* antigenic specificities, e.g. *H-2.33* and *H-2.2,* are determined by differences in the primary structures of the polypeptides. Recent sequence data indicate that the products of alleles at the *H-2K* and *H-2D* loci differ in multiple amino acids. These results also indicate that there is as much homology between the products of the *H-2K* and *H-2D* loci as there is between the products of different alleles at either single locus (cf. 8). This supports the prediction, based on serological data (9), that the *H-2K* and *H-2D* genes are products of a *gene duplication* event at some time during their evolution. The *H-2* polypeptides appear to be anchored in the lipid of the membrane by hydrophobic sequences at the carboxy-terminal end of the polypeptide (8). Associated with these polypeptides are carbohydrate groups that do not seem to vary from one *H-2* type to another, and a single β_2-microglobulin polypeptide. The β_2-microglobulin is a molecule that has substantial homology with, but is distinct from, the immunoglobulins. Its function in association with the *H-2* polypeptides is so far unknown.

For almost 40 years, from their initial discovery by Peter Gorer in 1936 (10) until 1974, there were no really significant clues to the biological function of the *H-2K*- and *H-2D*-gene products. In 1974, very important observations were made by Zinkernagel & Doherty (11) that directly implicated the *H-2* molecules in immune mechanisms. They found that effective cell-mediated killing reactions, or cytotoxity, against virus-infected cells expressing on their membranes new, virus-induced surface antigens, require very specific *H-2* compatibility. These observations

TABLE II

H-2 restrictions on cell-mediated cytotoxicity against virus-infected target cells[a]

Immune[b] Cells	Target Cells[c]		
	H-2k/H-2k	*H-2b/H-2b*	*H-2d/H-2d*
H-2k/H-2k	+	−	−
H-2b/H-2b	−	+	−
H-2d/H-2d	−	−	+

[a]After Zinkernagel & Doherty (11).
[b]Spleen cells from virus-infected mice.
[c]Virus-infected fibroblasts or culture lines;
+ = cytotoxicity,
− = no reaction.

are depicted in very simple fashion in Table II. Even though the cell-mediated cytotoxic reaction was expected to be directed against the new virus-induced antigen, immune cells capable of killing virus-infected cells of the *same H-2* type were unable to kill virus-infected cells of *other H-2* types, even though they were infected with the same virus. This implied either that compatibility for *H-2*-determined products is required for some obligatory cell-cell *interaction* between the killer cell and the target cell or that the *H-2* antigens are themselves involved in the *specificity* of recognition of the viral antigen. Similar results with chemically modified target cells were also reported by Shearer (12).

As discussed below, Katz and others (13, 14) had already at that time observed requirements for *H-2* compatibility for effective helper interactions between T and B lymphocytes. This re-

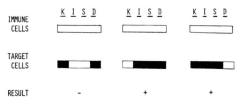

Figure 6. A schematic illustration of the evidence localizing *H-2*-linked restrictions on cell-mediated cytotoxicity reactions against virus-infected cells to the *K* and *D* regions.

3*

quirement had been shown to involve products of the *I* region. However, the restrictions on cell-mediated cytotoxicity were found to involve the *K*- and *D*-region products (15). This localization is depicted simply in Figure 6. In this diagram the open and shaded areas represent two different sets of genetic information in the indicated *H-2* regions.

In the first case, involving two recombinants, the immune cells and the virus-infected target cells have the *I* and *S* regions in common, but differ in the *K* and *D* regions. In this case, there is no cytotoxic reaction. On the other hand, if the immune cells and the target cells have in common *either* the *K* or the *D* region, effective killing takes place.

Several lines of evidence (not enumerated here, but see Chapter XIV) suggest that the role of the *H-2* products in this process involves a direct contribution to the antigenic site recognized by the receptor on the cytotoxic lymphocyte, as represented in Figure 7. It is postulated that the cytotoxic lymphocyte reacts with a virus-infected cell or neoplastic cell or any other cell expressing new surface antigens because the *H-2K*- or *H-2D*-gene product *associates* with the new antigen and forms an

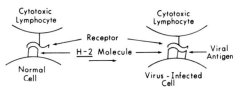

Figure 7. A schematic model of the "altered-self" recognition hypothesis for *H-2*-linked restrictions on cell-mediated cytotoxicity reactions against virus-infected cells.

"altered-self" site. This phenomenon is viewed as an expression of an *immune surveillance* mechanism whereby any cell expressing an altered-self determinant is rapidly recognized and destroyed by cytotoxic lymphocytes carrying receptors that may perhaps have unique specificity for altered-self structures.

This subject is dealt with in greater detail in Chapter XIV. It is intended here only to introduce the phenomenon in a general way. It should be strongly emphasized, however, that these observations are very important to the understanding of the normal biological function of the *H-2K*- and *H-2D*-gene products, and are particularly significant because they imply that these products, as well as the products of the other *H-2* regions, play a positive role in immune mechanisms, and may therefore contribute to MHC-associated resistance or susceptibility to disease.

The *S* region

The *S* region is defined by the *Ss-Slp* serum-protein variants (16). *Ss* refers to the so-called *serum serological* quantitative variation, *Slp* to the *sex-limited protein* allotype, so named because it is expressed only in males and is subject to rather direct testosterone regulation. Both of these traits involve variations in a specific class of serum β-globulins. The quantitative *Ss* variation is detected by immunodiffusion techniques with a

rabbit antiserum. Associated with some *H-2* haplotypes are *Ss*h alleles that determine a high level of this protein, with others an *Ss*l allele that determines a low level of the protein. The *Slp* variation is allotypic, detected with an antiserum produced in mice of the *Slp*-negative type (lacking the allotype) against serum from mice of the *Slp*-positive type. The presence of the allotype is determined by an *Slp*a allele, absence by the *Slp°* allele. An *Slpʷ* allele determines expression of the allotype that is not subject to testosterone regulation. The controlling gene or genes for the *Ss* and *Slp* traits map within the *H-2* complex, in the *S* region (16).

For many years the *Ss-Slp* variation provided a useful marker for genetic analysis of the *H-2* complex, but there was no clue to the function of the proteins or their relationship to other products of the *H-2* complex. However, in the past few years it has become clear that the *S* region controls one or more components of the complement system and recent data indicate that the *Ss-Slp* proteins are the mouse homologues of the human C4 component of complement. The first evidence relating complement variations to the *S* region was presented by Demant *et al.* in 1972 (17). They found differences in serum levels of total hemolytic complement that were linked to the *H-2* complex. Furthermore, as shown in Table III, those differences in total complement levels were also strongly correlated with differences in *Ss* level. The *H-2* haplotype with the highest complement level also has the highest *Ss* level, that with the lowest complement level has the lowest *Ss* level, and the two intermediate values are also correlated. Analyses of intra-*H-2* recombinants established that this

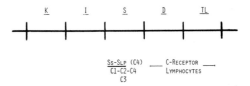

Figure 8. H-2-linked variations in complement functions.

complement variation is controlled by the *S* region.

Recently, Meo and others have identified the *Ss* and *Slp* proteins as mouse C4 (18, 19, 20). The discovery of MHC-associated complement variations has stimulated many further studies on associations of individual complement components with the *H-2* complex. The *H-2* associated variations described thus far are depicted in Figure 8. Associated with the *S* region are not only the *Ss-Slp* (C4) variation, but quantitative variations in *assayed* levels of individual components, C1, C2, and C4, all of which are correlated with differences in level of the *Ss* protein (21). Quantitative differences in level of C3, not *Ss* correlated, are also controlled by the *S* region (22). Associated with the *H-2* complex, but not with the *S* region, there are also developmental differences in numbers of complement-receptor lymphocytes (23). As will be noted in ensuing chapters, deficiencies of C2 and C4 and electrophoretic variation in properdin-pathway Factor B have all been shown to be linked to the HLA system. Thus, rather surprisingly, it has emerged that the *S* region, along with the *K* and *D* regions, join the *I* region in playing important roles in specific functions of the immune system. Once again, this has obvious implifications for resistance and susceptibility to disease.

TABLE III

H-2 associated complement variations

Haplotype	Total complement	Ss level
*H-2*ᵇ	1.0	1.0
*H-2*ᵈ	2.1	1.4
*H-2*ᵏ	0.5	0.1
*H-2*ʷ⁷	3.2	1.9

The *I* region

Of course, the *H-2*-gene complex has been implicated in immune mechanisms before, dating from the work of Lilly in 1966 (24) who demonstrated *H-2* linked control of susceptibility to Gross virus-induced leukemogenesis. Subsequently, following the demonstration of single-gene control of response to the linear amino acid homopolymer, poly-L-lysine, by Benacerraf *et al.* in the guinea pig (25), McDevitt *et al.* described genetic variation in response to the synthetic polypeptide antigen (T, G)-A--L, and showed that this variation is also controlled by a single mendelian genetic unit (26) closely associated with the *H-2* complex (27). Analyses of intra-*H-2* recombinants localized the controlling element to the *I* region (28). With time, genetically determined differences in responses to many antigens and susceptibility to a number of oncogenic viruses were found to be associated with the *H-2* complex (cf. 2, 3, 14). Studies to define the functional roles of the *I*-region products have also led to the recognition of a number of other kinds of traits that are associated with the *I* region. In addition to resistance to oncogenic viruses and immune response to specific antigens, the *I* region controls a variety of regulatory interactions among the cells of the immune system – T lymphocytes, B lymphocytes and macrophages (14, 29). In the transplantation context, the *I* region controls the principal factors that stimulate the MLR and determines one or more histocompatibility antigens, i.e. products that serve as targets for cell-mediated cytotoxicity reactions (cf. 2, 3). Finally, a set of serologically detected lymphocyte antigens, the immune-response-associated or Ia antigens, have been found to be controlled by the *I* region (cf. 2, 3, 4). Obviously these traits are not *necessarily* all controlled by discrete genes.

The observation most critical to the recognition of an immune response role of the *H-2* complex was the initial detection of the *H-2*-linked *Ir-1* genes. Properties of these genes have been reviewed elsewhere (14, 30). These genes control *H-2*-linked differences in capacity to respond to specific antigens. Capacity to respond is dominant. The response differences may be seen in the levels of antibodies produced against a specific antigen or in differences in intensity of strictly cell-mediated responses, such as graft rejection or *in vitro* T-cell proliferation in response to a specific antigen.

The *Ir-1* genes control differences in response to more than 30 different antigens. These multiple-response differences are undoubtedly determined by multiple genes, although it is not yet known whether this means a few genes or perhaps hundreds of genes. The relevant genes map inside the *H-2* complex in the *I* region. Recent findings in several laboratories have demonstrated that normal response to at least some antigens requires an interaction between dominant responder alleles at two discrete genetic loci, both located within the *H-2* complex (31). The functional basis for this interaction is not understood, but this observation implies that typical responses may require the interplay of two or more gene products, all determined by the *I* region. It is not yet proven that this is a general phenomenon applicable to all *H-2*-linked responses, but it may very possibly prove to be general.

The specific functional roles of the *Ir-1* genes and their products have not yet been resolved. Three possible functions have been suggested (30). The products might serve as the antigen receptors of T lymphocytes, they might determine normal immune responses by mediating regulatory interactions among B and T lymphocytes and macrophages, or they might function as self-recognition structures in an altered-self recognition mechanism, comparable to that described above for the *H-2K* and *H-2D* products. It should be emphasized that these possible functions are not mutually exclusive and that all three might apply to one or another of the various *I*-region gene products.

As noted above, the *Ir-1* genes control differences in responses to a variety of antigens. *Examples* of a number of such kinds of responses are listed in Table IV, including synthetic polypeptides, foreign protein antigens given in low doses, serum alloantigens and cellular alloantigens, including even an *H-2D* gene product. Most relevant in the context of MHC-disease relationships are the *H-2*-controlled differences in susceptibility to autoimmune thyroiditis induced by injection of thyroglobulin and to experimental autoimmune encephalomyelitis induced by injection of basic protein of myelin (32). These latter two categories may be

especially relevant to the mechanisms underlying HLA-disease associations.

Another key observation that led to recognition of a more specific functional role for the *I* region, was the finding by Kindred (13) that the antibody response to thymus-dependent anitgens, which involves a helper effect by T cells on antibody-producing B cells, requires *H-2* compatibility between the interacting T and B cells. This observation was extended by Katz *et al.* (cf. 14) in a cell-transfer system that measures the helper activity of T cells for B cells, with the very significant finding that the genetic basis for this compatibility requirement resides in the *I* region. These observations are illustrated in Figure 9. Again, the open and shaded areas represent different genetic information (different alleles) in the indicated regions. When the cooperating T cell and B cell are of completely different *H-2* types, no cooperation is observed. When they differ in the *K* and *I* regions, but are identical in the *S* and *D* regions, there is again no cooperation. However, when they are compatible in the *K* and *I* regions, effective cooperation does take place. This effect is localized in the *I* region, however, since compatibility for *K* and incompatibility for *I* results in no cooperation.

Space does not permit a detailed review of the many very interesting findings on lymphoid-cell interactions that were subsequently described by numerous workers. They include, in addition to the T-cell-helper effect on B

TABLE IV
Examples of some H-2-associated immune responses

Synthetic Polypeptides	Protein Antigens (Low Dose)
(T,G)-A--L GLΦ_5	Ovalbumin Lactate dehydrogenase
Serum Alloantigens	Cellular Alloantigens
IgG allotype *Slp* allotype	Male (H-Y) antigen *H-2.2* antigen
Oncogenic Viruses	Self Antigen
Gross virus Friend virus	Thyroglobulin Basic myelin protein

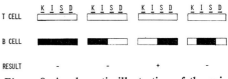

Figure 9. A schematic illustration of the evidence localizing *H-2*-linked factors mediating T-cell-B-cell cooperation to the *I* region.

cells, the effect of suppressor T cells on other T cells and the capacity of antigen-charged macrophages to induce the development of specific helper T cells. The specific basis for these interactions and the requirement for *I*-region compatibility is not yet understood. These phenomena may reflect a requirement for a very specific complementarity between the products of certain alleles at two or more closely linked, but discrete, loci within the *I* region, such that only certain combinations of products are capable of interaction. Alternatively, this may reflect a self-recognition mechanism analogous to that postulated for the *H-2K* and *H-2D* products. This problem remains to be resolved, but it is clear that these restrictions reflect a very significant functional role of the *I* region.

Another recent development relating to *I*-region functions and products has been the production of specific antisera that recognize *I*-region-determined lymphocyte-membrane structures (cf. 2). These structures, termed Ia or immune-response-associated antigens, are clearly concerned with immune functions. The antisera which recognize them are proving to be extremely useful as probes for studies of *I*-region-determined immune functions. These antisera are produced by using certain intra-*H-2* recombinants, such as those shown in Figure 10. Represented here are three recombinant haplotypes that differ only in the *I-A* subregion, or only in the *I-C* and *S* regions. (The *S* region plays no role in determination of Ia antigens, so it is irrelevant.) By reciprocal immunizations among the strains carrying such recombinant *H-2* types, it has been possible to produce many specific antisera that detect specific protein products of the *I-A* subregion and of the *I-C* subregion, as well as of two additional subregions, *I-J* and *I-E* (cf. 2, 4, 5).

The properties of these Ia antigens are summarized in Table V (33, 34). Because the recombinant strain combinations employed do not differ in their *K* or *D* regions, the alloantisera produced contain no anti-*H-2* antibodies, which had previously masked the existence of the Ia antigens. These antigens are expressed strongly on the majority of B cells, and less strongly on only certain subpopulations of T cells. *I*-region-controlled antigens are also expressed on macrophages, and on sperm and epidermal cells. Their role on the latter two cell types and the relationship of the antigens on these cells to the structures on lymphoid cells are not clear. They are not found on platelets, erythrocytes or many other tissues. To date, at least four discrete Ia-antigen molecules have been defined. These are under the control of four discrete Ia

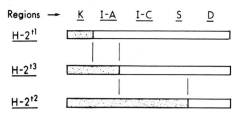

Figure 10. Three recombinant *H-2* types utilized for production of anti-Ia (immune-response-associated antigen) sera.

TABLE V

Properties of immune-response-associated (Ia) antigens

1. Detected by alloantisera that contain no anti-*H-2K* or *H-2D* antibodies.
2. Expressed on most B cells, certain subpopulations of T cells, and macrophages. Also on sperm and epidermal cells. Not expressed on platelets or erythrocytes.
3. Include at least four discrete molecules controlled by four discrete *I* subregions.
4. B-cell molecules are glycoproteins, mol.wt. 58,000, comprising two polypeptides of mol.wt. 25,000 and 33,000.
5. Antigenic variation resides in the polypeptides.

loci located in four different subregions of the *I* region. Biochemical characterizations of the molecules on B cells indicate that they are glycoproteins, with molecular weights of about 58,000 daltons, comprised of two discrete polypeptides with molecular weights of about 25,000 and 33,000 daltons. The antigenic variation resides in the polypeptide portion of the glycoprotein but it has not yet been determined whether one or the other or both of the polypeptides is controlled by the *I* region.

As stated above, Ia antigens are associated with four different *I* subregions. In Figure 11, certain of the key Ia specificities associated with each subregion are shown. Those associated with *I-A* and *I-C* were described first. The *I-J* and *I-E* subregions and their products have been defined within the past year (4, 5, 35).

Anti-Ia antibodies have proven to be very useful probes for the examination of the functions of *I*-region gene products. In a variety of assays of lymphocyte function, they have been shown to have the capacity to inhibit specific immune functions, without complement, i.e. without killing the cells. Such inhibition presumably involves steric blocking or interference with the normal biological functions of the Ia-antigen molecules. Control treatments with anti-*H-2* antibodies under the same conditions give no inhibition, indicating that the blocking is not due to nonspecific membrane perturbations. Such inhibition has,

TABLE VI
Roles of Ia antigens in immune functions

A. Anti-Ia inhibition of:

1. B-cell receptors for T-helper factors, Fc and LPS. B-cell MLR-stimulating antigens.

2. Antigen-induced T-cell proliferation.

3. Macrophage function in *in vitro* PFC response.

4. Soluble mediators from T cells (helper, suppressor) and macrophages (helper-inducer).

B. Anti-Ia cytotoxicity *vs:*

1. Suppressor T cells.

2. Concanavalin-A-responsive T cells.

as shown in Table VI, been demonstrated for the B-cell receptors for T-cell-helper factors (36) and for the Fc region of immunoglobulins (37), as well as the structures on B cells involved in mitogenic stimulation by LPS (38). Anti-Ia antibodies also specifically and rather completely block the structures that stimulate the mixed-leukocyte reaction (39), implying that the MLR-stimulating antigens are also Ia antigens. Anti-Ia antibodies block antigen-induced T-cell proliferation (40) and the role of the macrophage in *in vitro* immune-response assay systems (4). Anti-Ia sera have also been shown to react specifically with soluble T-cell-helper (36) and suppressor (35) factors and with factors produced by macrophages that induce the development of helper T cells (29). By the use of anti-Ia in the presence of complement, it has been demonstrated that *I*-region gene products are expressed on suppressor T cells (5) and on the T cells that respond to concanavalin A stimulation (4). There is thus no question that the cell-surface structures detected by these antisera play important roles in immune mechanisms involving B cells, T cells and macrophages, although the *precise*

I-A	I-B	I-J	I-E	I-C
2		(Ts)	22	6
4				7
11				21
20				

Figure 11. A genetic map of some key Ia specificities. Symbol Ts refers to an antigen of suppressor T cells.

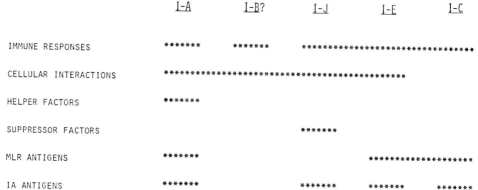

	I-A	I-B?	I-J	I-E	I-C
IMMUNE RESPONSES	*******	*******	******************************		
CELLULAR INTERACTIONS	**				
HELPER FACTORS	*******				
SUPPRESSOR FACTORS			*******		
MLR ANTIGENS	*******			********************	
IA ANTIGENS	*******		*******	*******	*******

Figure 12. Localization of immune-response-related traits to subregions of the *I* region of the *H-2*-gene complex.

roles of these structures remain to be defined.

In the past few years, a tremendous volume of information has accumulated with respect to the phenomena and products associated with the *I* region. It is impossible in such a brief review even to mention many important observations. Some of these will be discussed in greater detail in other chapters. Figure 12 is presented to summarize, in a relatively simple way, the most important immune-response-related functions or products of the *I* region and their genetic resolution to date. Immune responses have been associated with the *I-A* and *I-B* subregions and with a segment encompassed by the *I-J, I-E* and *I-C* subregions. The current data on cellular interactions have implicated all but the *I-C* region, but these must still be more specifically localized. Probably the genetic factors that control different sorts of cellular interactions (T-B, T-T, macrophage-T) will be found in different map positions. A clearer indication of this comes from work on the localization of genes producing soluble-helper factors, which have been localized in the *I-A* subregion (35, 36), and soluble suppressor factors (35), which have been localized to the *I-J* subregion. The major antigens sti-

mulating MLR are localized in the *I-A* subregion, and an additional factor (or factors) is associated with *I-E* and/or *I-C*. Although not yet definitively established, there is a strong presumption that the products that stimulate the MLR are products whose normal functions relate to specific immune mechanisms of B cells. It has been postulated that the MLR represents a discrete, but parallel, manifestation of an altered-self recognition phenomenon comparable to that described for the *H-2K* and *H-2D* products (41). Finally, the most specific molecular definition of *I*-region products to date has come through analyses of the Ia antigens (34). As indicated previously, at least four discrete products, controlled by four discrete subregions, have been identified. The product of the *I-J* subregion has been very specifically related to T-cell suppressor activity and this product is expressed on suppressor T cells and not on B cells (5). The products of the other three subregions are principally represented on B cells. Their specific functional roles are not yet so clearly defined, although the *I-A* region is apparently involved both in helper activity (35, 36) and in macrophage-T interactions (29), probably implying the action of at least two discrete genes.

Conclusion

To summarize, Figure 13 represents the simple map of the four major regions of the *H-2* complex, and their potential roles in mechanisms of disease resistance that might account for observations of MHC-disease associations can be considered again. As indicated earlier, the *K* and *D* regions appear to be involved in mechanisms of immune surveillance. A genetic defect in one of these products might lead to a breakdown in the immune-surveillance mechanism against cells expressing specific neoantigens, potentially resulting in a specific neoplastic disease or in progression of a specific viral disease. Diseases resulting from deficiencies of MHC-linked early-complement components, such as C2 and C4, have already been described in man. It seems obvious that genetically determined total deficiencies, partial deficiencies, or perhaps even subtle structural modifications of any of the complement components might potentially either result directly in disease or confer a predisposition to certain kinds of disease. Finally, as has been most clearly demonstrated with the *H-2* model, defects in any one of multiple genes in the *I* region which are concerned with lymphocyte regulation and/or antigen recognition might result in deficiencies in capacity to mount a specific immune response that could lead to susceptibility to the etiologic factor in a specific disease.

The most cogent new point to be made is that, whereas a few years ago associations of specific diseases with the MHC were *only* thought about in terms of *Ir*-gene defects, it now appears that the *entire* MHC may be involved in immune mechanisms. This means that a defect in *any* of the genes of the MHC may have the potential either to cause disease *directly* or to *predispose* for specific kinds of diseases. That fact will undoubtedly complicate the understanding of the functional bases for specific HLA-disease associations, but it also implies that the role of the MHC in disease will prove to be even more important than was previously imagined.

References

1. Frelinger, J. A. & Shreffler, D. C. (1975) The major histocompatibility complexes. In: *Immunogenetics and Immunodeficiency,* ed. Benacerraf, B., p. 81, Medical and Technical Publishing Co. Ltd., London.
2. Shreffler, D. C. & David, C. S. (1975) The *H-2* major histocompatibility complex and the *I* immune response region: genetic variation, function and organization. *Adv. Immunol.* 20, 125.
3. Klein, J. (1975) *Biology of the Mouse Histocompatibility-2 Complex.* Springer-Verlag, New York.
4. Shreffler, D. C., David, C. S., Cullen, S. E., Frelinger, J. A. & Niederhuber, J. E. (1975) *Cold Spring Harbor Symyposium on Quantitative Biology,* **41**, (in press).
5. Murphy, D., Herzenberg, L. A., Okumura, K., Herzenberg, A. & McDevitt, H. O. (1976) A new *I* subregion *(I-J)* marked by a locus *(Ia-4)* controlling surface determinants on suppressor T lymphocytes. *J. exp. Med.* 144, 699.
6. David, C. S., Stimpfling, J. H. & Shreffler, D. C. (1975) Identification of specificity H-2.7 as an erythrocyte antigen: control by an independent locus, *H-2G,* between the *S* and *D* regions. *Immunogenetics* 2, 131.

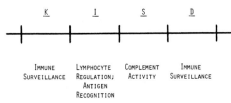

Figure 13. The principal genetic regions of the *H-2*-gene complex and their roles in conferring resistance to disease.

7. Nathenson, S. G. & Cullen, S. E. (1974) Biochemical properties and immunochemical-genetic relationship of mouse H-2 alloantigens. *Biochem. Biophys. Acta.* **344**, 1.

8. Nathenson, S. G., Brown, J. L., Ewenstein, B. M., Nisizawa, T., Sears, D. W. & Freed, J. H. (1976) *Cold Spring Harbor Symposium on Quantitative Biology* **41**, (in press).

9. Shreffler, D. C., David, C. S., Passmore, H. C. & Klein, J. (1971) Genetic organization and evolution of the mouse H-2 region: a duplication model. *Transplant. Proc.* **3**, 176.

10. Gorer, P. A. (1936) The detection of antigenic differences in mouse erythrocytes by the employment of immune sera. *Brit. J. exp. Pathol.* **17**, 42.

11. Zinkernagel, R. M. & Doherty, P. C. (1974) Restriction of in vitro T cell-mediated cytotoxicity in lymphocytic choriomeningitis within a syngeneic or allogeneic system. *Nature (Lond.)* **248**, 701.

12. Shearer, G. M., Rehn, T. G. & Garbarino, C. A. (1975) Cell-mediated lympholysis of trinitrophenyl-modified autologous lymphocytes. Effector cell-specificity to modified cell surface components controlled by the H-2K and H-2D serological regions of the murine major histocompatibility complex. *J. exp. Med.* **141**, 1348.

13. Kindred, G. & Shreffler, D. C. (1972) H-2 dependence of cooperation between T and B cells in vivo. *J. Immunol.* **109**, 940.

14. Benacerraf, B. & Katz, D. H. (1975) The nature and function of histocompatibility-linked immune response genes. In: *Immunogenetics and Immunodeficiency,* ed. Benacerraf, B., p. 117, Medical and Technical Publishing Co. Ltd., London.

15. Blanden, R. V., Doherty, P. D., Dunlop, M. B. C., Gardner, I. D., Zinkernagel, R. M. & David, C. S. (1975) Genes required for T cell-mediated cytotoxicity against virus-infected target cells are in the *K* or *D* regions of the *H-2* gene complex. *Nature (Lond.)* **254**, 269.

16. Shreffler, D. C. (1976) The *S* region of the mouse major histocompatibility complex *(H-2):* genetic variation and functional role in the complement system. *Transplant. Rev.* **32**, 140.

17. Demant, P., Capkova, J., Hinzova, E. & Varacova, B. (1973) The role of the histocompatibility-2-linked Ss-Slp region in the control of mouse complement. *Proc. nat. Acad. Sci. (Wash.)* **70**, 863.

18. Meo, T., Krasteff, T. & Shreffler, D. C. (1975) Immunochemical characterization of murine *H-2*-controlled Ss (serum substance) protein through identification of its human homologue as the fourth component of complement. *Proc. nat. Acad. Sci. (Wash.)* **72**, 4536.

19. Curman, B., Ostberg, L., Sandberg, L., Malmheden-Erikson, I., Stalenheim, G., Rask, L. & Peterson, P. A. (1975) H-2 linked Ss protein is C4 component of complement. *Nature (Lond.)* **258**, 243.

20. Lachmann, P. J., Grennan, D., Martin, A. & Demant, P. (1975) Identification of Ss protein as murine C4. *Nature (Lond.)* **258**, 242.

21. Goldman, M. B. & Goldman, J. N. (1975) Relationship of levels of early components of complement to the H-2 complex of mice. *Fed. Proc.* Vol. **34**, 979.

22. Ferreira, A. & Nussenzweig, V. (1975) Genetic linkage between serum levels of the third component of complement and the *H-2* complex. *J. exp. Med.* **141**, 513.

23. Gelfand, M. C., Sachs, D. H., Lieberman, R. & Paul, W. E. (197) Ontogeny of B lymphocytes. III. H-2 linkage of a gene controlling the rate of appearance of complement receptor lymphocytes. *J. exp. Med.* **139**, 1142.

24. Lilly, R. (1966) The inheritance of susceptibility of the Gross leukemia virus in mice. *Genetics* **53**, 529.

25. Kantor, F. S., Ojeda, A. & Benacerraf, B. (1963) Studies on artificial antigens. I. Antigenicity of DNP-polylysine and DNP copolymer of lysine and glutamic acid in guinea pigs. *J. exp. Med.* **55**, 55.

26. McDevitt, H. O. & Sela, M. (1965) Genetic control of the antibody response. I. Demonstration of determinant-specific differences in response to synthetic polypeptide antigens in two strains of inbred mice. *J. exp. Med.* **122**, 517.

27. McDevitt, H. O. & Tyan, M. L. (1968) Genetic control of the antibody response in inbred mice. Transfer of response by spleen cells and linkage to the major histocompatibility *(H-2)* locus. *J. exp. Med.* **128**, 1.

28. McDevitt, H. O., Deak, B. D., Shreffler, D. C., Klein, J., Stimpfling, J. H. & Snell, G. D. (1972) Genetic control of the immune response. Mapping of the *Ir-1* locus, *J. exp. Med.* **135**, 1259.

29. Erb, P. & Feldmann, M. (1975) The role of macrophages in the generation of T-helper cells. III. Influence of macrophage derived factors in helper cell induction. *Europ. J. Immunol.* **5**, 759.

30. Katz, D. H. & Benacerraf, B. (eds.) (1976) *The role of Products of the Histocompatibility Gene Complex in Immune Responses,* Academic Press Inc., New York.
31. Dorf, M. E. & Benacerraf, B. (1975) Complementation of *H-2* linked *Ir* genes in the mouse. *Proc. nat. Acad. Sci. (Wash.)* **72**, 3671.
32. Bernard, C. C. A. (1976) Experimental autoimmune encephalomyelitis in mice: Genetic control of susceptibility. *J. Immunogenetics* **3**, (in press).
33. David, C. S. (1976) Serologic and genetic aspects of murine Ia antigens. *Transplant. Rev.* **30**, 299.
34. Cullen, S. E., Freed, J. H. & Nathenson, S. G. (1976) Structural and serological properties of murine Ia alloantigens. *Transplant. Rev.* **30**, 236.
35. Tada, T., Taniguchi, M. & David, C. S. (1976) Properties of the antigen-specific suppressive T cell factor in the regulation of antibody response in the mouse. IV. Special subregion assignment of the gene(s) which codes for the suppressive T cell factor in the *H-2* histocompatibility complex. *J. exp. Med.* **144**, 713.
36. Munro, A. J. & Taussig, M. J. (1975) Two genes in the major histocompatibility complex control immune response. *Nature (Lond.)* **256**, 103.
37. Dickler, H. B. & Sachs, D. H. (1974) Evidence for identity or close association of the Fc receptor of B lymphocytes and alloantigens determined by the *Ir* region of the *H-2* complex. *J. exp. Med.* **140**, 779.
38. Niederhuber, J. E., Frelinger, J. A., Dugan, E., Coutinho, A. & Shreffler, D. C. (1975) Effects of anti-Ia serum on mitogenic response. I. Inhibition of the proliferative response to B cell mitogen, LPS, by specific anti-Ia sera. *J. Immunol.* **115**, 1672.
39. Meo, T., David, C. S. & Shreffler, D. C. 1976) *H-2*-associated MLR determinants: immunogenetics of the loci and their products. In: *The Role of Products of the Histocompatibility Gene Complex in Immune Responses,* p. 167, Academic Press Inc., New York.
40. Schwartz, R. H., David, C. S., Sachs, D. H. & Paul, W. E. (1976) T lymphocyte-enriched murine peritoneal exudate cells. III. Inhibition of antigen-induced T lymphocyte proliferation with anti-Ia antisera. *J. Immunol.* **117**, 531.
41. Nabholz, M. & Miggiano, V. (1976) The biological significance of the mixed leukocyte reaction. In: *B and T Cells in Immune Recognition,* eds. Loor, F. & Roelants, G. E., Wiley and Sons, Intern. Publ. Co., Chichester, England.

Associations Between HLA and Disease

Notes on methodology and a report from the HLA and Disease Registry

Arne Svejgaard & Lars P. Ryder

Introduction

There are two major different approaches to studying whether a genetic trait, or more generally a genetic system, in this case the HLA system, is related to a disease or a condition. One of these consists of population studies in which the frequencies of HLA characters in a group of unrelated patients are compared with the corresponding frequencies in a group of healthy controls. The other is to study families in order to see if affected relatives share HLA haplotypes more often than expected according to the general genetic rules. Each of the two approaches gives different kinds of information: the population studies give, strictly speaking, only information about association (in the statistical sense) between the markers employed and the disease, while the family studies can reveal genetic linkage between the marker locus (loci) and a major disease-controlling gene. Association and linkage are two different concepts; association between two characters can, in principle, occur without linkage between the corresponding loci, and linkage between two loci does not imply association between corresponding characters. However, association may, under various conditions, be found between some alleles at two closely linked loci, which is a well-known feature of the HLA system (1, 2). Population studies are, in general, much easier to perform, but they have one major drawback: the HLA characters under study may not include that (or those) which is (are) truly responsible for disease susceptibility. Thus, if an association is found, it may be due to linkage disequilibrium between HLA factors which makes it difficult to determine the degree to which HLA is involved in disease susceptibility or resistance. In the extreme case, the truly responsible HLA factor may be so loosely (or not at all) associated with the HLA factors studied that a connection may go entirely undetected. In such cases, family studies may reveal a relationship, but such studies are, of course, limited to families with more than one affected member and these may well represent a biased sample of patients. Moreover, family studies are often hampered by problems due to incomplete penetrance and varying age at onset.

Family studies are dealt with elsewhere in this book by Kidd *et al.* (3) and Thomson & Bodmer (4). In this chapter, only population studies will be examined. In the first part there is a more general discussion of how these studies are performed and the implica-

Tissue-Typing Laboratory of the Blood-Grouping Department, State University Hospital of Copenhagen, Denmark.

46

tions of the HLA and disease associations in terms of diagnosis; how it can be decided which HLA characters are most strongly associated with a disease; and whether an association primarily concerns a specific HLA haplotype. In the final part of the chapter, the results of combined calculations are given on most of the association data that was available at the International HLA and Disease Registry in Copenhagen.

General discussion on HLA and disease association studies

Population studies

The basic material for these studies consists of the HLA phenotypes in a group of unrelated patients and in a group of unrelated control individuals of the same homogeneous ethnic origin. Due to the extreme polymorphism of HLA, virtually all phenotypes are very rare, and a comparison of all occurring phenotypes would, in general, not be very informative. Accordingly, the analysis is usually reduced to a comparison of the frequencies of the individual HLA characters in patients with those in controls. For each character (HLA antigen), a 2×2 table is set up as illustrated in Table I, and an investigation is made into whether there is a statistically significant deviation between the frequencies in patients and controls.

This can be done by Fisher's exact test or by various approximations, for example, the classical chi-square test. The latter test is not completely reliable when one or more of the expected entries in the 2×2 table is small (<5). (For a more detailed description of methods of analysis, the reader is referred to references 6–10).

It is important to distinguish between the statistical significance and the strength of an association. The *strength* can be measured by the so-called cross-product ratio ($=$ incidence ratio) which, for diseases of low frequencies in the population, is the *relative risk* of developing a disease when an antigen is present in an individual relative to the risk when it is lacking. As shown in Table I, the relative risk is simply esti-

TABLE I

Detection of association – the 2×2 table

| Group | No. of individuals | | Total |
	HLA-B8 positive	HLA-B8 negative	
Juvenile diabetes	38 (44.7 %)	47	85
Controls	467 (23.7 %)	1500	1967
Total	505 (24.6 %)	1547	2052

Strength of the association: Relative risk $= \dfrac{38 \times 1500}{47 \times 467} = 2.60$

Statistical significance:
χ^2 with Yate's correction for discountinuity $= 18.19$, which for one degree of freedom corresponds to p $= 10^{-5}$ (two sided).
Fisher's exact p $= 3 \times 10^{-5}$ (one sided)

Data from Nerup *et al.* (5)

mated by the cross-product ratio of the entries in the 2×2 table. A relative risk higher than one (a positive association) is seen when an antigen is more frequent in the patients than in the controls, whereas a risk below unity (a negative association) reflects decreased frequency in the patients. One reason for distinguishing between the statistical significance and the strength is that they do not always parallel each other. For example, a relative risk may well deviate strongly from unity in the absence of statistical significance when the number of patients and/or controls is small. In contrast, when many subjects have been studied, a relative risk deviating only slightly from unity may do so in a statistically highly significant way. The relative risk may further be considered a measure of the biological significance.

It is worth noting that it is in general more difficult to obtain statistical significance for decreased relative risks than for increased ones. This is true when the controls outnumber the patients and the control antigen frequency is below 50 per cent. This fact should not be misinterpreted to mean that the number of controls should be kept low: on the contrary, it is always advantageous to have a large control population. But it is more difficult (i.e. more patients are needed) to demonstrate that an antigen confers resistance than to demonstrate susceptibility. For example, if only 50 patients have been studied, it is virtually impossible to demonstrate a decrease of a control antigen frequency from ten to five per cent irrespective of how many controls are available; it can only be done by increasing the number of patients studied.

Combination of data

When several sources of data are available (i.e. several 2×2 tables for a given antigen), it is possible to make combined estimates of a supposedly common relative risk by special formulae developed by Woolf (7) and Haldane (8) which are discussed elsewhere (9, 10). This is obviously a great advantage because more accurate estimates of the relative risks can thus be made, and at the same time a more valid picture of the statistical significance can be obtained. Naturally, data obtained in different races should not be pooled without comment.

Evaluating the statistical significance

Usually, the frequencies of 20 or more HLA antigens are compared between the patients and controls and, accordingly, there is a considerable possibility that one of these antigens will by chance deviate significantly at the 0.05 probability level. The easiest way of overcoming this problem is to correct the ordinary p values for the number of comparisons made by multiplying them with the number of antigens studied. The p values thus obtained are often referred to as 'corrected p values' (pc). Another possibility is, of course, to use conservative p values. For example, if 25 antigens have been studied, a true probability of one per cent would correspond to a p value of $0.01/25 = 4 \times 10^{-4}$. It may be worth noting that these procedures are somewhat conservative but this seems fair as there is no reason to accept too many 'false' associations.

The above correction is only necessary in the first study when there is no *a priori* expectation that a specific antigen will deviate. It is not suggested that the correction be used in subsequent studies aiming at proving or disproving the deviation of a specific antigen, but it must be done when combined estimates of the statistical significance are made from all available data.

Analysis of more detailed phenotype data

When an association with one or more antigens has been established, additional valuable information can usually be obtained by analysis of more detailed phenotype data. This information relates to topics such as susceptibility *vs.* resistance and dominance *vs.* recessivity.

Antigens belonging to the *same segregant series,* A, B, C, or D, behave as is controlled by allelic genes, and accordingly, when one of these antigens occurs with increased (or decreased) frequency, it must be expected, that the other antigens from the same series are decreased (or increased). Therefore, it is possible that confusion might arise as to which antigen shows the 'true' association, positive or negative. There has been little difficulty up to now in this respect but the situation may arise, in particular when primary decreases of one or a few antigens are involved. When determining whether a negative association is stronger than a positive one, it can be done by comparing the reciprocal of the relative risk for the negative association with the risk for the positive one; for example, in psoriasis vulgaris, the relative risks for HLA-B13-, BW17-, and BW37-positive individuals are 4.7, 4.7, and 6.4 respectively, while the risks for HLA-B7 and B8 positives are 0.41 and 0.47 respectively. The reciprocals of the two latter values are 2.4 and 2.1; these negative associations are weaker than the positive ones and accordingly it seems likely that the decreases in B7 and B8 are secondary to the increases of the three former antigens.

Whether one is dealing with primarily increased or decreased frequencies naturally refers to the problem of whether *susceptibility* or *resistance* is at hand. It seems fair to state that most associations detected so far reflect susceptibility associated with one or a few antigens. The next problem to be solved concerns *dominance vs. recessivity* and is dealt with in detail by Thomson & Bodmer in this volume. Here it suffices to say that recessivity would betray itself by a high proportion of homozygotes among the affected individuals, and this would be true even if a marker which is associated with the character truly responsible for the association is dealt with.

In some diseases, more than one antigen from the same segregant series show positive associations; apart from psoriasis vulgaris mentioned above, this is also true for juvenile diabetes mellitus, in which the HLA-B8 and BW15 antigens of the B series are both increased in most Caucasian populations studied. Naturally, when the relative risk for B8 alone is estimated, this antigen is compared also with BW15 which in itself shows an increased risk, and thus, a true picture is not given for either of these two antigens by looking at them separately. Evidence has been provided (11) by analysing the detailed phenotype data that there is considerably increased risk for *B8/BW15* heterozygotes compared with other B8- or BW15-positive individuals. In Table II, the authors have analysed their data together with phenotype data kindly submitted by Mayr (12) and Woodrow (13). The increased risk for *B8/BW15* heterozygotes is outstanding and present in all three sources of data. It is important to note that the risks for individuals who are most likely homozygous for *B8* or *BW15* are not nearly as high. If they were, it might have been argued that the extraordinary increase of *B8/BW15* heterozygotes was

TABLE II
Risk of juvenile diabetes for various HLA-B phenotypes

HLA-B phenotype	Relative risk		Significance	
	Estimate	95 % Limits	Relative risk	Heterogeneity
BW15,x	2.5	1.8 → 3.4	10^{-7}	>.05
BW15	2.1	0.8 → 5.2	>.05	≥.05
B8,x	2.5	2.0 → 3.3	<10^{-10}	>.05
B8	3.1	2.0 → 4.8	10^{-6}	>.05
B8,BW15	9.8	6.0 →16.0	<10^{-10}	>.05
Others	1.0			

Calculation based on three different studies on a total of 490 patients and 2,792 controls (5, 12, 13).
'x' indicates the presence of an HLA-B antigen different from B8 and BW15.
The phenotypes 'BW15' and 'B8' indicate absence of other HLA-B antigens. All comparisons were made between the phenotype in question and the group of other phenotypes.

due to the possibility that *B8* and *BW15* were both associated with the same gene on another HLA locus closely linked to the B locus, and that this gene conferred a recessive susceptibility to juvenile diabetes. In this case, however, *B8* and *BW15* homozygotes would frequently be homozygous for the supposed disease gene as well and should also show a greater risk. It may be argued that some of these 'homozygotes' are in fact heterozygous and carry a *'blank' (null)* allele of the B series. However, the frequency of this allele is very low (3.1 per cent in Danes (14)), and it can be estimated that about two thirds of the 'homozygotes' are truly homozygous for *B8* and *BW15*. The possibly slightly increased risks for *B8* and *BW15* homozygotes compared with heterozygotes not carrying both may easily be explained by the fact that the B8- and BW15-associated HLA-D antigens, DW3 and DW4 respectively, are more strongly associated with the disease than B8 and BW15 themselves (cf. below and 15): *B8* homozygotes have a higher chance of being DW3 positive than *B8* heterozygotes, and the same is true for *BW15* homozygotes with respect to DW4.

The above observations are most easi-ly interpreted by assuming that there is one *B8*-associated *HLA* gene which by itself confers an increased risk of diabetes and another *BW15*-associated gene which also does, and when the two are present together they act together to further increase the risk. As pointed out by Ceppellini (personal communication), this is an example of overdominance (if the genes in question are on the same locus) or epistasis (if they are not), and not one of recessivity. It is worth noting that overdominance or epistasis may, to a large extent, simulate recessivity in family analyses, and thus the authors' findings are in agreement with those obtained by Thomson & Bodmer (4) using the sib-pair method of Day & Simons (16) although Thomson & Bodmer reach another conclusion.

When two normally associated antigens from *different series,* for example, HLA-B8 and DW3, are both increased, it is naturally important to investigate which of them shows the strongest association. This can again be done by comparing the magnitudes of the relative risk for these two antigens. However, it is generally difficult to obtain statistical significance between two risks, and instead the authors suggest testing the presence *vs.* absence of one of the

TABLE III
Detection of the stronger association

Group		No. of Individuals			Relative risk	Fisher's p
		DW3 pos.	DW3 neg.	Total		
HLA-B8 pos.	Juvenile diabetes	15 (100 %)	0	15 ⎫	indef.	0.020
	Controls	26 (72 %)	10	36 ⎭		
HLA-B8 neg.	Juvenile diabetes	6 (22 %)	21	27 ⎫	4.7	0.015
	Controls	7 (6 %)	114	121 ⎭		
		B8 pos	B8 neg.	Total		
DW3 pos.	Juvenile diabetes	15 (71 %)	6	21 ⎫	0.67	
	Controls	26 (79 %)	7	33 ⎭		
DW3 neg.	Juvenile diabetes	0 (0 %)	21	21 ⎫	0.0	
	Controls	10 (8 %)	114	124 ⎭		

Data from Thomsen *et al.* (15, 17).

antigens in patients and controls in individuals with and without the other antigen. An example of this procedure for juvenile diabetes is shown in Table III, and it appears that DW3 is significantly increased both in B8-positive and in B8-negative patients compared with the corresponding controls. In contrast, B8 has approximately the same frequency in DW3-positive patients and controls, and in DW3-negative patients and controls. Accordingly, DW3 is more strongly associated with juvenile diabetes than B8, and the increase of the latter is simply secondary to that of DW3.

Does an association primarily concern certain haplotypes?

This is a difficult question to answer, but the following procedure is proposed. If the assumption is that the *HLA-A1, B8, DW3* haplotype is more strongly associated with a DW3-associated disease than other *DW3*-carrying haplotypes, then A1 and B8 should occur together more often in DW3-positive patients than in DW3-positive controls. This can be tested in a 2×2 table as illustrated in Table IV. There is no evi-

TABLE IV

Association between HLA-A1 and B8 in DW3 -positive patients with juvenile diabetes and in DW3-positive controls

Group	No. of Individuals with Phenotype		
	HLA-A1, B8	Others	Total
Patients	23 (59 %)	16	39
Controls	25 (74 %)	9	34
Total	48 (66 %)	25	73

Fisher's p = 0.14
Data from Thomsen *et al.* (17)

dence of an association and the authors conclude that the association is not specific for the *A1,B8,DW3* haplotype, and their impression is that the association concerns all *DW3*-carrying haplotypes equally. Obviously, this is not easy to prove except by extensive family studies with unequivocal establishment of many patients' HLA genotypes. Terasaki & Mickey (18) developed a special formula for estimating haplotype frequencies from phenotype data on unrelated patients and provided some evidence that certain haplotypes may confer higher susceptibility than others for some diseases. However, the crucial problem is the significance testing, and for most diseases, it has not been shown that one specific haplotype is more involved than others.

Nevertheless, there is one condition in which one haplotype is outstanding. As discussed by Dupont *et al.* (19), deficiency for the second component of complement, C2, is very strongly associated with *HLA-DW2* which, in the general population, occurs most often on *B7*-carrying haplotypes; however, in haplotypes carrying the C2-deficiency gene and the *DW2* gene, *B18* is by far the most common HLA-B allele. Although there is a weak association between B18 and DW2 in the general population, the *B18, DW2* haplotype is much more strongly associated with C2 deficiency than other DW2-carrying haplotypes. It is uncertain whether the association between AW25 and B18 in C2 deficiency is stronger than in controls where there is also a similarly very strong association. The very high proportion of DW2 homozygotes among C2-deficient individuals reflects the well-known fact that C2 deficiency is a recessive condition.

Another good candidate for special haplotype involvement is the *HLA-A3, B14* haplotype in haemochromatosis (20). However, this has as yet only been shown in one population and needs confirmation in others.

Notes on the diagnostic value of HLA typing

At the time of writing, the strongest case for the diagnostic use of HLA typing concerns investigation of HLA-B27 in suspected ankylosing spondylitis. However, as pointed out by Brewerton & Albert (21), even in that disease HLA typing is probably used too much at the moment. Nevertheless, there is little doubt that HLA typing has its place in some cases, and it is also likely to become valuable in other diseases when

B-lymphocyte typing becomes easier. The point the authors would like to emphasize here is that the value of HLA typing in diagnosis largely depends on the *a priori* probability (based on clinical and other findings) that a given patient has the disease (22). The following formulae can be used for estimating the *a posteriori* probabilities of the disease when HLA typing has been done:

(I) the probability of the disease, if the patient has the disease-associated antigen is:

$$p_{D/A+} = h_p \cdot p_a / [h_p \cdot p_a + h_c(1 - p_a)];$$

(ii) the probability of the disease if this antigen is absent is:

$$p_{D/A-} = (1 - h_{\ddot{p}}) \, p_a / [(1 - h_p) \, p_a + (1 - h_c)(1 - p_a)];$$

where $h_{\ddot{p}}$ and h_c are the frequencies of the antigen in patients and controls, respectively, and p_a is the *a priori* probability. In fact, these formulae can be used in general to evaluate the importance of a diagnostic test: h_c is the frequency of 'false positives' and $1 - h_p$ that of 'false negatives'.

Table V illustrates how the *a priori*

TABLE V
Diagnostic value.
HLA-B27 is a diagnostic criterium for ankylosing spondylitis (AS) with:
9 % false positives
10 % false negatives

A priori probability (%) of AS	A posteriori probability (%) of AS	
	Pat. B27 pos.	Pat. B27 neg.
20	72	3
50	91	12
80	98	34

Note: B27 cannot distinguish between AS and Reiter's syndrome or other reactive arthropathies.

probabilities of ankylosing spondylitis influence the *a posteriori* probabilities after HLA typing. It would appear that

HLA typing gives most information when the *a priori* probability is between, say, 20 and 70 per cent. The authors are well aware that it is often difficult to establish an *a priori* probability; and it should also be noted that HLA typing naturally cannot distinguish between ankylosing spondylitis and reactive arthritis – if this distinction is to be made.

Pitfalls in HLA and disease studies

There are several possibilities of drawing false conclusions from HLA and disease studies. Apart from the statistical problems discussed above, erroneous statements may be due to special selection of patients and/or controls and to technical typing difficulties. These problems have been discussed in detail elsewhere (11), and here attention will be drawn to some of the pitfalls which may arise due to a biased ascertainment of patients. For diseases which do not always need hospital care there is a considerable possibility that the cases studied represent the more severe ones. Retrospective studies of lethal disease are likely to include a high proportion of long-term survivors and an association found in retrospective studies may well reflect increased survival value (23) and not susceptibility to the disease. An increased survival value is obviously of great interest, but the distinction between prospective and retrospective studies should be kept in mind. Finally, it should be noted that spurious associations may arise if inbred populations are studied, and in studies of populations which show stratification, i.e. which have not yet reached equilibrium after racial admixture, for example, the American Blacks.

THE DATA

In Table VI, the results are given of combined calculations on most of the data available at the HLA and Disease Registry. The data include those found in the literature and unpublished data submitted to the registry. Most of the latter will probably be published elsewhere by the authors in question. The data treated in the report (24) prepared prior to the First International Symposium on HLA and Disease are included in the present calculations. In addition, the authors have tried to incorporate as much as possible of the data which have been received during or after the symposium. However, it appeared an impossible task to include all these new data within the time limits given, and accordingly, selections have been made, and these have been based on the following rules: the authors have preferentially included, (i) new data concerning diseases not previously studied, (ii) data concerning diseases for which only few patients had previously been reported, or where (iii) doubtful or negative associations had previously been found, and (iv) data on non-Caucasians. However, studies concerning only few patients were often excluded, and when earlier abundant studies of many patients had shown definite associations (e.g. psoriasis), new data were not included (but it is only a matter of time before this will be done). Nevertheless, when it was decided to include new data on a disease, the authors tried to treat all new data.

In general, the principles have been followed which were outlined in the earlier report (24) which discusses the problems arising from things such as lack of control groups, double or triple publication of the same data, different diagnostic criteria, different subdivisions of diseases, and antigen 'splits'.

Calculations were made according to the method of Woolf as modified by Haldane (for details see 9, 10). In the first report (24), the individual data were included from all studies reported for all deviating antigens. Space does not allow this to be done here. Table VI gives only the results of combined calculations and when there is little doubt as to which antigen(s) show(s) the 'primary' association(s), only the results for this (or these) antigen(s) are given; for example, in the HLA-B27-association arthropathies the 'secondary' decreases of most of the other HLA-B series antigens are not included.

The general cut-off point for including an antigen has been a p value of 4×10^{-4}, roughly corresponding to a corrected p value of 0.01 if 25 antigens have been studied. Naturally, this is a rather conservative approach, but it was felt that if a higher p value were used, too many false associations would be included, and it is justified because the individual chapters of this book discuss the doubtful, but perhaps true, associations in detail. Even with the authors' conservative approach, some of the associations given may be due to chance but they would appear to be rather few. Occasionally, antigens not passing the above test are also given, when they have been of special interest, and accordingly, the p values should always be consulted.

The analyses have, in general, concerned all HLA-A and -B antigens reported; the C-series antigens have only been reported in a few studies and have not been subject to a complete analysis. On the other hand, the authors have

54

tried to include all HLA-D data available, and the results of these are given when they were found relevant in terms of HLA-B associations. Too few data are as yet available on B-lymphocyte typing to justify combined analyses, and the corresponding data are only quoted in the chapters dealing with the various disease groups.

Table VI gives the results for the diseases grouped according to the chapters of this book: rheumatology, neurology, dermatology, endocrinology, gastroenterology, allergology, immunopathology, malignant diseases, and other diseases, in that order.

For each group, *the first part of the Table* gives a serial number, the diseases studied (with names and extended WHO code numbers), the reference numbers, and the antigens deviating; the direction of the deviation is indicated with upward or downward arrows for increased and decreased frequencies respectively. References indicated by an asterisk contain HLA-D data. In general, only antigens differing significantly at the arbitrary p value of less than 4×10^{-4} are given. Data on antigens in bold face are given in detail in the second part of the Table (cf. below). When no antigens passed the significance test, the minimum and maximum number of patients reported for the disease in question are given. The minimum numbers refer to antigens which have only been studied in a limited number of patients. The number of studies is usually, but not always, identical to the number of references. If not otherwise stated, the information concerns Caucasians only. When data on other ethnic groups are available they are given separately with a separate serial number.

In *the second part of the Table,* the data on the antigens in bold face in the first part are given in more detail under the same serial number as in the first

part. For each antigen, the authors have given, (i) the number of studies, (ii) the total number of patients studied, (iii) the minimum and maximum frequencies (percentages) of the antigen in the various patient groups studied (range-%-positive), (iv) the total number of controls, (v) the range-%-positive in controls, (vi) the combined estimate of the relative risk, (vii) the significance of the deviation from unity, and (viii) the significance of heterogeneity between relative risks of the individual studies concerning the antigen. The p values in the last two columns have been calculated from the chi-square values by approximation formula; when only one study is available, Fisher's exact p (one sided) is given, and there is, of course, no heterogeneity. Other p values are 'two sided' and all are given in floating-point notation, for example p = 3.2E–06 means $p = 3.2 \cdot 10^{-6}$; they have not been multiplied by the number of antigens studied. Significant heterogeneity may reflect differences between the various studies concerning patient selection (e.g. diagnostic criteria, prospective and retrospective studies), environmental and genetic factors in general, and serological difficulties, or it may result from chance variations.

The references relating to Table VI are given below and in order to save space, only the name of the first author is given when published data are concerned; in this case a '+ +' after the reference indicates that additional data have been submitted to the registry by these investigators and these data are also included in the calculations. For unpublished data, the names of all investigators and their location (city and/or country) are given; data received during or after the First International Symposium on HLA and Disease (Paris, June 1976) are indicated by '§'; in many cases, abstracts of these data can be found in ref. 25; for data received earlier, the year of receipt is indicated. This study was financed in part by grants from the Danish Medical Research Council, the Danish Blood Donor Foundation, the Danish Rheumatoid Association, the EEC, and WHO.

The authors are extremely grateful to colleagues from all over the world who have submitted data to the the registry. They would also like to thank Mrs. Elly Andersen and Mrs. Elisabeth Schacht for their expert secretarial assistance.

TABLE VI
Rheumatology

ANKYLOSING SPONDYLITIS (WHO: 712,490)
1. European and North American Caucasians (5, 45, 46, 52, 62, 72, 73, 95, 153, 155, 184, 202, 209, 251, 256, 258, 263, 271, 321, 326)
            A1↓, A2↑, B5↓, B7↓, B8↓, B12↓, B27↑
2. Indians (Haida, British Columbia) (105)   **B27↑**
3. American Blacks (155)   **B27↑**
4. Persians (71)   **B27↑**
5. Japanese (285, 297)   **B27↑**
6. REITER's DISEASE (WHO: 136,010) (1, 2, 5, 48, 62, 202, 207, 333, 336)   **B27↑**
7. YERSINIA ARTHRITIS (WHO: 714,991) (1, 2, 117)   **B27↑**
8. SALMONELLA ARTHRITIS (WHO: 714,992) (92, 129)   **B27↑**
  PSORIATIC ARTHRITIS (WHO: 696,090)
9. Central (48, 88, 147, 200, 263)   **B13↑, B27↑, BW38↑**
10. Peripheral (48, 88, 147, 200, 263)   **B17↑, B27↑, BW38↑**
11. Unspecified (48, 149, 337)   **B13↑, B17↑, B27↑**
12. FROZEN SHOULDER (WHO: 717,190) (51)   **B27↑**
13. JUVENILE ARTHRITIS (WHO: 712,090)
  (50, 102, 119, 220, 242, 267, 303, 326)   **B27↑, BW15↑**
  ACUTE ANTERIOR UVEITIS (WHO: 366,000)
14. Caucasians (29, 47, 48, 183)   **B27↑**
15. Japanese (94), 25 patients studied   n.s.d.
  RHEUMATOID ARTHRITIS (WHO: 712,390)
16. Caucasians (41, 96, 131, 139, 174, 184, 222, 271, 282, 315*)   **A2↑, B27↑, DW4↑**
17. Japanese (212), 34 patients studied   n.s.d.
17a. Mixed (298*)   **DW4↑**
18. RHEUMATIC FEVER AND/OR RHEUMATIC HEART DISEASE (WHO: 390,990)
  (54, 85, 172), 109–235 patients studied   n.s.d.
  RHEUMATIC HEART DISEASE (WHO: 391,000)
19. Caucasians (20, 144, 172, 327)   **A2↑**
20. Mexicans (108), 48 patients studied   n.s.d.
21. CHONDROCALCINOSIS (WHO: 722,990) (97, 224) 13–42 patients studied   n.s.d.
22. PAGET's DISEASE (WHO: 721,990) (64, 199), 46–140 patients studied   n.s.d.
  CALCIFICATION OF POSTERIOR LONGITUDINAL LIGAMENT (WHO: 733,000)
23. Japanese (3), 50 patients studied   n.s.d.
24. GOUT (WHO: 274,000) (271), 66 patients studied   n.s.d.

Serial no.	HLA	No. of studies	Patients Total	Patients % pos-range	Controls Total	Controls % pos-range	Relative risk	Relative risk	Heterog.
ANKYLOSING SPONDYLITIS									
1.	A2	14	664	47–68	6236	42–57	1.55	2.3E–07	>.05
1.	B27	21	967	71–100	7879	3–12	90.09	<1E–10	>.05
2.	B27	1	17	100	222	51	34.38	1.7E–05	

56

3. B27	1	23	48	60	2	36.49	8.5E–07	
4. B27	1	25	92	400	3	349.59	4.4E–28	
5. B27	2	63	67–92	167	0–2	324.49	<1E–10	>.05

REITER's DISEASE

6. B27	8	321	65–100	5517	4–14	35.89	<1E–10	2.7E–02

YERSINIA ARTHRITIS

7. B27	2	116	58–76	2293	9–14	17.59	<1E–10	>.05

SALMONELLA ARTHRITIS

8. B27	2	18	60–69	1987	8–10	17.57	3.1E–10	>.05

PSORIATIC ARTHRITIS

9. B13	4	86	9–37	996	4–8	4.79	7.7E–08	>.05
9. B27	5	97	17–58	1071	4–14	8.58	<1E–10	>.05
9. BW38	2	44	17–27	416	3–3	9.09	5.6E–07	>.05
10. BW17	4	121	6–35	996	4–9	5.84	<1E–10	>.05
10. B27	5	168	7–24	1071	4–14	2.50	3.5E–04	>.05
10. BW38	2	87	7–18	416	3–3	4.52	3.2E–04	>.05
11. B13	2	104	9–18	2405	4–7	2.86	5.4E–04	>.05
11. BW17	2	104	25–25	2405	8–8	3.80	6.9E–08	>.05
11. B27	3	115	27–91	2480	4–12	4.45	<1E–10	2.3E–04

FROZEN SHOULDER

12. B27	1	38	42	216	10	6.34	6.9E–06	

JUVENILE RHEUMATOID ARTHRITIS

13. B27	8	487	15–57	4792	6–14	4.51	<1E–10	2.0E–05
13. BW15	7	433	4–49	4478	8–26	1.84	1.2E–05	>.05

ACUTE ANTERIOR UVEITIS

14. B27	3	291	37–58	1533	7–10	9.43	<1E–10	3.4E–03

RHEUMATOID ARTHRITIS

16. A2	10	831	49–67	6372	42–58	1.45	1.9E–06	>.05
16. B27	9	769	4–49	6258	5–14	1.81	1.3E–06	1.1E–02
16. DW4	1	38	45	157	17	3.9	5.5E–04	
17a. DW4	1	43	72	45	13	16.8	1.5E–08	

RHEUMATIC HEART DISEASE

19. A2	4	276	57–65	3509	46–55	1.68	1.2E–04	>.05

Neurology

MULTIPLE SCLEROSIS (WHO: 340,000)
1. Caucasians (8, 24, 69, 111*, 142, 209*, 211, 225*, 227*, 231*, 238*, 257, 292, 300*, 317*)
   A2↓, **B7**↑, B12↓, **DW2**↑
2. American Blacks (78*)   **B7**↑, **DW2**↑
3. OPTIC NEURITIS (WHO: 367,020) (209*, 262*)   **B7**↑, **DW2**↑
4. SUBACUTE SCLEROSING PANENCEPHALITIS (SSPE) (WHO: 323,090)
   (163, 166), 60 patients studied   n.s.d.
5. AMYOTROPHIC LATERAL SCLEROSIS (WHO: 348,090)
   (7, 232), 25–69 patients studied   n.s.d.
   MYASTHENIA GRAVIS (WHO: 733,090)
6. Caucasians (14, 17, 93, 145, 209*, 237*, 309)   A1↑, B7↓, **B8**↑, **DW3**↑
7. Japanese (3, 214, 216, 324)   **B12**↑
8. PARALYTIC POLIOMYELITIS (WHO: 41,990) (69, 141, 235, 338)   **BW16**↑
9. NEUROMYELOPATHY IN VITAMIN B12 DEFICIENCY (WHO: 263,800)
   (127), 16 patients studied   n.s.d.
10. CHORIORETINITIS (WHO: 366,030) (30), 48 patients studied   n.s.d.

11. RETINITIS CENTRALIS SEROSA (WHO: 366,031) (30), 67 patients studied n.s.d.
12. MORBUS EALES (WHO: 378,990) (30), 48 patients studied n.s.d.
13. SCHIZOPHRENIA (WHO: 295,000) (15, 79, 135, 198, 293) **A28↑, B5↑**
14. MANIC DEPRESSIVE DISORDER (WHO: 296,000) (15, 21, 110, 134, 283) **BW16↑**
15. HARADA's DISEASE
    Japanese (310, 335*) **LD-Wa↑**

Serial no.	HLA	No. of studies	Patients Total	Patients % pos-range	Controls Total	Controls % pos-range	Relative risk	Relative risk	Heterog.
								Significance	
MULTIPLE SCLEROSIS									
1.	B7	12	2351	12–46	12767	14–30	1.73	<1E–10	>.05
1.	DW2	7	734	47–70	1095	15–31	4.3	<1E–10	>.05
2.	B7	1	31	36	268	16	2.91	1.1E–02	
2.	DW2	1	31	35	34	0	indef.	9.5E–05	
OPTIC NEURITIS									
3.	B7	2	84	33–39	2067	27–29	1.58	>.05	≥.05
3.	DW2	2	84	40–50	232	18–30	2.9	6.9E–05	>.05
MYASTHENIA GRAVIS									
6.	B8	5	259	38–65	1881	18–31	4.40	<1E–10	>.05
6.	DW3	2	110	25–36	164	14–19	2.3	5.6E–03	>.05
7.	B12	4	186	8–38	599	8–17	2.04	7.7E–04	9.4E–03
PARALYTIC POLIOMYELITIS									
8.	BW16	2	78	12–15	5269	3–5	4.28	2.9E–06	>.05
SCHIZOPHRENIA									
13.	A28	5	261	0–19	3172	6–10	2.25	3.9E–05	1.4E–02
MANIC DEPRESSIVE DISORDER									
14.	BW16	5	266	0–14	3909	4–12	2.29	6.4E–05	>.05
HARADA's DISEASE									
15.	LD-Wa	1	33	67	81	12	10.5	2.9E–07	

Dermatology

PSORIASIS VULGARIS (WHO: 696,000)
1. Caucasians (147, 150, 185, 221, 273, 299, 304) A3↓, B7↓, B8↓, **B13↑, BW17↑, BW37↑**
2. Japanese (3, 205, 323) **A1↑, B13↑, BW↑**
   PSORIASIS UNSPECIFIED (WHO: 696,000) A1↓, A2↓, B7↓, B8↓,
3. Caucasians (13, 26, 112*, 164, 257, 272, 276, 329, 332) **B13↑, B16↑, BW17↑, LD-E1↑**
4. Japanese (217), 47 patient studied n.s.d.
5. PUSTULAR PSORIASIS (WHO: 696,100) (146, 304) **B27↑**
6. DERMATITIS HERPETIFORMIS (WHO: 693,990)
   (44, 152, 248, 274, 296*, 314*, 328) A1↑, A2↑, **B8↑, DW3↑**
   PEMPHIGUS (WHO: 694,000)
7. Caucasians (151, 162, 248) **A10↑**
8. Japanese (122) **A10↑**
   BEHCET's DISEASE (WHO: 136,020)
9. Caucasians (56, 69, 80, 104, 252) **B5↑**
10. Japanese (94, 212, 226, 229, 311) **B5↑**
11. RECURRENT APHTHOUS STOMATITIS (WHO: 528,290)
    (55, 76, 133, 239), 100–242 patients studied n.s.d.
12. RECURRENT HERPES LABIALIS (WHO: 54,000) (255) **A1↑, B8↑**

13. SCLERODERMA (WHO: 734,000) (32, 34, 69) 25–187 patients studied   n.s.d.
14. ATOPIC DERMATITIS (WHO: 691,000) (161, 306) 42–87 patients studied   n.s.d.
15. VITILIGO (WHO: 709,010) (128, 246) 51–141 patients studied   n.s.d.
16. ALOPECIA AREATA (WHO: 704,000) (156)   **B12↑**
17. ACNE CONGLOBATA (WHO: 706,000) (266), 65 patients studied   n.s.d.
18. LICHEN PLANUS (696,490) (176, 249, 265), 43–182 patients studied   n.s.d.
19. KELOID AND HYPERTROPHIC SCARS (WHO: 701,390)
    (170), 40 patients studied   n.s.d.
20. HAILEY-HAILEY's DISEASE (WHO: 694,040) (148), 9 patients studied   n.s.d.

Serial no.	HLA	No. of studies	Patients Total	Patients % pos-range	Controls Total	Controls % pos-range	Relative risk	Significance Relative risk	Heterog.
PSORIASIS VULGARIS									
1.	B13	8	688	2–34	5601	2–9	4.67	<1E–10	>.05
1.	B17	8	688	12–36	5601	4–11	4.69	<1E–10	>.05
1.	BW37	3	220	4–16	1029	1–3	6.35	7.3E–08	>.05
2.	A1	3	206	6–14	572	0–1	10.50	3.2E–09	>.05
2.	B13	3	206	6–11	572	1–3	3.20	8.6E–04	>.05
2.	BW37	1	100	16	355	1	19.67	1.6E–07	
PSORIASIS UNSPECIFIED									
3.	B13	9	920	7–27	7738	1–8	3.89	<1E–10	6.9E–03
3.	BW16	3	274	11–22	3857	3–5	4.11	1.9E–09	>.05
3.	BW17	9	920	10–50	7738	1–9	5.10	<1E–10	7.7E–03
3.	LD-E1	1	69	22	226	5	5.3	8.0E–05	
PUSTULAR PSORIASIS									
5.	B27	2	47	13–56	1867	8–14	3.73	1.8E–04	4.3E–02
DERMATITIS HERPETIFORMIS									
6.	B8	7	269	58–87	4081	17–33	8.74	<1E–10	3.9E–04
6.	DW3	2	66	62–93	293	19–20	13.5	<1E–10	8.5E–03
PEMPHIGUS									
7.	A10	4	81	10–61	1556	8–20	2.80	1.5E–04	>.05
8.	A10	1	19	42	77	11	6.04	2.8E–03	
BEHCET's DISEASE									
9.	B5	5	102	18–86	1360	9–25	7.43	<1E–10	7.7E–03
10.	B5	5	183	64–84	1052	31–46	4.30	<1E–10	>.05
RECURRENT HERPES LABIALIS									
12.	A1	1	90	56	606	25	3.72	1.3E–08	
12.	B8	1	90	33	606	17	2.48	3.5E–04	
ALOPECIA AREATA									
16.	B12	1	47	38	326	15	3.60	2.55E–04	

Endocrinology

JUVENILE/INSULIN-DEPENDENT DIABETES (WHO: 250,001)
1. European and American Caucasians   A1↑, A11↓, B5↓, B7↓, **B8↑**, **B18↑**
    (23, 53, 59, 63, 89, 130, 159, 177, 191, 240, 280, 291, 313*)   **BW15↑**, **DW3↑**, **DW4↑**
2. Jews (99)   **B8↑**

3. Japanese (3), 44 patients studied — n.s.
   DIABETES MELLITUS – UNSPECIFIED
4. Japanese (94), 54 patients studied — n.s.
   MATURITY-ONSET DIABETES (WHO: 250,002)
5. Caucasians (59, 63, 291, 313), 28–210 patients studied — n.s.
6. Japanese (3, 259), 54–128 patients studied — n.s.
   THYROTOXICOSIS (WHO: 242,090)
7. Caucasians (12*, 115, 218, 268, 277, 319*, 330) — B8↑, DW3↑
8. Japanese (94, 114, 212) — BW35↑
8a. Newfoundlanders (86) — B8↑
   HASHIMOTO's THYROIDITIS (WHO: 245,030)
9. Caucasians (191, 251, 331), 24–91 patients studied — n.s.
10. Japanese (94, 212), 60–95 patients studied — n.s.
10a. Newfoundlanders (87), 73 patients studied — n.s.
11. **SUBACUTE THYROIDITIS (WHO: 245,020)** (11*, 182, 222) — BW35↑, DW1↑
12. **IDIOPATHIC ADDISON's DISEASE (WHO: 255,100)** (179, 313*) — B8↑, DW3↑
13. **ADRENOCORTICAL HYPERFUNCTION (WHO: 258,000)** (167) — A1↑, A3↓

Serial no.	HLA	No. of studies	Patients Total	Patients % pos--range	Controls Total	Controls % pos--range	Relative risk	Significance Relative risk	Heterog.
	JUVENILE/INSULIN-DEPENDENT DIABETES								
1.	B8	13	1200	19–55	6856	2–29	2.42	<1E–10	>.05
1.	B18	12	1088	5–59	5856	5–50	1.65	1.3E–06	>.05
1.	BW15	13	1200	4–50	6856	2–26	1.89	<1E–10	2.2E–02
1.	DW3	1	42	50	157	21	3.8	3.0E–04	
1.	DW4	1	79	42	157	19	3.5	5.6E–05	
2.	B8	1	50	18	500	6	3.30	7.5E–03	
	THYROTOXICOSIS								
7.	B8	7	550	25–47	5188	16–27	2.34	<1E–10	>.05
7.	DW3	2	112	52–54	202	16–21	4.4	4.9E–09	>.05
8.	BW35	3	154	0–57	644	5–20	3.68	3.0E–09	>.05
8a.	B8	1	47	57	128	26	3.82	1.2E–04	
	SUBACUTE THYROIDITIS								
11.	BW35	3	80	63–73	2512	9–14	16.81	<1E–10	>.05
11.	DW1	1	24	33	157	19	2.1	>.05	
	IDIOPATHIC ADDISON's DISEASE								
12.	B8	2	52	20–69	2417	18–24	3.88	7.3E–06	7.4E–03
12.	DW3	1	30	70	157	21	8.8	3.4E–07	
	ADRENOCORTICAL HYPERFUNCTION								
13.	A1	1	100	49	352	28	2.45	9.4E–05	
13.	A3	1	100	9	352	26	.29	9.5E–05	

Gastroenterology

1. **COELIAC DISEASE (WHO: 269,000)** (4, 69, 82, 84, 154*, 159, 178, 251, 253, 274, 297, 302) — A1↑, A9↓, B7↓, B8↑, BW35↓, DW3↑

   ULCERATIVE COLITIS (WHO: 563,190)
2. Caucasians (9, 19, 40, 103, 173, 325), 42–224 patients studied — n.s.
3. Japanese (322) — B5↑

4. CROHN's DISEASE (WHO: 563,010) (9, 19, 40, 103, 173, 254, 318, 325)
   62–298 patients studied   n.s.d.
5. PERNICIOUS ANAEMIA (WHO: 281,000) (107, 126, 190, 334, 339)   **B7↑**
6. ATROPHIC GASTRITIS (WHO: 535,000) (331)   **B7↑**
7. AUTOIMMUNE CHRONIC ACTIVE HEPATITIS (WHO: 571,931)
   (28, 91, 175, 180, 193, 195, 228*, 261)   A1↑, **B8↑**, **DW3↑**
   HEPATITIS B ASSOCIATED CHRONIC ACTIVE HEPATITIS (WHO: 571,932)
8. Caucasians (28, 91)   **B18↑**
8a. Japanese (213), 96 patients studied   n.s.d.
   HEALTHY HBsAg CARRIERS (WHO: 70,001)
9. Caucasians (27, 118, 136, 281)   **BW41↑**
10. Australian Aborigines (38)   **BW15↓**
11. ACUTE HEPATITIS (WHO: 570,000) (82, 91), 100–224 patients studied   n.s.d.
12. PRIMARY BILIARY CIRRHOSIS (WHO: 571,900) (261) 17 patients studied   n.s.d.
   HEPATITIS UNSPECIFIED (WHO: 573,030)
13. Japanese (94), 72 patients studied   n.s.d.
14. IDIOPATHIC HAEMOCHROMATOSIS (WHO: 273,290) (39, 286)   A3↑, **B14↑**

Serial no.	HLA	No. of studies	Patients		Controls		Relative risk	Relative risk	Heterog.
			Total	% pos-range	Total	% pos-range			
	COELIAC DISEASE								
1.	B8	11	505	45–89	5003	11–29	8.63	<1E–10	>.05
1.	DW3	1	28	96	100	27	73.	<1E–10	
	ULCERATIVE COLITIS								
3.	B5	1	44	73	271	41	3.80	6.3E–05	
	PERNICIOUS ANAEMIA								
5.	B7	6	251	26–52	1506	19–34	1.70	4.5E–04	5.0E–02
	ATROPHIC GASTRITIS								
6.	B7	1	27	37	395	19	2.55	2.7E–02	
	AUTOIMMUNE CHRONIC ACTIVE HEPATITIS								
7.	B8	8	339	9–68	3830	8–24	2.85	<1E–10	3.3E–05
7.	DW3	1	38	68	91	24	6.8	3.2E–06	
	HEPATITIS B ASSOCIATED CHRONIC ACTIVE HEPATITIS								
8.	B18	2	109	16–25	5302	9–10	2.58	7.8E–05	>.05
	HEALTHY HBsAg CARRIERS								
9.	BW41	1	42	12	500	1	11.16	3.3E–05	
10.	BW15	2	92	10–19	227	38–45	0.29	1.6E–04	>.05
	IDIOPATHIC HAEMOCHROMATOSIS								
14.	A3	2	80	76–78	299	27–31	8.34	<1E–10	>.05
14.	B14	1	51	25	204	3	9.23	3.1E–06	

Allergology

1. GRASS POLLINOSIS (WHO: 507,080) (137), 48 patients studied   n.s.d.
2. DUST ALLERGY (WHO: 692,910) (233, 279)   **AW33↑**
3. SILICOSIS (WHO: 515,090) (116), 75 patients studied   n.s.d.
4. ALLERGY TO INSULIN (WHO: 962,390) (22), 44 patients studied   n.s.d.
5. RAGWEED
   (see chapter on ALLERGOLOGY)

Serial no.	HLA	No. of studies	Patients		Controls		Relative risk	Significance	
			Total	% pos-range	Total	% pos-range		Relative risk	Heterog.
	DUST ALLERGY								
2.	AW33	1	60	20	300	2	11.68	1.39E–06	

Immunopathology

SYSTEMIC LUPUS ERYTHEMATOSUS (WHO: 734,190)
1. Caucasians (18, 77, 106, 113, 120, 157, 219, 308)   **B5↑, B8↑**
2. Japanese (94, 125, 214), 39–128 patients studied   n.s.d.
3. American Blacks (120), 71 patients studied   n.s.d.
   SARCOIDOSIS (WHO: 135,990)
4. Caucasians (123, 165, 234), 130–262 patients studied   n.s.d.
5. Japanese (3, 94), 45–117 patients studied   n.s.d.
6. SICCA SYNDROME (WHO: 734,900) (58, 101, 132*, 302)   **B8↑, DW3↑**
   CHRONIC GLOMERULONEPHRITIS (WHO: 582,000)
7. Caucasians (140, 201), 183–890 patients studied   n.s.d.
8. Japanese (75), 59–248 patients studied   n.s.d.
9. POLYMYALGIA RHEUMATICA (WHO: 446,310) (264), 50 patients studied   n.s.d.
   THROMBOANGITIS OBLITERANS (WHO: 443,190)
10. Japanese (3, 160), 30–90 patients studied   n.s.d.
    AORTITIS (WHO: 446,000)
11. Japanese (3), 31 patients studied   n.s.d.
12. HORTON's DISEASE (TEMPORAL ARTERITIS) (WHO: 446,300)
    (278), 61 patients studied   n.s.d.
13. ACQUIRED HAEMOLYTIC ANAEMIA (WHO: 283,090)
    (69), 36 patients studied   n.s.d.
14. IDIOPATHIC THROMBOCYTOPENIC PURPURA (WHO: 287,090)
    (69), 48 patients studied   n.s.d.
15. COMPLEMENT DEFICIENCIES
    (see chapter on IMMUNOPATHOLOGY)

Serial no.	HLA	No. of studies	Patients		Controls		Relative risk	Significance	
			Total	% pos-range	Total	% pos-range		Relative risk	Heterog.
	SYSTEMIC LUPUS ERYTHEMATOSUS								
1.	B5	6	325	11–34	3185	11–15	1.83	5.8E–05	4.5E–02
2.	B8	8	424	19–48	4361	12–23	2.11	<1E–10	>.05
	SICCA SYNDROME								
6.	B8	4	127	38–58	2637	21–31	3.15	2.5E–10	>.05
6.	DW3	1	29	69	58	10	19.	4.1E–08	

Malignant diseases

1. MALIGNANT MELANOMA (WHO: 172,990)
    (16, 57, 60, 67, 168, 290, 312), 54–514 patients studied   n.s.d.
    MAMMARY CARCINOMA (WHO: 174,990)
2. Caucasians (31, 61, 65, 143, 186, 230, 312), 233–966 patients studied   n.s.d.

3. Japanese (94), 22 patients studied   n.s.d.

4. RETINOBLASTOMA (WHO: 190,030) (43, 269)   **B12↓, BW35↑**

5. TROPHOBLASTIC NEOPLASIA (WHO: 634,290)
   (171, 204), 53–151 patients studied   n.s.d.

6. CANCER OF THE CERVIX (WHO: 180,090) (158), 69–121 patients studied   n.s.d.

7. CANCER OF THE COLON (WHO: 153,000) (67), 75 patients studied   n.s.d.

8. MYCOSIS FUNGOIDES (WHO: 202,190) (181), 19 patients studied   n.s.d.
   BURKITT's LYMPHOMA (WHO: 202,991)

9. African Blacks (37, 70, 74), 106 patients studied   n.s.d.

10. MULTIPLE MYELOMA (WHO: 203,990)
    (25, 138, 187, 294), 14–149 patients studied   n.s.d.

11. HODGKIN's DISEASE (WHO: 201,990)
    The references are given in ref. no. 305, except reference no. 121

12. ACUTE LYMPHATICA LEUKAEMIA   **A2↑, B12↑**
    The references are given in ref. no. 305. Note the heterogeneity

13. OTHER LEUKAEMIAS
    Combined calculations not yet performed; probably no significant deviations,
    see references nos. 68, 69, 206
    NASOPHARYNGEAL CARCINOMA

14. Tunisians (33), 109 patients studied   n.s.d.

15. Chinese (287, 288, 289)   Sin-2

| Serial no. | HLA | No. of studies | Patients | | Controls | | Relative risk | Significance | |
			Total	% pos- -range	Total	% pos- -range		Relative risk	Heterog.
RETINOBLASTOMA									
4.	B12	2	128	10–17	740	25–28	.37	1.1E–03	>.05
4.	BW35	2	128	0–25	740	11–23	2.35	1.9E–03	3.3E–02
HODGKIN's DISEASE									
11.	A1	17	1509		5464		1.42	5.1E–08	>.05
11.	B5	17	1508		5474		1.59	3.7E–07	4.0E–02
11.	B8	17	1510		5475		1.33	5.3E–05	>.05
11.	B18	12	1165		3677		1.85	7.0E–08	>.05
ACUTE LYMPHATICA LEUKAEMIA									
12.	A2	10	527		3215		1.34	3.0E–03	2.3E–03
12.	B12	10	527		3215		1.24	4.6E–02	3.1E–04

Other diseases

1. DOWN's SYNDROME (WHO: 759,000) (275), 76 patients studied   n.s.d.
2. CONG. HEART MALFORMATION (WHO: 746,000) (49)   **A2↑**
3. PYLORIC STENOSIS (WHO: 537,000) (66), 104 patients studied   n.s.d.
4. POLYCYSTIC KIDNEY DISEASE (WHO: 753,000) (42, 69)   **B5↑**
5. SPINA BIFIDA (family studies) (6, 36)   n.s.d.
6. BRACHYMETACARPY (259), 8 patients studied   n.s.d.
7. HARE-LIP CLEFT PALATE (family studies) (243, 244)   n.s.d.
8. CYSTIC FIBROSIS (family studies) (169, 241)   n.s.d.
9. HAEMOPHILIUS INFLUENZA, TYPE b (WHO: 39,920)
   (250), 65 patients studied   n.s.d.
10. MONONUCLEOSIS (WHO: 75,000) (270, 320), 40–150 patients studied   n.s.d.
    LEPRA (WHO: 30,000)

11. Amharas (316), 39 patients studied		n.s.d.
12. Indians (196), 49 patients studied		n.s.d.
13. Mixed (294), 82 patients studied		n.s.d.
14. ACUTE APPENDICITIS (WHO: 540,000) (202)		**B5↓, B12↑, B27↓**
15. CONG. RUBELLA (WHO: 761,390) (124), 58 patients studied		n.s.d.
16. ASBESTOSIS (WHO: 515,290) (188, 197)		**B27↑**
17. FARMER's LUNG (90), 20 patients studied		n.s.d.
18. CRYPTOGENIC FIBROSING ALVEOLITIS (81)		**B12↑**
19. ESSENTIAL HYPERTENSION (WHO: 401,990) (100, 189), 144–255 patients studied		n.s.d.
20. ISCHAEMIC HEART DISEASE (WHO: 412,990) (189) 233 patients studied		n.s.d.
GLAUCOMA (WHO: 375,000)		
21. Caucasians (10, 194, 284), 41–137 patients studied		n.s.d.
22. Japanese (3), 52 patients studied		n.s.d.
23. PARODONTITIS (WHO: 523,590) (245, 312), 251 patients studied		n.s.d.
24. AZOOSPERMY (WHO: 606,990) (35), 39 patients studied		n.s.d.
25. von WILLEBRANDT's DISEASE (WHO: 286,390) (109, 208), 28–62 patients studied		n.s.d.
26. FAMILIAL MEDITERRANEAN FEVER (98), 67 patients studied		n.s.d.

Serial no.	HLA	No. of studies	Patients		Controls		Significance		
			Total	% pos-range	Total	% pos-range	Relative risk	Relative risk	Heterog.
CONG. HEART MALFORMATION									
2.	A2	1	50	80	314	44	4.92	1.3E–06	
POLYCYSTIC KIDNEY DISEASE									
4.	B5	2	106	23–32	637	13–13	2.64	2.5E–04	>.05
APPENDICITIS ACUTA									
14.	B5	1	696	28	1085	37	.68	1.7E–04	
14.	B12	1	696	31	1085	18	2.00	6.3E–10	
14.	B27	1	696	5	1085	11	.47	2.8E–05	
ASBESTOSIS									
16.	B27	2	78	18–27	265	5–10	3.69	2.8E–04	>.05
CRYPTOGENIC FIBROSING ALVEOLITIS									
18.	B12	1	15	80	616	30	9.39	1.1E–04	

References to table VI

1. Aho, K. et al. (1975) Ann. Rheum. Dis., Suppl. 34, 29.
2. Aho, K. et al. (1974) Arthr. & Rheum. 17, 521.
3. Aizawa, M. (Hokkaido) (1976§).
4. Albert, E. D. et al. (1973) Transplant. Proc. 5, 1785.
5. Amor, B. et al. (1974) Nouv. Presse Med. 3, 1373.
6. Amos, D. B. et al. (1975) Transplant Proc. 7, 93.
7. Antel, J. P. (1976) Arch. Neurol. 33, 423.
8. Arnason, B. G. W. et al. (1974) J. Neurol. Sci. 22, 419.
9. Asquith, P. et al. (1975) Lancet i, 113.
10. Aviner, Z. et al. (1976) Tissue Antigens 7, 193.
11. Bech, K., Nerup, J., Thomsen, M., Platz, P., Ryder, L. P., Svejgaard, A., Siersbæk-Nielsen, K. & Hansen, J. Mølholm (Copenhagen/Denmark) (1976§).
12. Bech, K., Lumholz, B., Nerup, J., Thomsen, M., Platz, P., Ryder, L. P., Svejgaard, A., Siersbæk-Nielsen, K. & Han-

sen, J. Mølholm (Copenhagen/Denmark) (1976§).

13. Beckman, L. et al. (1974) Hum. Heredity 24, 496.
14. Behan, P. O. et al. (1973) Lancet ii, 1033.
15. Bennahum, D. A., Troup, G. M., Rada, R. T., Kellner, R. & Kyner, W. T. (USA) (1976§).
16. Bergholtz, B., Brennhovd, I., Klepp, O., Kaakinen, A. & Thorsby, E. (Norway) (1976§).
17. van den Berg-Loonen, E., Engelfriet, C. P., Nijenhuis, L. E., Feltkamp, T. E. W., Oosterhuis, H. J. G. H., Galema, J. M. D., van Rijn, A. C. M., Verheugt, F. W. H., Kortbakken, M., van Rossum, A. L. & van Loghem, J. J. (1973), submitted to Tissue Antigens.
18. van den Berg-Loonen, E. M., Svaak, A. J. G., Nijenhuis, L. E., Feltkamp, T. E. W. & Engelfriet, C. P. (the Netherlands) (1976§).
19. Bergman, L. et al. (1976) Tissue Antigens 7, 145.
20. Berning, J., Thomsen, M., Hansen, P. F. & Olesen, K. H. (Copenhagen/Denmark) (1975).
21. Bertelsen, A. & Kissmeyer-Nielsen, F. (Denmark), submitted in 1975.
22. Bertrams, J. & Grüneklee, D. (Germany) (1976§).
23. Bertrams, J. et al. (1976) Tissue Antigens 8, 13.
24. Bertrams, J. & Kuwert, E. (1974). Thesis.
25. Bertrams, J. et al. (1972) Tissue Antigens 2, 41.
26. Bertrams, J. et al. (1973) 5th Int. Congr. Soc. Human Blood Group Science in View of Forensic Aspects, Amsterdam.
27. Bertrams, J. et al. (1974) German Soc. Blood Transf. and Immunhematol., Berlin.
28. Bertrams, J. et al. (1974) Z. Immun Forsch. 146, 300.
29. Bertrams, J. et al. (1975) Z. Immun Forsch. 148, 389.
30. Bertrams, J., Spitznas, M., Rommelfanger, M. & Kuwert, E. (Germany) (1976§).
31. Bertrams, J. et al. (1975) Z. Krebsforsch. 83, 219.
32. Betuel, H. et al. (France) (1976§).
33. Betuel, H. et al. (1975) Int. J. Cancer 16, 249.
34. Birnbaum, N. S., Rodnan, G. P., Rabin, B. S. & Bassion, S. (1976), submitted to Tissue Antigens.
35. Bisson, J. P., David, G., Kolevsky, P., Hors, J. & Dausset, J. (France) (1976§).
36. Bobrow, M. et al. (1975) Tissue Antigens 5, 234.
37. Bodmer, J. G. et al. (1975) Tissue Antigens 5, 63.
38. Boettcher, B., Hay, J., Watterson, C. A., Bashir, H., MacQueen, J. M. & Hardy, G. (1976) J. Immunogenet., (in press).
39. Bomford, A., Eddleston, A. L. W. F., Williams, R., Kennedy, L. & Batchelor, J. R. (United Kingdom) (1976§).
40. Boné, J. & Kissmeyer-Nielsen, F. (Denmark) (1976§).
41. Brackertz, D. et al. (1973) Z. Immunforsch. 146, 108.
42. Braun, W. E., Grecek, D., Vidt, D. & Nakamoto (USA) (1976§).
43. Braun, W. E. & Price, R. L. (USA) (1976§).
44. Braun, W. E., Roberts-Thomson, I. C. & Morris, P. J. (1976), submitted to Gastroenterology.
45. Brautbar, C., Porat, S., Nelken, D., Gabriel, K. R. & Cohen, T. (Israel) (1976§).
46. Brewerton, D. A. et al. (1973) Lancet i, 904.
47. Brewerton, D. A. et al. (1973) Lancet ii, 994.
48. Brewerton, D. A. & James, D. C. O. (1975) Sem. Arthr. & Rheum. 4, 191.
49. Buc, M. et al. (1975) Tissue Antigens 5, 128.
50. Buc, M. et al. (1974) Tissue Antigens 4, 395.
51. Bulgen, D. Y. et al. (17976) Lancet i, 1042.
52. Calin, A. et al. (1974) Lancet i, 874.
53. Cathelineau, G. et al. (1976) Nouv. Presse Med. 5, 586.
54. Caughey, D. E. et al. (1975) J. Rheumatol. 2, 319.
55. Challacombe, S. J., Batchelor, J. R., Kennedy, L .A. & Lehner, T. (United Kingdom) (1976§).
56. Chamberlain, M. A. (1975) Ann Rheum. Dis. Suppl. 34, 53.
57. Clark, D. A. et al. (1974) Israel J. Med. Sci. 10, 836.
58. Clough, J. D., Aponte, C. J. & Braun, W. R. (USA) (1976§).
59. Contu, L., Puligheddu, A., Mura, C. & Gabbas, A. (Italy) (1976§).
60. Cordon, A. L. (1973) Lancet i, 938.
61. Cordon, A. L. & James, D. C. O. (1973) Lancet ii, 565.
62. Cross, R. A. et al. (1975) Aust. N. Z. J. Med. 5, 108.
63. Cudworth, A. G. & Woodrow, J. C. (1975) Diabetes 24, 345++.

64. Cullen, P. *et al.* (1976) *Tissue Antigens* **7**, 55.
65. Darke, C. (Wales) – data submitted to the registry in 1975.
66. Darke, C. *et al.* (1976) *Tissue Antigens* **7**, 189.
67. Darke, C. (Wales) (1976§).
68. Dausset, J. *et al.* (1974) *Clin. Immunol. Immunopathol.* **3**, 127.
69. Dausset, J. & Hors, J. (1975) *Transplant. Reviews* **22**, 44.
70. Dausset, J. *et al.* (1975) *Tissue Antigens* **5**, 48
71. Davatchi, F., Nikbin, B. & Ala, F. (Iran) (1976§).
72. de Deuxchaisnes, C. N. *et al.* (1974) *Lancet* **i**, 1238.
73. Dick, H. M. *et al.* (1975) *Tissue Antigens* **5**, 26.
74. Dick, H. M. *et al.* (1975) *Tissue Antigens* **5**, 52.
75. Dohi, K. & Fukuda, Y. (Hiroshima) (1976§).
76. Dolby, A. E. (Wales) data submitted to the registry in 1975.
77. Dostal, C., Ivanyi, D., Macurova, H., Hana, I. & Strejcek, I. (1976) submitted to Ann. Rheum. Dis.
78. Dupont, B., Lisak, R. P., Jersild, C., Hansen, J. A., Silberberg, D. H., Whitsett, C., Zwieman, B. & Ciongoli, K. (USA) submitted to Transplant. Proc.
79. Eberhard, G. *et al.* (1975) *Neuropsychobiol.* **1**, 211.
80. Ersoy, F., Berkel, A. I., Pirat, T. & Kazokoglu, H. (Turkey) (1976§).
81. Evans, C. C. & Evans, J. M. (1975) *Lancet* **ii**, 975.
82. Evans, D. A. P. (1973) *Lancet* **ii**, 1096.
83. Faber, V., Nielsen, L. Staub & Jersild, C. (Copenhagen/Denmark), 1972.
84. Falchuk, Z. M. *et al.* (1972) *J. Clin. Invest.* **51**, 1602.
85. Falk, J. A. *et al.* (1973) *Tissue Antigens* **3**, 173.
86. Farid, N. R. *et al.* (1975) *Int. Arch. Allergy Appl. Immun.* **49**, 837.
87. Farid, N. R. *et al.* (1976) *Tissue Antigens* **8**, 181.
88. Feldmann, J. L. *et al.* (1976) *Nouv. Presse Med.* **5**, 477.
89. Finkelstein, S. *et al.* (1972) *Tissue Antigens* **2**, 74.
90. Flaherty, D. K. *et al.* (1975) *Lancet* **ii**, 507.
91. Freudenberg, J. *et al.* (1973) *Klin. Woch.* **51**, 1075.
92. Friis, J. & Svejgaard, A. (1974) *Lancet* **i**, 1350.
93. Fritze, D. *et al.* (1974) *Lancet* **i**, 240.
94. Fukunishi, T. (Nishinomiya/Japan) (1976§).
95. Gaucher, A., Faure, G., Netter, P. & Pourel, J. (France) (1976§).
96. Gaucher, A., Faure, G., Netter, P., Pourel, J., Raffoux, C. & Streiff, F. (France) (1976§).
97. Gaucher, A., Faure, G., Netter, P., Pourel, J., Raffoux, C., Streiff, F., Tongio, M. M. & Mayer, S. (France) (1976§).
98. Gazit, E., Orgad, S. & Pras, M. (1976) submitted to Tissue Antigens.
99. Gazit, E., Sartani, A., Mizrachi, Y. & Ravid, M. (Israel) (1976§).
100. Gelsthorpe, K. *et al.* (1975) *Lancet* **i**, 1039.
101. Gershwin, M. E. *et al.* (1975) *Tissue Antigens* **6**, 342.
102. Gibson, D. J. *et al.* (1975) *New Eng. J. Med.* **293**, 636.
103. Gleeson, M. H. *et al.* (1972) *GUT* **13**, 438.
104. Godeau, P., Torre, D., Campinchi, R., Bloch-Michel, E., Schmid, M., Nunez-Roldan, A., Hors, J. & Dausset, J. (France) (1976§).
105. Gofton, J. P. *et al.* (1975) *J. Rheumatol.* **2**, 319.
106. Goldberg, M. A. *et al.* (1976) *Arthr. & Rheum.* **19**, 129.
107. Goldstone, A. H. *et al.* (1976) *Clin. Exp. Immunol.* **25**, 352.
108. Gorodezky, C., Sergio, U. L. & Escobar-Gutierrez, A. (Mexico) (1976§).
109. Goudemand, J., Mazurier, C, & Parquet-Gernez, A. (France) (1976§).
110. Govaerts, A., Mendlewicz, J. & Verbanck, P. (Belgium) data received 1976.
111. Grosse-Wilde, H., Bertrams, J., Schuppien, W., Netzel, B. & Kuwert, E. K. (Germany) (1976§).
112. Grosse-Wilde, H., Wüstner, B., Albert, E. D., Kuntz, B., Netzel, B., Scholz, S. & Braun-Falco, O. (Germany) (1976§).
113. Grumet, F. C. *et al.* (1971) *New Eng. J. Med.* **285**, 193.
114. Grumet, F. C. *et al.* (1975) *Tissue Antigens* **6**, 347.
115. Grumet, F. C. *et al.* (1974) *J. Clin. Endocrin. & Metabolism* **39**, 1115.
116. Gualde, N., de Leobardy, J., Seruzay, B. & Malinvaud, G. (France) (1976§).
117. Gylding-Sabroe, J. & Svejgaard, A. (Copenhagen/Denmark), 1975.
118. Gyódi, E., Penke, S., Novak, E. & Hollan, S. R. (1973) *Haematol.* **7**, 199.
119. Hall, M. A. *et al.* (1975) *Ann. Rheum. Dis. Suppl.* **34**, 36.

120. Hansen, J. A., Rothfield, N. F., Jersild, C., Wernet, P., McLean, R., Good, R. A. & Dupont, B. (1976) submitted to Clin. Immunol. & Immunopath.

121. Hansen, J. A., Young, C. W., Whitsett, C., Case, D. C., Jersild, C., Good, R. A. & Dupont, B. (1976) *Buffalo Symp. HLA & Malign.*

122. Hashimoto, K., Miki, Y., Nakata, S., Shirakura, R. & Mori, T. (Osaka) (1976§).

123. Hedfors, E. & Möller, E. (1973) *Tissue Antigens* 3, 95.

124. Honeyman, M. C. *et al.* (1975) *Tissue Antigens* 5, 12.

125. Horiuchi, Y. (Tokyo) (1976§).

126. Horton, M. A. & Oliver, R. T. D. (1976) *Tissue Antigens* 7, 239.

127. Horton, M. A. & Oliver, R. T. D. (United Kingdom) (1976§).

128. Howitz, J. C. & Svejgaard, A. (Copenhagen/Denmark) (1976.

129. Håkansson, U. *et al.* (1975) *Tissue Antigens* 6, 366.

130. Illeni, M. T., Pellegris, G., del Guercio, M. J., Tarantino, A., Busetto, F., Pietro, C. di, Clerici, E., Garotta, G. & Chiumello, G. (Italy) (1976§).

131. Isomäki, H. *et al.* (1975) *Ann. Clin. Res.* 7, 138.

132. Ivanyi, D. *et al.* (1975) *Tissue Antigens* 7, 45.

133. Ivanyi, D. & Zabrodsky, S. (Czechoslovakia) (1976§).

134. Ivanyi, D., Zemek, P. & Ivanyi, P. (Czechoslovakia) (1976§).

135. Ivanyi, D. *et al.* (1976) *Tissue Antigens* 8, 217.

136. Jeannet, M. & Farquet, J. J. (1974) *Lancet* ii, 1383.

137. Jeannet, M., Girard, J. P., Varonier, H. S., Mirimanoff, P. & Joye, P. (Switzerland) (1976§).

138. Jeannet, M. & Magnin, C. (1976) *Europ. J. Clin. Invest.* 2, 39.

139. Jeannet, M., Vischer, T. & Grob, P. (Switzerland) (1976§).

140. Jensen, H. *et al.* (1975) *Tissue Antigens* 6, 368.

141. Jersild, C., Larsen, E. Errebo, Dupont, B., Thomsen, M. & Svejgaard, A. (Copenhagen/Denmark) (1973).

142. Jersild, C. *et al.* (1975) *Transplant. Rev.* 22, 148.

143. de Jong-Bakker, M. *et al.* (1974) *Europ. J. Cancer* 10, 555.

144. Joysey, V. C., Bullman, W. & Roger, J. H. (United Kingdom) (1976§).

145. Kaakinen, A. *et al.* (1975) *Tissue Antigens* 6, 175.

146. Karvonen, J. (1975) *Ann. Clin. Res.* 7, 301.

147. Karvonen, J. *et al.* (1976) *Ann. Clin. Res.* 6, 304.

148. Karvonen, J. & Tiilikainen, A. (1976) *Tissue Antigens* 8, 277.

149. Kastelan, A., Jajic, I., Kerhin, V. & Balog, V. (Yugoslavia) (1976§).

150. Kastelan, A., Jajic, I., Kerhin, V. & Balog, V. (Yugoslavia) (1976§).

151. Katz, S. I. *et al.* (1973) *Arch. Dermatol.* 108, 53.

152. Katz, S. I. *et al.* (1972) *J. Clin. Invest.* 51, 2977.

153. Keuning, J. J. *et al.* (1974) (quoted in Ceppellini, R. & van Rood, J. J.) *Sem. Hematology* 11, 233.

154. Keuning, J. J. *et al.* (1976) *Lancet* i, 506.

155. Khan, M. A., Braun, W. E., Kushner, I., Grecek, D. E., Muir, W. B. & Steinberg, A. G. (USA) (1976§).

156. Kianto, U., Reunala, T., Karvonen, J., Lassus, A. & Tiilikainen, A. (Finland) (1976§).

157. Kissmeyer-Nielsen, F. *et al.* (1975) *Transplant. Rev.* 22, 146.

158. Koenig, U. D. & Müller, N. (Germany) (1976§).

159. Koivisto, V. A., Kuitunen, P., Tiilikainen, A. & Åkerblom, H. K. (1976) submitted to Diabete et Metabolisme.

160. Kozaki, M. (Tokyo) (1976§).

161. Krain, L. S. & Terasaki, P. I. (1973) *Lancet* i, 1059.

162. Krain, L. S. *et al.* (1973) *Arch. Dermatol.* 108, 803.

163. Kreth, H. W. *et al.* (1975) *Lancet* ii, 415.

164. Krulig, L. *et al.* (1975) *Arch. Dermatol.* 111, 857.

165. Kueppers, F. *et al.* (1974) *Tissue Antigens* 4, 56.

166. Kurent, J. E. *et al.* (1975) *Lancet* i, 927.

167. Lada, G., Gyódi, E. & Glaz, E. (Hungary) (1976§).

168. Lamm, L. U., *et al.* (1974) *Cancer* 33, 1458.

169. Lamm, L. U. *et al.* (1975) *Ann. Hum. Genet. (Lond.)* 38, 383.

170. Laurentaci, G. & Dioguardi, D. (Italy) (1976§).

171. Lawler, S. L. *et al.* (1971) *Lancet* ii, 834.

172. Leirisalo, M., Tiilikainen, A. & Laitinen, O. (Finland) (1976§).

173. Lewkonia, R. M. *et al.* (1974) *Lancet* i, 574.

174. Lies, R. B. *et al.* (1972) *Arthr. Rheum.* 15, 524.

175. Lindberg, J. *et al.* (1975) *Brit. Med. J.* **4**, 77.
176. Lowe, N. J. *et al.* (1976) *Brit. J. Dermatol.* **95**, 169.
177. Ludvigson, J., Säfwenberg, J. & Heding, L. G. (1976++) submitted to Diabetologia.
178. Ludwig, H. *et al.* (1974) *J. Immunogenet.* **1**, 91.
179. Ludwig, H. *et al.* (1975) *Z. Immun. Forsch.* **149**, 423.
180. Mackay, I. R. & Morris, P. J. (1972) *Lancet* **ii**, 793.
181. Mackie, R. *et al.* (1976) *Lancet* **i**, 1179++.
182. Majsky, A. & Feiz, C. (1976) *Tissue Antigens* (in press).
183. Mapstone, R. & Woodrow, J. C. (1975) *Brit. J. Ophtal.* **59**, 270.
184. Marcolongo, R. & Contu, L. (1974) *Nouv. Presse Med.* **3**, 2023.
185. Marcusson ,J. *et al.* (1975) *Acta Dermatovener.* **55**, 297.
186. Martz, E. & Benacerraf, B. (1973) *Tissue Antigens* **3**, 30.
187. Mason, D. Y. & Cullen, P. (1975) *Tissue Antigens* **5**, 238.
188. Matej, H., Lange, A. & Smolik, R. (Poland) (1976§).
189. Mathews, J. D., England, J., Shaw, J. & Mathieson, I. D. (Australia) (1976§).
190. Mawhinney, H. *et al.* (1975) *Clin. exp. Immunol.* **22**, 47.
191. Mayr, W. (Austria) data submitted in February/1976.
192. Mayr, W. (Austria) data submitted in April/1976.
193. Mayr, W. (Austria) data submitted in February/1976.
194. Mayr, W. *et al.* (Austria) data submitted in April/1976.
195. Mazzilli, M. C., Trabace, S., Raimondo, F. di, Visco, G. & Gandini, E. (Italy) (1976§).
196. Mehra, N. K., Dasgupta, A., Ghei, S. K. & Vaidya, M. C. (India) (1976§).
197. Marchant, J. A. *et al.* (1975) *Brit. Med. J.* **i**, 189.
198. Mercier, P., Kieffer, N., Julien, R. & Sutter, J. M. (France) (1976§).
199. Mercier, P. & Seignalet, J. (1975) submitted to Tissue Antigens.
200. Metzger, A. *et al.* (1975) *Arthr. Rheum.* **18**, 111.
201. Mickey, M. R. *et al.* (1970) *Histocompatibility Testing 1970*, pp. 237–242, (Munksgaard, Copenhagen).
202. Mills, D. M. *et al.* (1975) *JAMA* **231**, 268.
203. Minev, M. & Tzekov, G. (Bulgaria) (1976§).
204. Mittal, K. K. *et al.* (1975) *Tissue Antigens* **6**, 57.
205. Miyajima, T. (Chiba/Japan) (1976§).
206. Morris, P. J. (1974) *Contemporary Topics in Immunobiology*, vol. 3. Plenum Press, N.Y., London, pp. 141–169.
207. Morris, R. *et al.* (1974) *New Eng. J. Med.* **290**, 554.
208. Müller, N., Budde, U. & Etzel, F. (Germany) (1976§).
209. Möller, E. *et al.* (1975) *Histocompatibility Testing 1975*, pp. 778–781, (Munksgaard, Copenhagen).
210. Möller, E. *et al.* (1976) *Tissue Antigens* **7**, 39.
211. Naito, S. *et al.* (1972) *Tissue Antigens* **2**, 1.
212. Nakagawa, J. (Kyoto/Japan) (1976§).
213. Nakagawa, J. *et al.* (Kyoto/Japan) (1976§).
214. Nakagawa, J., Ikehara, Y. & Fukase, M. (Kyoto/Japan) (1976§).
215. Nakagawa, J., Ikehara, Y., Ito, K. & Fukase M. (Kyoto/Japan) (1976§).
216. Nakata, S. *et al.* (Osaka/Japan) (1976§).
217. Nakata, S., Shirakura, R., Matsuyama, M., Hirose, H. & Mori, T. (Osaka/Japan) (1976§).
218. Nelson, S. D. & Pollet, J. E. (1975) *Tissue Antigens* **5**, 38.
219. Nies, K. M. *et al.* (1974) *Arthr. Rheum.* **17**, 397.
220. Nissilä, M. *et al.* (1975) *New Eng. J. Med.* **292**, 430.
221. Nyfors, A. & Svejgaard, A. (1976) *Acta Dermatovener.* **56**, 235.
222. Nyulassy, S. *et al.* (1975) *Tissue Antigens* **6**, 105++.
223. Nyulassy, S. *et al.* (1974) *Lancet* **i**, 450, 1974.
224. Nyulassy, S. *et al.* (1976) *Arthr. Rheum.* **19**, 391.
225. Oger, J., Sabouraud, O., Fauchet, R., Genetet, N. & Genetet, B. (France) (1976§).
226. Ohno, S. *et al.* (1975) *Amer. Ophthalmol.* **80**, 636.
227. Opelz, G., Terasaki, P., Myers, L., Ellison, G., Ebers, G., Zabriskie, J., Weiner, H., Kempe, H. & Sibley, W. (1976) submitted to Tissue Antigens.
228. Opelz, G., Vogten, A. J. M., Summerskill, W. H. J., Schalm, S. W. & Terasaki, P. I. (1976) submitted to Tissue Antigens.
229. Orita, K. & Matsuo, Y. (Okayama/Japan) (1976§).

230. Patel, R. *et al.* (1972) *Amer. J. Surg.* **124**, 31.
231. Paty, D. W. *et al.* (1974) *Canad. J. Neurol. Sci.* **i**, 211++.
232. Pedersen, L., Platz, P., Jersild, C. & Thomsen, M. (1976) *J. Neurol. Sci.* (in press).
233. Perrin-Fayolle, M., Betuel, H., Biot, N. & Grosclaude, M. (France) (1976§).
234. Persson, I. *et al.* (1975) *Tissue Antigens* **6**, 50.
235. Pietsch, M. C. & Morris, P. J. (1974) *Tissue Antigens* **4**, 50.
236. Pirskanen, R. *et al.* (1972) *Ann. Clin. Res.* **4**, 304.
237. Pirskanen, R. (1976) *Ann. N.Y. Acad. Sci.* **274**, 451–460, 1976.
238. Platz, P. *et al.* (1974) *Proc. Roy. Soc. Med.* **67**, 1133.
239. Platz, P., Ryder, L. P. & Donatsky, O. (1976) *Tissue Antigens* **8**, 279.
240. Pointel, J. P., Raffoux, C., Janot, C., Sauvanet, J. P., Drouin, P., Streiff, F. & Debry, G. (France) (1976§).
241. Polymenidis, Z. (1973) *Lancet* **ii**, 1452.
242. Rachelefsky, G. S. *et al.* (1974) *New Eng. J. Med.* **290**, 892.
243. Rapaport, F. T. *et al.* (1973) *Transplant. Proc.* **5**, 1817.
244. Rapaport, F. T. *et al.* (1975) *Transplant. Proc.* **5**, 1823.
245. Reinholt, J., Bay, I. & Svejgaard, A. (1976) *J. Dental Res.* (in press).
246. Retornaz, G. *et al.* (1976) *Brit. J. Dermatol.* **95**, 173.
247. Retornaz, G., Betuel, H. & Thivolet, J. (France) (1976§).
248. Reunala, T. *et al.* (1976) *Brit. J. Dermatol.* **94**, 139.
249. Risum, G., Paulli, H. P. & Svejgaard, A. (Copenhagen/Denmark) (1975).
250. Robbins, J. B. *et al.* (1973) *Ann. Int. Med.* **78**, 259.
251. van Rood, J. J. *et al.* (1975) *Transplant. Rev.* **22**, 75.
252. Rosselet, E. *et al.* (1976) *Ophthalmologia* **172**, 116.
253. Rotthauwe, H. W. *et al.* (1976) *Deutsche Med. Woch.* **101**, 849.
254. Russell, A. S. *et al.* (1975) *Amer. J. Digest. Dis.* **20**, 359.
255. Russell, A. S. & Schlaut, J. (1975) *Tissue Antigens* **6**, 257.
256. Russell, A. S. *et al.* (1974) *J. Rheum.* **1**, 203.
257. Russell, T. J. *et al.* (1972) *New Eng. J. Med.* **287**, 738.
258. Sachs, J. A. *et al.* (1975) *Tissue Antigens* **5**, 120.
259. Saint-Hillier, Y. *et al.* (1976) *Nouv. Presse Med.* **5**, 1003.
260. Sakurami, T., Nabeya, N., Nagaoka, K., Kurahachi, H., Kuno, S., Nose, Y., Sumitomo, K. & Tsuji, K. (Tokai/Japan) (1976§).
261. Salaspuro, M., Tiilikainen, A., Makkonen, H. & Sipponen, P. (Finland) (1976§).
262. Sandberg-Wollheim, M. *et al.* (1975) *Acta Neurol. Scand.* **52**, 161.
263. Sany, J. *et al.* (1975) *Rev. Rheum. Osteo-Articul.* **42**, 451.
264. Sany, J., Seignalet, J., Serre, H. & Lapinski, H. (France) (1976§).
265. Saurat, J. H., Lemarchand, F., Hors, J., Nunez-Roldan, A., Gluckman, E., Cosnes, A., Puissant, A. & Dausset, J. (France) (1976§).
266. Schackert, K. *et al.* (1974) *Arch. Dermatol.* **110**, 468.
267. Schaller, J. G. *et al.* (1976) *J. Pediatrics* **88**, 927.
268. Schernthaner, G., Ludwig, H., Mayr, W. R. Höfer, R. (Austria) (1976§).
269. Schildberg, P. *et al.* (1973) *Arch. Klin. exp. Ophthal.* **186**, 33.
270. Schiller, J. & Davey, F. R. (1974) *A.J.C.P.* **62**, 325.
271. Schlosstein, L. *et al.* (1973) *New Eng. J. Med.* **288**, 704.
272. Schoefinius, H. H. *et al.* (1974) *New Eng. J. Med.* **291**, 51.
273. Schunter, F. & Schieferstein, G. (1974) *Der Hautarzt* **25**, 82.
274. Seah, P. P. *et al.* (1976) *Brit. J. Dermatol.* **94**, 131.
275. Segal, D. J. *et al.* (1975) *Humangenetik* **27**, 45.
276. Seignalet, J. *et al.* (1974) *Tissue Antigens* **4**, 59.
277. Seignalet, J. *et al.* (1975) *Rev. Franc. Transf.* **17**, 305.
278. Seignalet, J., Janbon, C., Sany, J., Janbon, F., Bidet, J. M., Brunel, M., Jourdan, J. & Bussiere, J. L. (France) (1976§).
279. Seignalet, J., Levallois, C., Lapinski, H. & Jean, R. (France) (1976§).
280. Seignalet, J. *et al.* (1975) *Tissue Antigens* **6**, 272.
281. Seignalet, J. *et al.* (1974) *Nouv. Rev. Fr. d'Hematol.* **14**, 89.
282. Seignalet, J. *et al.* (1974) (Montpellier).
283. Shapiro, R. W. *et al.* (1976) *Arch. gen. psychiatry* **33**, 823.
284. Shin, D. H., Becker, B. & Bell, C. E. (USA) (1976§).

69

285. Shirakura, R., Nakata, S., Matsuyama, M., Hirose, H. & Mori, T. (Osaka/Japan) (1976§).

286. Simon, M. *et al.* (1976) *GUT* **17**, 332.

287. Simons, M. J. *et al.* (1975) *Histocompatibility Testing 1975*, pp. 809–812, (Munksgaard, Copenhagen).

288. Simons, M. J. *et al.* (1974) *Int. J. Cancer* **13**, 122.

289. Simons, M. J. *et al.* (1975) *Lancet* **i**, 142.

290. Singal, D. P. *et al.* (1974) *Transplantation* **18**, 186.

291. Singal, D. P. & Blajchman, M. A. (1973) *Diabetes* **22**, 429.

292. Smeraldi, E. (1972) *Boll. 1st Sieroter (Milan)* **51**, 220.

293. Smeraldi, E. *et al.* (1976) *Tissue Antigens* **8**, 191.

294. Smith, G. *et al.* (1974) *Tissue Antigens* **4**, 374.

295. Smith, G. *et al.* (1975) *Vox Sang.* **28**, 42.

296. Solheim, B. G. *et al.* (1976) *Tissue Antigens* **7**, 57.

297. Sonozaki, H. *et al.* (1975) *Tissue Antigens* **5**, 131.

298. Stastny, P. (1976) *J. Clin. Invest.* **57**, 1148.

299. Stenzky, V., Nagy, E. & Ladanyi, E. (1976) *Derm. Mschr.* **162**, 35++.

300. Stewart, G. J., Basten, A., Guinan, J., Bashir, H., Cameron, J. & McLeod, J. G. (1976) submitted to J. Neurol. Sci.

301. Stokes, P. L. *et al.* (1973) *GUT* **14**, 627.

302. Sturrock, R. D. *et al.* (1974) *Ann. Rheum. Dis.* **33**, 165.

303. Sturrock, R. D. & Dick, H. M. (1974) *J. Rheum.* **1**, 269.

304. Svejgaard, A. *et al.* (1974) *Brit. J. Dermatol.* **91**, 145.

305. Svejgaard, A. *et al.* (1975) *Transplant. Rev.* **22**, 3.

306. Svejgaard, E. & Svejgaard, A. (Copenhagen), 1974.

308. Szegedi, G. & Stenzky, V. (1973) *Haematologia* **7**, 211++.

309. Säfwenberg, J. *et al.* (1973) *Tissue Antigens* **3**, 465.

310. Tagawa, Y., Sugiura, S., Yakura, H., Wakisaka, A., Aizawa, M. & Itakura, K. (1976) *New Eng. J. Med.* **295**, 173++.

311. Takano, M. *et al.* (1976) *Tissue Antigens* **8**, 95.

312. Takasugi, M. *et al.* (1973) *Cancer Res.* **33**, 648.

312. Terasaki, P. & Kaslick, R. S. (1975) *Tissue Antigens* **5**, 286.

313. Thomsen, M. *et al.* (1975) *Transplant. Rev.* **22**, 125.

314. Thomsen, M. *et al.* (1976) *Tissue Antigens* **7**, 60.

315. Thomsen, M., Sørensen, S. F., Platz, P., Ryder, L. P. & Svejgaard, A. (Copenhagen/Denmark) (1976).

316. Thorsby, E. *et al.* (1973) *Tissue Antigens* **3**, 373.

317. Thorsby, E., Helgesen, A., Solheim, B. G. & Vandvik, B. (Norway) (1976§).

318. Thorsby, E. & Lie, S. O. (1971) *Transplant. Proc.* **3**, 1305.

319. Thorsby, E. *et al.* (1975) *Tissue Antigens* **6**, 54.

320. Ting, A. *et al.* (1973) *Ser. Immunbiol. Standard.* **18**, 276.

321. Truog, P. *et al.* (1975) *Histocompatibility Testing 1975*, pp. 788–796 (Munksgaard, Copenhagen).

322. Tsuchiya, M., Yoshida, T., Asakura, H., Hibi, T., Ono, A. & Mizuno, Y. (Tokyo/Japan) (1976§).

323. Tsuji, K. *et al.* (1976) *Tissue Antigens* **8**, 29.

324. Tsuji, K. (Tokai/Japan) (1976§).

325. Vachon, A., Gebuhrer, L. & Betuel, H. (France) (1976§).

326. Veys, E. M. *et al.* (1976) *Tissue Antigens* **8**, 61.

327. Ward, G. *et al.* (1976) *Tissue Antigens* **7**, 227.

328. White, A. G. *et al.* (1973) *Brit J. Dermatol.* **89**, 133.

329. White, S. H. *et al.* (1972) *New Eng. J. Med.* **287**, 740.

330. Whittingham, S. *et al.* (1975) *Tissue Antigens* **6**, 23.

331. Whittingham, S. *et al.* (1975) *Clin. exp. Immunol.* **19**, 289.

332. Woodrow, J. C. *et al.* (1975) *Brit. J. Dermatol.* **92**, 427.

333. Woodrow, J. C. *et al.* (1974) *Tissue Antigens* **4**, 533.

334. Wright, J. P., Callender, S. T. E., Grumet, F. C., Payne, R. O. & Taylor, K. B. (USA) (1976§).

335. Yakura, H. *et al.* (1976) *Tissue Antigens* **8**, 35.

336. Zachariae, H. *et al.* (1975) *Scand. J. Rheum.* **4**, 13.

337. Zachariae, H. *et al.* (1974) *Acta Dermatovener.* **54**, 443.

338. Zander, H., Grosse-Wilde, H., Scholz, S., Kuntz, B., Netzel, B. & Albert, E. D. (Germany) (1976§).

339. Zittoun, R. *et al.* (1975) *New Eng. J. Med.* **293**, 1324.

References

1. Payne, R. (1977) The HLA complex: Genetics and implications in the immune response, p. 20.
2. Bodmer, W. F. & Thomson, G. (1977) Population genetics and evolution of the HLA system, p. 280.
3. Kidd, K. K., Bernoco, D., Carbonara, A. O., Daneo, V., Steiger, U. & Ceppellini, R. (1977) Genetic analysis of HLA-associated diseases: the "illness-susceptible" gene frequency and sex ratio in ankylosing spondylitis, p. 72.
4. Thomson, G. & Bodmer, W. F. (1977) The genetic analysis of HLA and disease associations, p. 84.
5. Nerup, J., Platz, P., Andersen, O. O., Christy, M., Lyngsøe, J., Poulsen, J. E., Ryder, L. P., Nielsen, L. Staub, Thomsen, M. & Svejgaard, A. (1974) HL-A antigens and Diabetes Mellitus. *Lancet* **ii**, 864–866.
6. Armitage, P. (1971) *Statistical Methods in Medical Research*, Blackwell, Oxford.
7. Woolf, B. (1951) On Estimating the Relation between Blood Group and Disease. *Ann. hum. Genet.* **19**, 251–253.
8. Haldane, J. B. S. (1948) The number of genotypes which can be formed with a given number of genes. *J. Genet.* **49**, 117–119.
9. Svejgaard, A., Jersild, C., Nielsen, L. Staub & Bodmer, W. F. (1974) HL-A antigens and disease. Statistical and genetical considerations. *Tissue Antigens* **4**, 95–105.
10. Ryder, L. P. & Svejgaard, A. (1976) Histocompatibility associated diseases. In: *B and T cells in immune reaction*, eds. Loor, F. & Roelants, G. E., John Wiley & Sons Limited, England, (in press).
11. Svejgaard, A., Platz, P., Ryder, L. P., Nielsen, L. Staub & Thomsen, M. (1975) HL-A and disease asociations – a survey. *Transplant. Rev.* **22**, 3–43.
12. Mayr, W. (1976) Personal communication.
13. Woodrow, J. C. (1976) Personal communication.
14. Nielsen, L. Staub, Jersild, C., Ryder, L. P. & Svejgaard, A. (1975) HL-A antigen, gene, and haplotype frequencies in Denmark. *Tissue Antigens* **6**, 70–76.
15. Thomsen, M., Platz, P., Andersen, O. Ortved, Christy, M., Lyngsøe, J., Nerup, J., Rasmussen, K., Ryder, L. P., Nielsen, L. Staub & Svejgaard, A. (1975) MLC typing *in juvenile Diabetes Mellitus and Idiopathic Addison's Disease. Transplant. Rev.* **22**, 125–147.
16. Day, N. E. & Simons, M. J. (1976) Disease susceptibility genes – their identification by multiple case family studies. *Tissue Antigens* **8**, 109–119.
17. Thomsen, M., Christy, M., Nerup, J., Platz, P., Ryder, L. P. & Svejgaard, A. (1976,) unpublished.
18. Terasaki, P. I. & Mickey, M. R. (1975) HL-A haplotypes of 32 diseases. *Transplant. Rev.* **22**, 105–119.
19. Dupont, B., Good, R. A., Hauptmann, G., Schreuder, I. & Seligmann, M. (1976) Immunopathology, immunodeficiencies and complement deficiencies, (this volume).
20. Simon, M., Bourel, M., Fauchet, R. & Genetet, B. (1976) Association of HLA-A3 and HLA-B14 antigens with Idiopathic Haemochromatosis. *GUT* **17**, 332–334.
21. Brewerton, D. A. & Albert, E. (1976) Rheumatology, p. 94.
22. Katz, M. A. (1974) A probability graph describing the predictive value of a highly selective diagnosis test. *New Eng. J. Med.* **291**, 1115–1116.
23. Falk, J. & Osoba, D. (1971) HL-A antigens and survival in Hodgkin's Disease. *Lancet* **ii**, 1118–1121.
24. Ryder, L. P. & Svejgaard, A. (1976) Associations between HLA and Disease. Report from the HLA and Disease Registry of Copenhagen.
25. Dausset, J., Svejgaard, A., Degos, L., Hors, J. & Ryder, L. P. (Eds.) *HLA and Disease*, Abstracts, INSERM, Paris 1976.

Genetic Analysis of HLA-Associated Diseases: The »Illness-Susceptible« Gene Frequency and Sex Ratio in Ankylosing Spondylitis

K. K. Kidd[1], D. Bernoco[2], A. O. Carbonara[3], V. Daneo[4], U. Steiger[5] & R. Ceppellini[2]

Introduction

Diseases which show familial concentration but do not show simple Mendelian patterns are difficult to describe unambiguously in genetic terms (Kidd & Cavalli-Sforza (1), Kidd & Spence (2)). In fact, familial concentration is not even proof that genetic factors are relevant to the disease. On the other hand, provided that one is willing to consider population stratification to be a genetic (albeit population-genetic/social) phenomenon, a population study can provide evidence for a genetic component. A significant association of any disease with a good genetic marker, such as an HLA antigen, is *per se* evidence that a genetic element exists in

the etiopathogenesis of that disease. However, unless the marker itself is clearly of etiologic significance, the interpretation of the association in genetic terms will not be clear. With HLA-associated diseases both of the above complications exist; diseases being studied usually do not show simple Mendelian patterns and there are, at present, no known pathological alleles at the HLA loci (with the single exception of the C2 and C4 amorph mutants (3, 4) that can explain the significant, but not complete, association of the illness with particular allele and/or haplotypes. Since HLA markers (antigens) are co-dominant traits with full penetrance for their serological expression, several reasons for the incomplete association of the disease with the antigen can be given. One explanation is linkage to (or hitchhiking within) the HLA region of a gene directly responsible for the disease (that is, an "Illness-susceptibility" allele, hereafter abbreviated to *Is*). At the moment the best candidates may be the

[1] Department of Human Genetics, Yale University School of Medicine, Connecticut, U.S.A.
[2] Basel Institute for Immunology, Basel, Switzerland.
[3] Istituto di Genetica Medica, Torino, Italy.
[4] Centro di Reumatologia, Ospedale S. Giovanni Battista, Torino, Italy.
[5] Rheumatology Department, University Clinics of Basel, Basel, Switzerland.

hypothesized Ir (immune response) genes, but other possible polymorphisms, such as hormone receptors, should also be considered (5). A second explanation is epistasis, as in the typical case of antigen Lewis b (6). Ragweed-pollen allergy is possibly due to epistasis between the ability to recognize a pollen determinant, due to an HLA-linked Ir gene, and the high level phenotype for IgE (7–10), although conflicting evidence exists (11, 12). Another explanation, not necessarily in contrast with the others, is "incomplete penetrance" (lack of the phenotype expression expected for a given genotype) of the HLA-antigen allele in regard to illness susceptibility (if directly responsible) or of the linked Is allele.

Because the diseases that are being considered are already known to show no simple Mendelian pattern, incomplete penetrance in some form is a likely and almost necessary component in any genetic explanation. Such incomplete penetrance may be caused by a variety of factors, both genetic and environmental. On the genetic side, besides the simplest case mentioned above of epistatic interaction with a single major locus, polygenic inheritance, with only one of the many loci linked to the HLA system, is another purely genetic situation. Environmental explanations would include, for instance, a triggering infectious disease and also some "familial" factors, such as cohabitation with relatives sharing not only a similar genotype but also similar conditions of housing and habits of living.

Existence of environmental variation dilutes out the degree to which genetic factors determine the variation in the population for presence or absence of a trait or illness. The relative amount of genetic variation is frequently expressed as heritability (h^2), the ratio of the genetic variance in the population

to the total variance for the trait. The authors feel that heritability ignores some typical and most interesting features of human genetics, for example, possible modes of gene action and the difficult distinction between biological and cultural inheritance. Thus, when applied to human diseases, *heritability* is often a misnomer. Therefore, the authors will not use it. A more detailed discussion of the inappropriateness of heritability in human genetics is given in Matthysse & Kidd (13).

Family data on diseases are rarely not insufficient to be informative; population association data of a disease and a marker locus are often not readily interpretable in genetic terms. The authors wish to show that family data on both a disease and an associated (HLA) marker can be used to gain a clearer

TABLE I

Criteria followed in Basel and Torino for diagnosis of Ankylosing Spondylitis[1]

Subjective and functional
    (a) limitation of motion of lumbar spine[2]
    (b) history of persistent pain
    (c) chest expansion $\leq$ 3 cm (measured at fourth intercostal space)

X-ray grading (each side graded separately)
    0: normal
    1: doubtful changes
    2: minimal definite change
    3: moderate or advanced sacroiliitis with erosion, evidence of sclerosis, widening, narrowing or partial ankylosis
    4: total ankylosing

Definite AS: grade 3–4 X-ray, bilateral, plus at least one clinical sign; grade 3–4 unilateral or grade 2 bilateral plus a+c or b+c

Probable AS: grade 3–4 bilateral in absence of any clinical sign

To maximize penetrance: all individuals $\leq$ 20 years of age were excluded

To maximize homogeneity: all cases with complications were excluded

1) As recommended by Gofton *et al* (18)
2) As recommended by Macrae & Wright (19)

understanding of the genetics of the disease. Ankylosing spondylitis (AS) is a paradigmatic model because AS is the disease that shows the highest relative risk with an HLA antigen (14, 15). Family data have been collected in Torino (TO) (16) and Basel (BS) (17) on 53 index or primary cases who had at least one first-degree relative that could be examined as completely as the proband, according to a rigid application of the criteria in Table 1 (18, 19). Two groups of normal controls were also examined with the same diagnostic criteria: (a) a selected sample of B27-positive individuals who had not reported subjective symptoms nor had been in any way aware of being affected by AS; and (b) a selected sample of B27-negative individuals, mostly chosen for being B7-positive because of the well-known crossreactivity between these two B antigens. All data in the two studies (BS and TO) were collected without communication between the rheumatologists, the HLA typists, and the statisticians until the work had been completed.

Results and Discussion

The diagnostic criteria listed in Table I were followed in both the Basel and Torino studies. Table II presents the data for the primary cases (probands) and population controls. A preponderance of males among ankylosing spondylitis patients is found, as has been reported in other studies. The preponderance of males in the normal control populations reflects the male preponderance among employees of Hoffman-LaRoche in Basel and in the blood-donor panel in Torino. These controls give the B27-antigen frequency in the population. Through some difference exists between Basel and Torino, the increased frequency of B27 among AS patients is spectacular and highly significant, as reported in all previous studies (see 14, 15). From the data on first-degree relatives, presented in Table III, the familiality of ankylosing spondylitis is obvious. The two control populations included in Table III were examined using the same diagnostic criteria. These data confirm the low incidence of AS in a non-B27 population and the high frequency of affected individuals (7 out of 43 = 16 %) among the "normal" B27-positive controls, using a more rigorous diagnostic examination than in the report by Calin & Fries (20). Only one of the affected first-degree relatives, a mother, did not have B27; however, in that family the proband's *Is B27* haplotype came from the father, who was also AS

TABLE II

Number studied, sex, and B27-phenotype frequency in patients (primary cases) and controls studied in Basel (BS) and Torino (TO)

Number studied	Sex		Class	Area	B27 frequency
	M	F			
58	48	10	AS patients	BS	0.93
623	459	164	Normal controls[1]	BS	0.100
21	20	1	AS patients	TO	0.90
1428	980	448	Normal controls[2]	TO	0.043

[1] random employees of Hoffman-La Roche
[2] random blood donors

TABLE III
Familiality of Ankylosing Spondylitis

Area	Primary case No.	Type	First-Degree Relatives Type	No.	Normal B27+	B27−	Affected B27+	B27−
BS	7	Parent	Child	13	4	7	2	0
BS	15	Sib	Sib	32	13	13	6	0
BS	18	Child	Parent	27	10	9	8	0
BS			All	72	27	29	16	0
TO	3	Parent	Child	5	4	1	0	0
TO	11	Sib	Sib	15	6	4	5	0
TO	9	Child	Parent	16	6	7	2	1
TO			All	36	16	12	7	1
BS + TO combined			All	108	43	41	23	1
BS	147	Non-B27 controls			−	146	−	1
BS	43	"Normal" B27 controls			36	−	7	−

affected. Also worth noting is that one affected individual (B7+) was found among the non-B27 controls. Thus, to the best diagnostic criteria accepted today, ankylosing spondylitis can occur, albeit rarely, in the absence of the antigen B27.

Tables IV and V show that the preponderance of affected males among probands neither occurs among the "normal" B27+ controls nor among the first-degree relatives; Calin & Fries (20) also found essentially equal frequencies of affected males and females

TABLE IV
Frequency of Females (ff) in Ankylosing Spondylitis

Area	Class of Data	Total	Number Males	Females	ff
BS	Primary cases	58	48	10	0.17
BS	Secondary cases	72	8/33 [1]	8/39 [1]	0.46 [2]
BS	"Normal" B27+	43	5/34 [1]	2/9 [1]	0.60 [2]
TO	Primary cases	21	20	1	0.05
TO	Secondary cases	36	4/19 [1]	4/17 [1]	0.53 [2]

[1] Ratio of number affected by AS to total number studied
[2] ff corrected for a 1:1 sex ratio in sample

TABLE V
Frequency of Affected Relatives according to Sex [1]

		Primary Cases Males ($n = 33$)	Females ($n = 8$)
All First-degree relatives	Males	$9/41 = 0.22 \pm 0.06$	$3/11 = 0.27 \pm 0.13$
	Females	$11/42 = 0.26 \pm 0.07$	$1/14 = 0.07 \pm 0.07$

[1] Values given as number affected/total = mean ± standard error
x^2 (3 d. f.) = 2.3 g   P = 0.50

in their study. The family data also show that AS is as frequent, within the statistical limits of the small sample, among the relatives of female probands as of male probands, suggesting that there is no "hereditary" component to any hypothesized sex limitation or greater male susceptibility. An obvious conclusion is that the male preponderance among AS patients is not a reflection of a truly greater incidence among males. Possible explanations for this could be greater severity in males, a greater tendency for the diagnosis to be made in males, and a greater tendency for males to seek treatment. Whatever the explanation, the "fact" that males are more frequently affected with AS than females is probably not true in an absolute sense.

Genetic Analyses

Analyses of family data normally involve testing the goodness of fit of different genetic hypotheses (models) to the observed data. The two models most commonly used in human genetics are the simple extremes of single major locus (SML) and multifactorial-polygenic (MF) inheritance (see Matthysse & Kidd (12) for a review of these two models). One major problem with these models is that they are statistically indistinguishable and agreement cannot be tested when family incidence data are used without additional sources of genetic information (1, 21). Nonetheless, both models have been applied to the AS family data to see whether the results would be biologically reasonable.

The single parameter of the MF model needing estimation is the genetic correlation among relatives. This correlation is often translated into an heritability (h^2) value; however, the correlation or heritability does not apply to the measured trait, in this case ankylosing spondylitis, but to a hypothetical underlying continuous and normally distributed variable called "liability to disease". The general incidence of the illness and the frequency of affected first-degree relatives are the necessary data for estimating the correlation. The generally accepted population prevalence for AS is about 0.5 % for males and considerably less for females. The average incidence among first-degree relatives is 0.22 ± 0.04. These values give an estimate of the tetrachoric correlation (1) of about 0.65, a nonsensical result according to the MF model, for which the theoretical maximum is 0.50, i.e. $h^2 = 100 \%$. However, the general incidence estimate is based on the frequency of patients seeking treatment and not upon a complete diagnostic survey of the population using both functional tests and X-rays. In fact, primary and secondary cases are usually ascertained according to widely different criteria. The authors' finding that 16 % of a sample of B27+ individuals were affected suggests that the population prevalence may be about 1.5 % for both males and females. Using this value for the incidence in the population and 0.22 for the frequency of affected first-degree relatives, the correlation coefficient is lower but still above 0.50 – the heritability (h^2) is > 100 %. Such high correlations are often interpreted as suggesting that a locus of major effect is involved.

Methods for using family data to estimate the parameters of the SML model are extensively discussed elsewhere (1, 2, 13, 21, 22). To save space the model and methods will not be discussed here. Analyses show that no solution is possible for an incidence of the disease in the population of less than 1.0 %. However, the closest solution to the data (using the method of Suarez et al. (22)) predicts a population incidence for AS

TABLE VI
Genetic Analysis of Ankylosing Spondylitis by the Method of Thomson & Bodmer (23)

Basic Values:

q = frequency of *HLA-B27* allele *(B27)* = 0.048

$f(M|Ill)$ = frequency of the marker (B27) phenotype among ill (AS) patients =
73/79 = 0.924 $\pm$ 0.030

krec. = $1 - \sqrt{1-f(M|Ill)}$ = 0.724

kdom. = $(1 - (1-f(M|Ill))/(1-q))$ = 0.920

Observed genotype distribution in AS patients (primary cases only)

	B27/B27	B27/ –	– / –	
BS	3	51	4	
TO	0	19	2	
Totol	3	70	6	

Expected genotype distributions

Recessive hypothesis	41.5	31.5	6	X^2_1 = 82.5
				$p \ll 0.0001$
Dominant hypothesis	3.5	69.5	6	X^2_1 = 0.075
				p = 0.78

of about 1.6 % and frequencies of AS among first-degree relatives of about 22 %, essentially the same as the "adjusted" values used for the MF model. This SML "solution" predicts a gene frequency of 1.8 % for the *Is* allele and penetrances (that is, risks of actually contracting the illness) of < 0.001, 0.43, and > 0.995 for the homozygous "normal" *(is/is)*, heterozygous *(is/Is)*, and homozygous "susceptible" *(Is/Is)* genotypes, respectively. The predicted genotypic composition of the population of affected individuals is about 3 % homozygous "normal" (i.e. phenocopies), 95 % heterozygous, and 2 % homozygous "susceptible". Although there is no way to test this model statistically using the available data, the SML results, in combination with the unrealistically high correlations of the MF model, strongly suggest that a single locus hypothesis is the more likely one. This "conclusion" is independent of the association of AS with B27.

Thomsen & Bodmer (23) (largely reprinted in this volume) have developed a method for testing two simple models that assumes linkage disequilibrium with a co-dominant marker. Their method is based only on the genotype distribution among affected probands and does not utilize family data. This makes it useful in practice since, unfortunately, family data are at present not generally available for HLA-associated diseases. In Table VI data are organized appropriately and the results of the analysis by the Thomson & Bodmer method are presented. The analysis strongly rejects the recessive hypothesis and is in almost exact agreement with the dominant hypothesis. Thus, AS appears to be due to an illness-susceptibility allele at a locus closely linked to the HLA-B locus and susceptibility seems to be inherited in a dominant fashion. The linkage disequilibrium estimate, measured in this analysis as k (= 0.928), is a very high value, providing indirect proof that tight linkage is responsible for the strong population association.

As explained by Kidd & Ceppellini (24), it is possible to modify the Thomson & Bodmer method to incorporate estimates of the frequency of the disease among individuals with the marker and of the "penetrance", that is, the frequency of the illness among those with the susceptibility allele. Utilizing whichever model fits the data, it is then possible to estimate all four haplotype frequencies. Though more exact treatments are possible, the low frequencies of the marker allele (B27) and the illness (AS) allow a simplified calculation for the dominant model, as outlined in Table VII. The estimates for the penetrance and the haplotype frequencies agree well with the SML solution obtained without consideration of the HLA association.

Some caveats about the penetrance estimate are very important in evaluating these results. It is impossible to generalize from this penetrance estimate to families not ascertained through a proband. The value of 0.38 is not significantly less than 0.5, the approximate value expected in families if an allele at an independent locus were also required for development of the illness. Probands, being affected, would be carriers for both alleles; because of independent segregation, only about half of the first-degree relatives with the *Is* allele at the main locus would also have the necessary allele at the second. Thus, the family estimate of penetrance will be an overestimate for an unrelated group of individuals. The accuracy of the estimate depends on the degree of epistasis and, if epistasis exists, on the frequencies of the interacting alleles.

Another caveat about the family estimate of penetrance is that it includes recombination that seperates the marker from the susceptibility allele.

Even an exact calculation of the penetrance from family data would include corrections for the age of onset distribution (only roughly done in this study by limiting consideration to adult relatives) and for the probability of ascertainment, which is determined by the number of affected individuals in a family. In spite of these potential biasses, not all of which operate in the same direction, the penetrance estimate is roughly consistent with the population and control data. From what is known about AS, it is very unlikely to be as high as 100 %, and the "normal" B27+ control data show that it cannot be below 16 %.

The estimated frequency of the haplotype *m Is* is too low (0.002) to explain the 4 % of AS patients who lack the B27 marker, even if the "penetrance"

TABLE VII

Summary of a simplified Bayesian probability analysis for Ankylosing Spondylitis

M = marker allele for B27 antigen; frequency of M = 0.048 ± 0.01
I = allele for illness susceptibility
A. observed frequency of M among AS patients = 0.92 ± 0.03 = Pr (M|I) = Pr (M|AS)
B. observed frequency of AS amond M+ (B27+) population = 0.16 ± 0.06 = Pr (AS|M)
C. observed frequency of AS among M+ (B27+)
   first-degree relatives of probands = "penetrance" = 0.38 ± 0.06 = Pr (AS|I)
   Therefore, Pr (I|M) = 0.16/0.38 = 0.42
   and   Pr (I) = Pr (I|M) . Pr (M) /Pr (M|I) = 0.022
   It follows that:
   x_1 = freq. (MI haplotype) = Pr (I|M) . Pr (M) = 0.020
   x_2 = freq. (Mi) = Pr (M) − x_1 = 0.028
   x_3 = freq. (mI) = Pr (I) − x_1 = 0.002
   x_4 = freq. (mi) = 1 − x_1 − x_2 − x_3 = 0.950
   $\Delta = x_1 x_4 − x_2 x_3 = 0.019$

for that haplotype were 100 %. Sampling error in the estimate of the penetrance or in the frequency of affected individuals who are B27 negative might have produced this apparent discrepancy. However, the SML solution discussed earlier predicted about 3 % phenocopies, a value in close agreement.

Conclusions

Though mathematical genetics has many limitations when applied to familial traits that are not obviously Mendelian, it becomes a powerful tool when a marker locus can also be studied in those families. The authors have shown that the oft-mentioned preponderance of affected males is found neither in families of AS patients nor in population surveys and one must conclude that the apparent sex limitation is mainly due to ascertainment. Susceptibility to AS is inherited as an autosomal dominant. The locus seems to be tightly linked to HLA-B. According to this model, the susceptibility allele has a gene frequency of about 2 %. Also, it is in strong linkage disequilibrium with the allele determining HLA-B27: nearly all (93 %) of the haplotypes with the *is* allele also carry the *B27* allele. The majority (62 %) of the carriers of the *Is* allele do not develop AS. As repeatedly mentioned, this incomplete penetrance may be due to environmental factors or to epistasis with an allele at an independent locus.

Obviously, this is a formal explanation with a strong heuristic component. Tests of these conclusions will have to be based on additional family studies of B27-negative AS probands, of female AS probands and of relatives of different degrees.

Acknowledgement

The part of the work done in Torino was supported by C.N.R. grant "Centro di Studio per l'Istocompatibilità a l'Immunogenetica". The analyses were supported in part by N.I.H. grant NS 11786.

References

1. Kidd, K. K. & Cavalli-Sforza, L. L. (1973) An analysis of the genetics of schizophrenia. *Soc. Biol.* **20**, 254–265.
2. Kidd, K. K. & Spence, M. A. (1976) Genetic analyses of pyloric stenosis suggesting a specific maternal effect. *J. med. Genetics* **13**, 290–294.
3. Agnello, V. M., de Bracco, M. E. & Kunkel, H. J. (1972) Hereditary C2 deficiency with some manifestations of systemic lupus erythematosus. *J. Immunol.* **108**, 873–881.
4. Hauptmann, G., Grosshause, E., Heid, E., Mayer, S. & Basset, A. (1976) Lupous érythémateaux aigu avec deficit complet de la fraction C4 du complément. *La Nouv. Presse Méd.* **3**, 881–885.
5. Ceppellini, R. (1971) Old and new facts and speculations about transplantation antigens of man. In: *Progress in Immunology I*, ed. Amos, D. B., p. 973. Academic Press Inc., New York.
6. Ceppellini, R. (1959) Physiological genetics of human blood factors. In: *Ciba Foundation symposium on Biochemistry of Human Genetics,* eds. Wolstenholme, G. E. W. & O'Connor, C. M., Churchill, London.
7. Blumenthal, M. N., Amos, D. B., Noreen, H., Mendell, N. R. & Yunis, E. J. (1974)

79

Genetic mapping of Ir locus in man: Linkage to second locus of HL-A. *Science* **184**, 1301–1303.

8. Levine, B. B., Stember, R. H. & Fotino, M. (1972) Ragweed hay fever: Genetic control and linkage to HL-A haplotypes. *Science* **178**, 1201–1203.

9. Marsh, D. G. & Bias, W. B. (1974) Control of specific allergic response in man: HL-A-associated and IgE-regulating genes. *Fed. Proc.* **33**, 774.

10. Marsh, D. G., Bias, W. B. & Ishizaka, K. (1974) Genetic control of basal serum immunoglobulin E level and its effect on specific reaginic sensitivity. *Proc. nat. Acad. Sci. (Wash.)* **71**, 3588–3592.

11. Bias, W B. & Marsh, D. G. (1975) HL-A linked antigen E immune response genes: An unproven hypothesis. *Science* **188**, 375 –377.

12. Black, P. L., Marsh, D. G., Jarrett, E., Delespesse, G. J. & Bias, W. B. (1976) Family studies of association between HLA and specific immune responses to highly purified pollen allergens. *Immunogenetics* **3**, 349–368.

13. Matthysse, S. W. & Kidd, K. K. (1976) Estimating the genetic contribution to schizophrenia. *Amer. J. Psychiatry* **133**, 185–191.

14. Brewerton, D. A., Caffrey, M., Hart, F. D., James, D. C. O., Nicholls, A. & Sturrock, R. D. (1973) Ankylosing spondylitis and HL-A 27. *Lancet* **i**, 904–907.

15. Schlosstein, L., Terasaki, P. I., Bluestone, R. & Pearson, C. M. (1973) High association of an HL-A antigen, W27, with ankylosing spondylitis. *New. Eng. J. Med.* **288**, 704.

16. Daneco, V., Migone, N., Modeno, V., Bianchi, S. D., Alfieri, G., Diotallevi, P., Carbona, A. O. & Piazza, A. (1976) Family studies and HLA typing in ankylosing spondylitis and sacroiliitis. *J. Rheumatol.*, (in press).

17. Truog, P., Steiger, U., Contu, L., Galfre, G., Trucco, M., Bernoco, D., Bernoco, M., Birgen, I., Dolivo, P. & Ceppellini, R. (1975) Ankylosing spondylitis (AS): A population and family study using HL-A serology and MLR. In: *Histocompatibility Testing 1975,* ed. Kissmeyer-Nielsen, F., p. 788–796. Munksgaard, Copenhagen.

18 Gofton, I. P., Bennett, P. H., Bremmer, I. M., Bywaters, E. G. L., Calabro, J. I., McEwan, C. & Martel, W. (1966) Population studies of rheumatic diseases, p. 456. *Proc. 3rd International Symposium,* New York.

19. Macrae, I. F. & Wright, U. (1969) Measurement of back movement. *Ann. rheum. Dis.* **28**, 584.

20. Calin, A. & Fries, J. F. (1975) Striking prevalence of ankylosing spondylitis in "healthy" W27 positive males and females. *New Eng. J. Med.* **293**, 835–839.

21. Reich, T., James, J. W. & Morris, C. A. (1972) The use of multiple thresholds in determining the mode of transmission of semi-continuous traits. *Ann. Hum. Genetics* **36**, 163–184.

22. Suarez, B. K., Reich, T. & Trost, J. (1976) Limits of the general two allele single locus model in genetic explanations. *Ann. Hum. Genetics,* (in press).

23. Thomson, G. & Bodmer, W. F. (1977) The genetics of HLA and disease association. In: *Measuring Selection In Natural Populations,* eds. Barndorff-Nielsen, O., Christiansen, F. B. & Fenchel, T. Munksgaard, Copenhagen, (in press).

24. Kidd, K. K. & Ceppellini, R. (1977) A bayesian method for estimation of HLA -associated illness-susceptibility (Is) allele frequencies. I. Dominant susceptibility. In: *HLA and Disease,* eds. Dausset, J. & Svejgaard, A., p. 81, Munksgaard, Copenhagen.

A Bayesian Method for Estimation of HLA-Associated Illness-Susceptibility (Is) Allele Frequencies. I. Dominant Susceptibility

Kenneth K. Kidd[1] & Ruggero Ceppellini[2]

Introduction

Thomson & Bodmer (1) present two types of genetic analysis for disease phenotypes associated with a genetic marker. Their first method utilizes the marker phenotype frequency in a population of unrelated affected individuals; the second is derived from more general models by Day & Simons (2) and utilizes the frequencies of the number of marker chromosomes (haplotypes) shared by affected sib pairs. Both methods involve tests for specific models of inheritance of illness susceptibility (Is) – recessive or rare dominant. Green & Woodrow (3) have also produced an analysis utilizing frequencies of shared chromosomes among affected siblings to test the null hypothesis of there being no association between marker locus and illness. None of these papers considers direct estimates of the haplotype frequencies, though Thomson & Bod-

mer (1) consider indirect estimates for their recessive model applied to data on pairs of affected siblings. Direct estimates are possible when certain types of data are available: (a) the frequency of illness among individuals with the associated marker, $f(Ill \mid M)$; and (b) the "penetrance" or frequency of the illness among those with the susceptibility genotype.

The general importance of these types of data, particularly estimating penetrance from family data, has been recognized in the design of the study of ankylosing spondylitis in Basel and Torino (Ceppellini, personal communication). Suitable data are consequently already available for ankylosing spondylitis; they may soon be collected for other HLA-associated illnesses. $f(Ill \mid M)$ can be collected using the same criteria for diagnosis as in probands and relatives and should be less subject to bias and uncertainty than estimates of the frequency of the illness in the general population. The penetrance can be estimated in many ways, but the simp-

[1] Department of Human Genetics, Yale University School of Medicine, Connecticut, U.S.A.
[2] Basel Institute for Immunology, Basel, Switzerland.

lest and most common is the proportion of affected individuals among relatives who carry the same marker chromosome (for the dominant model) or marker chromosomes (recessive model) as the proband. These estimates, combined with the marker allele frequency and the frequency of the marker phenotype among affected individuals, can be used to calculate haplotype frequencies. These types of data should become available before sufficient pairs of affected sibs have been studied for the other types of analysis, especially if the association is strong and illness susceptibility is dominant.

Method

A more exact and general treatment of the dominant and recessive models, utilizing the additional types of data and considering more precise estimates of penetrance (involving correction for age-of-onset variation and for ascertainment biasses) will be presented elsewhere. Only the simplified dominant model, as can be used for ankylosing spondylitis, is presented here. This approximate analysis is possible whenever both the marker allele and the Is allele have a low frequency in the population. The general method is based on the Bayesian probability.

$$Pr(Is) = \frac{Pr(Is|M) \cdot Pr(M)}{Pr(M|Is)}, \qquad (1)$$

i.e., that the frequency or probability of the Is genotype is equal to the frequency of the Is genotype among individuals with the marker phenotype multiplied by the frequency of the marker phenotype, and the product divided by the frequency of the marker among affected individuals. This assumes that illness occurs among some fraction of those carying the Is genotype but is otherwise independent of the presence of the marker.

The frequency of the marker, $Pr(M)$, is estimated from population surveys independent of studies of disease association. The frequency of the marker among affected persons, $Pr(M|Ill) = Pr(M|Is) = f(M|Ill)$, is the estimate used to show association and used in the initial tests of Thomson & Bodmer (their "FAD"). The third quantity in Equation 1, $Pr(Is|M)$, can be estimated from

$$Pr(Is|M) = \frac{Pr(Illness|M)}{Pr(Illness|Is)}, \qquad (2)$$

i.e., from the frequency of illness among those with the marker, $f(Ill|M)$ divided by the penetrance. Thus, the frequency of the Is genotype is a function of estimable values.

For the dominant model with the additional simplifying assumption that the phenotype frequency is twice the allele frequency, for both the marker and Is allele, Equation 1 roughly estimates the Is-allele frequency by using the marker allele frequency for $Pr(M)$. The four haplotype frequencies are then estimated as follows:

x_1 = freq. (M Is haplotype) =
$$Pr(Is|M) \cdot Pr(M)$$
x_2 = freq. (M is haplotype) =
$$Pr(M) - x_1$$
x_3 = freq. (m Is haplotype) =
$$Pr(Is) - x_1$$
x_4 = freq. (m is haplotype) =
$$1. - x_1 - x_2 - x_3.$$

This simplified form of the analysis is used by Kidd et al. (4) on data in ankylosing spondylitis. The error, when compared with a more exact analysis using the same data, is not detectable to three decimal places.

Acknowledgement

The work was supported in part by grant NS 11786 from the N.I.H., U.S. Public Health Service.

References

1. Thomson, G. & Bodmer, W. F. (1976) The genetics of HLA and disease association. In: *Measuring Selection in Natural Populations,* eds. Barndorff-Nielsen, O., Christiansen, F. B. & Fenchel, T. Munksgaard, Copenhagen, (in press).
2. Day, N. E. & Simons, M. J. (1976) Disease susceptibility genes – their identification by multiple case family studies. *Tissue Antigens* 8, 109–119.
3. Green, J. R. & Woodrow, J. C. (1976) Sibling method for detecting HLA linked genes in disease. (Submitted for publication.)
4. Kidd, K. K., Bernoco, D., Carbonara, A. O., Daneo, V, Steiger, U. & Ceppellini, R. (1977) Genetic analysis of HLA associated diseases: the "illness susceptible" gene frequency and sex ratio in ankylosing spondylitis. In: *HLA and Disease,* eds. Dausset, J. & Svejgaard, A. Munksgaard, Copenhagen, p. 72.

The Genetic Analysis of HLA and Disease Associations

Glenys Thomson & Walter Bodmer

Introduction

If associations between HLA and disease are not due to the direct effects of the serologically determined HLA antigens but, as suggested by McDevitt and Bodmer (7, 8) and others, to the effects of closely linked loci, which we shall refer to simply as disease susceptibility or 'disease' loci, then there must be significant linkage disequilibrium (that is non-random association of alleles – see other articles in this volume) between the alleles at these disease loci and those at the HLA-A, B, C and D loci. The stronger associations of the B and D loci with diseases imply that the 'disease' loci are probably closer to these two loci than to A or C. This follows from the fact that the effects of all mechanisms known to create linkage disequilibrium decrease steadily with increasing recombination fraction, other things being equal. So, for this reason, one is more likely to observe linkage disequilibrium between closely linked loci than between more loosely linked loci (see Bodmer and Thomson, Chapter XV). Associations due to linkage disequilibrium are likely to be much more complex than those resulting from a simple direct antigenic effect, and may vary substantially from one population to another with variation in haplotype frequencies. Even if a disease

Genetics Laboratory, Department of Biochemistry, University of Oxford, South Parks Road, Oxford, England.

susceptibility is associated with the effects of a gene in the HLA region this will not show up as a population association with the serologically detected antigens unless the disease susceptibility locus and the HLA antigen loci are in significant linkage disequilibrium.

The diseases under consideration are ones which do not show simple Mendelian segregation, but nevertheless in many cases have an obvious inherited component. The evidence that heredity plays some part comes from the usual observation that the incidence of the disorder is higher among the relatives of affected individuals than it is in the general population (see previous chapter by Cepellini, Kidd et al.). Several different modes of transmission have been proposed to explain the inheritance patterns of these types of diseases. These range from single locus two-allele models with variable penetrance in one or all genotypes to multifactorial models in which many genes of small effect and environmental sources of variance play a role. Attempts to distinguish between the two modes of transmission using family data have generally not been very successful (Smith (10), Kidd and Cavalli-Sforza (6)). Despite this, we shall in this paper consider only disease susceptibility models where there is a single 'disease' locus with a major detectable effect. The model does not exclude the possibility that other genes

84

are involved in the disease, but assumes that there is a single locus with a major effect. It is, however, difficult to explain the associations on a multifactorial basis with no detectable major effect of an HLA linked gene. So throughout the following we will consider models with such single 'disease' loci.

Two methods will be outlined in this paper which make it possible to discriminate between dominant and recessive modes of inheritance of 'disease' genes. The first involves looking at HLA genotype frequencies amongst diseased individuals. The second looks at the HLA similarity of affected sib pairs.

Antigen Genotype Frequencies Amongst the Diseased

A simple two locus disease association model is considered. The first locus, denoted A, is the antigen locus. The two alleles A and a denote the presence or absence of a particular antigen. The second locus, denoted D, with alleles D and d, is the disease susceptibility locus and henceforth we shall often refer to this simply as the 'disease' locus. (The use of the letters A and D here should not be confused with the loci HLA-A and HLA-D of the HLA system. The letters A for antigen locus and D for 'disease' locus have been used because the appropriate subscripts then make it easier to recognise whether we are talking about 'disease' gene frequencies or antigen frequencies). There are four possible gametic types or haplotypes namely AD, Ad, aD and ad, whose frequencies are denoted by x_1, x_2, x_3 and x_4 respectively. The gametic frequencies can be written in two forms.

The first notation is the well-known formulation in terms of gene frequencies and linkage disequilibrium, namely,

$$x_1 = f(AD) = p_A p_D + D$$
$$x_2 = f(Ad) = p_A p_d - D \qquad (1)$$
$$x_3 = f(aD) = p_a p_D - D$$
$$x_4 = f(ad) = p_a p_d + D$$

(see Chapter XV), where pA, pD are the frequencies of the alleles A and D respectively, etc. and $D = x_1 x_4 - x_2 x_3$

is the coefficient of linkage disequilibrium.

The second notation, which turns out to be the most useful when discussing disease associations, is in terms of gene frequencies and the ratio of antigen presence to absence (k : 1-k) in gametes containing the 'disease' allele D, namely

$$x_1 = f(AD) = k p_D$$
$$x_2 = f(Ad) = p_A - k p_D \qquad (2)$$
$$x_3 = f(aD) = (1-k) p_D$$
$$x_4 = f(ad) = p_a - (1-k) p_D$$

Here k is just the proportion of disease gene, D, bearing haplotypes which also carry the antigen gene, A. The two notations are completely interchangeable since it easily can be shown that

$$k = p_A + \frac{D}{p_D} \qquad (3)$$

It should be remembered that the maximum and minimum values D can take are a function of the gene frequencies. Similar limits apply for the variable k. The appropriate limits are given below.

$$\max(-p_A p_D, -p_a p_d) < D < \min (p_A p_d, p_a p_D) \qquad (4)\,(i)$$

$$\frac{\max (0, 1-p_a)}{p_D} < k < \frac{\min (1, p_A)}{p_D} \qquad (4)\,(ii)$$

TABLE I

Variables in the 'disease' gene models

pA	– antigen gene frequency. Know from population data
pD	– 'disease' gene frequency
D or k	– association of antigen and 'disease' loci
x	– proportion of susceptibles who get disease
R	– recombination fraction between the two loci

Dominant or recessive 'disease' gene.

For the dominant model individuals with 'disease' genotypes *DD* and *Dd* are susceptibles and *dd* individuals are non-susceptibles. For the recessive model only *DD* individuals are susceptibles and *Dd* and *dd* individuals are non-susceptibles. The frequencies of individuals in these classes in a population cannot be directly determined since it is not possible to establish the disease susceptibility status of an individual. However, by making the assumption that a proportion x of susceptibles get the disease then tables of the expected proportion of individuals with given disease status versus presence or absence of a particular antigen at one of the HLA loci can be constructed.

In the two models of disease association we have a number of variables involved in these calculations. These variables are listed in Table 1. The expected values of various quantities which are observable in the population, in terms of the unknown variables under the two models of dominant and recessive disease genes, can be calculated as described by Thomson and Bodmer (12).

It turns out that the expected antigen genotype frequencies amongst diseased individuals provide a simple test to determine whether a set of observed genotype frequencies is compatible with a recessive mode of inheritance of the 'disease' gene, or with a dominant mode of inheritance, (provided in the dominant case the 'disease' gene frequency p_D is small).

Let F denote the observed frequency of diseased individuals who have the antigen of interest. We can estimate the parameter k (as defined in equations 2 and 3) in terms of F. For the recessive case this can be shown to be given by

$$k_{rec} = 1 - \sqrt{1 - F} \qquad (5)$$

while the expected antigen genotype frequencies amongst diseased individuals are given by

$$\begin{array}{ccc} AA & Aa & aa \\ \overline{k^2} & \overline{2k(1-k)} & \overline{(1-k^2)} \end{array} \qquad (6)$$

where, as before, *A* denotes presence of the antigen of interest and *a* its absence. For the dominant case, with small 'disease' gene frequency it can be shown that

$$k_{dom} = 1 - (1 - F)/p_a \qquad (7)$$

where p_a denotes the frequency of the allele *A* and $p_a = 1 - p_A$. In this case the expected antigen genotype frequencies are

$$\begin{array}{ccc} AA & Aa & aa \\ \overline{k(1-p_a)} & \overline{kp_a + (1-k)p_A} & \overline{(1-k)p_a} \end{array} \qquad (8)$$

So for a given incidence of an antigen amongst the diseased we can calculate the expected antigen genotype frequencies amongst diseased under recessive and dominant modes of inheritance of the 'disease' genes and then check whether the observed population values are compatible or not with either mode of inheritance. In simple terms, the basis of the test is as follows. If a 'disease' gene is recessive then a high association of the disease with a particular antigen must imply a high frequency of individuals homozygous for the corresponding gene amongst the diseased. If the 'disease' gene is dominant then the majority of affected individuals will be heterozygous for the gene determining the relevant antigen.

These tests have been applied to data on ankylosing spondylitis patients from the Oxford file. Twenty-three patients with a definite diagnosis of ankylosing spondylitis were HLA typed (5). Of the 23 patients only 1 lacked the antigen HLA-B27, 21 were confirmed heterozygotes and 1 was a suspected homozygote for HLA-B27 having no other detectable antigen at the B locus. The expected number of individuals in these three classes under recessive and dominant modes of inheritance of 'disease' genes are given below, using the formulae of equations (5) to (8):

Expected	AA	Aa	aa	
Recessive	14.4	7.6	1.0	krec = 0.791
Dominant	.8	21.2	1.0	kdom = 0.955
Observed	1.0	21.0	1.0	

A X^2 goodness of fit of the observed values to the expected in each case shows that the observations are certainly not compatible with a recessive mode of inheritance ($X^2 = 36.13$, p<< .001) but are compatible with a dominant 'disease' gene with low frequency ($X^2 = .0642$).

It turns out that these tests only have strong discriminatory powers in cases where the frequency of the antigen amongst deseased, F, is large compared to the frequency of the antigen in the general population. The exact limits on the variables have not been determined and it remains to be seen how useful the tests will be in general. The problem is that, although a number of associations of diseases with HLA have been found, the majority of the associations are probably not strong enough to allow these tests to discriminate between the two modes of inheritance. However, as more loci are determined within the HLA region, and in particular, as 'typing' methods for Ir and Ia genes are found, it is possible that stronger associations for certain diseases will be found so that the above tests would then become generally applicable.

Multiple Case Family Studies

The use of multiple case family studies to try and detect the effects of HLA linked 'disease' genes has been investigated by Cudworth and Woodrow (3), Bobrow et al. (1), Day and Simons (4) and others. Day and Simons (4) developed a technique for studying the inheritance pattern of HLA haplotypes in sibs who are both affected by a disorder. Their models are more general than those considered in the previous section but the basic assumption is the same, namely that there is a disease susceptibility locus effectively within the HLA region. By looking at inheritance patterns within families we know that the disease susceptibility gene will be inherited with the HLA haplotype, discounting the possibility of recombination, which is rare within the HLA region and can often be detected and so eliminated from the analyses. Thus, the basis of multiple case family studies is to use HLA haplotypes as markers to trace the inheritance pattern of closely linked disease susceptibility genes. This is an approach which is similar, in some respects, to Penrose's (9) sib-pair linkage test.

We assume that the parents carry four different HLA haplotypes between them and these are used as markers. For each possible disease and haplotype combination of the parents the relative likelihood of getting a sib pair with the disease can be calculated. Thus, for each parental arrangement, the probabilities of the affected sib pairs having both, one or no HLA haplotypes in common can be calculated. Using all this information one can then calculate the overall probability of an affected sib pair having both, one or no haplotypes in common, denoted by X, Y and Z respectively. Values of X, Y and Z, the probabilities for the three classes of af-

TABLE II

The probabilities of an affected sib pair sharing both, one or no HLA haplotypes (X, Y and Z respectively) for various values of the disease susceptibility gene frequency pD, for the recessive case.

p_D	X (share both haplotypes)	Y (share one haplotype)	Z (share no haplotypes
.0	1.0	.0	.0
.05	.907	.091	.002
.1	.827	.165	.008
.15	.756	.227	.017
.2	.694	.278	.028
.25	640	.320	.040
.3	.592	.355	.053
.35	.549	.384	.067
.4	.510	.408	.082
.45	.476	.428	.096
.5	.445	.444	.111
.55	.416	.458	.126
.6	.391	.469	.140
.65	.367	.478	.155
.7	.346	.484	.170
.75	.326	.490	.184
.8	.309	.494	.198
.85	.292	.497	.211
.9	.277	.499	.224
.95	.263	.5	.237
1.0	.25	.5	.25

TABLE III

As for Table II for the dominant case

p_D	X (share both haplotypes)	Y (share one haplotype)	Z (share no haplotypes)
.0	.5	.5	.0
.05	.460	.495	.045
.1	.428	.491	.081
.15	.401	.488	.111
.2	.377	.387	.136
.25	.358	.486	.156
.3	.341	.485	.174
.35	.326	.485	.189
.4	.313	.486	.201
.45	.302	.487	.211
.5	.293	.488	.219
.55	.284	.489	.227
.6	.277	.490	.323
.65	.271	.492	.237
.7	.265	.494	.241
.75	.261	.495	.244
.8	.257	.497	.246
.85	.254	.498	.248
.9	.252	.499	.249
.95	.25	.5	.25
1.0	.25	.5	.25

fected sib pairs, given for different values of the disease gene frequency p_D and assuming the same model as used in the previous section, are given in Table 2 for the recessive and Table 3 for the dominant case. (See Thomson and Bodmer, (12), for further details).

Thus if, for example, data are available on the HLA types of a number of affected sib pairs, Tables 2 and 3 can be used to compare the observed frequencies of the proportions with none, one or two haplotypes in common with those expected for the dominant and recessive models for different disease gene frequencies p_D The simple basis of this test for a dominant versus a recessive disease gene is that in the recessive case, for small values of p_D one expects the proportion of sib pairs with both haplotypes in common to be substantially greater than that with one or none. On the other hand, in the dominant case the expected proportion of sibs with one haplotype in common is always greater than that sharing both, though for low disease gene frequencies the two values are nearly the same. Thus, for example, when the disease gene frequency $p_D = 0.1$, in the recessive case the respective frequencies of sib pairs sharing both or sharing one haplotype are 0.827 and 0.165, while for the dominant case they are 0.428 and 0.491.

As an example of the application of these results let us consider Cudworth and Woodrow's family data on juvenile diabetes melitus. They considered 15 affected sib pairs and found that 10 of these shared both HLA haplotypes, 4 had one haplotype in common and 1 sib pair had no haplotypes in common. From Table 2 we see that these observed values of X, Y, Z (10/15 = 0.667, 4/15 = 0.267, and 1/15 = 0.066) are quite consistent with a recessive mode of inheritance and a 'disease' gene with frequency of about $p_D = 0.20$. (The expected values in this case are 0.694, 0.278 and 0.028 resceptively). With the small sample size a dominant mode of inheritance cannot be completely ruled out although the results are much more compatible with a recessive mode of inheritance, because of the high frequency of sib pairs sharing both HLA haplotypes. It must be stressed that the data is insufficient at the present time to reach any firm conclusions about the mode of inheritance. It will be very interesting to obtain further HLA data on affected sib pairs to see if the suspected recessive mode of inheritance for juvenile diabetes mellitus can be confirmed. We should also point out that the methods and results discussed by Ryder and Svejgaard in a previous chapter are not necessarily at all in disagreement with the present approach.

If sufficient numbers of affected sib pairs are available this method provides a very powerful test for discriminating between dominant and recessive modes of inheritance of 'disease' genes, provided the 'disease' gene frequencies are fairly small. Appropriate data from all HLA associated diseases should provide very useful information for this test, without the need for more family data, which is often hard to obtain.

One further aspect of this approach is that once the mode of inheritance of a disease has been determined it then becomes possible to consider environmental and other non-HLA linked genetic factors predisposing individuals to disease. This can be done as follows. Suppose, as seems likely, that susceptibility to juvenile diabetes mellitus is determined by a recessive gene. If this is the case then we know that if an individual has juvenile diabetes then all their HLA identical sibs are disease susceptible. Environmental or non-HLA linked genetic differences experienced by HLA identical sibs, of whom one has juvenile diabetes mellitus and the other does not, can then give clues as to environmental or other genetic factors predisposing individuals to the disease.

Estimation of the »Disease« Gene Frequency, p_D, and Penetrance Factor, x

The two methods outlined above should usually enable one to distinguish between dominant and recessive modes of inheritance of HLA linked 'disease' genes. Once the mode of inheritance of the disease has been determined it is then of interest, to calculate the frequency of the 'disease' gene p_D and the penetrance factor x, and so the complete set of haplotype frequencies. There are various lines of approach to take in looking at this problem, as outlined below:

(1) When looking at the antigen genotype frequencies amongst diseased the estimate of k obtained for the relevant model allows an estimate of the maximum possible value of the 'disease' gene frequency, p_D, to be made. Thus, from equation 4(ii) we know

$$k < \frac{p_A}{p_D} \tag{9}$$

and so using an estimate of p_A from the appropriate population data we can obtain an upper limit on p_D.

For example, using the data on ankylosing spondylitis, which for a dominant model gave k = 0.955, and assuming a B27 gene frequency of $0.0357 = p_A$ we have

$$p_D < \frac{p_A}{k} = \frac{0.0357}{0.955} = 0.037,$$

giving an upper limit of 3.7 % for the disease gene frequency.

(2) Once the appropriate mode of inheritance has been determined from affected sib pair data the relevant 'disease' gene frequency p_D can be obtained from Table 2 or Table 3, as was done with Cudworth and Woodrow's (3) data.

(3) The frequency of a disease in the population (FDP) is a function of x and p_D. Thus, for the dominant model

$$FDPdom = x(1-p^2_D),$$
$$\text{where } p_d = 1-p_D \tag{10}$$

since a proportion $1-p^2_D$ of the population carry the disease gene $_D$, and of these a proportion x will be affected. Similarly, for the recessive model

$$FDPrec = xp^2_D \tag{11}$$

So, if an estimate of p_D has been obtained, say from affected sib pair data, then an estimate of x can be obtained, using equations (10) and (11). It is often difficult to obtain accurate estimates of the population incidence of diseases. However, since it should be possible to get reasonable estimates of the 'disease' gene frequency p_D, this method at least allows one to determine the order of magnitude of the penetrance factor x. For example, in the case of juvenile diabetes the population incidence of the disease appears to be between 0.1 % and 0.5 %. Using the gene frequency of 0.2 obtained from Cudworth and Woodrow's data and equation (11), this gives a value for x between $\frac{0.001}{(0.2)^2}$ and $\frac{0.005}{(0.2)^2}$, namely between 0.025 and 0.125. These are substantially lower estimates of penetrance than those previously quoted for a postulated recessive juvenile diabetes gene (see e.g. Caballi-Sforza and Bodmer (2)). They are, however, subject to a considerable margin of error as the gene frequency estimates could, by chance, easily be too high by a factor of 2, which would, for example, bring the upper limit of 0.125 to about 0.5, a value well above previous estimates of penetrance. The estimation of the disease incidence is a major problem when, as in all such situations, the disease has a variable manifestation. Mostly the incidence is likely to be underestimated in the population at large, since only the more severe cases are likley to be brought to the clinicians' attention. In families, on the other hand, once an affected individual has been identified, the other members of the family are likely to be more intensively investigated, so uncovering milder cases of the disease. This will tend to lead, necessarily, to a relatively higher estimate of incidence from family data than from general population data.

(4) Finally, another approach is to use data on the familial incidence of a disease to obtain direct estimates of the penetrance x, as discussed by Thomson, Bodmer and Bodmer (11). Then, given estimates of the disease incidence, equations (10) and (11) can be used to obtain estimates of p_D, the disease gene frequency. Thus, for the recessive model with incomplete penetrance, the expected frequency of diseased offspring when neither of the parents is diseased is simply about ¼x, since almost all such matings must be Dd x Dd when p_D is small, giving ¼DD offspring of which a proportion x are affected. It is, for example, from the observed incidence in such matings that previous estimates of the penetrance of the presumed recessive juvenile diabetes gene have been obtained. In the dominant model, with incomplete penetrance the frequency of diseased amongst offspring of matings between a diseased and a normal parent

is $\quad \dfrac{x(1-p_D p^2_d)}{1-p^2_d} \sim \frac{1}{2}x \quad$ (12)

when pD is small, since then nearly all such matings are Dd x dd giving ½Dd offspring of whom x are affected.

Alternatively, as suggested by Thomson, Bodmer and Bodmer (11), one can estimate x as the proportion of individuals with the appropriate antigen genotype (AA for the recessives and AA or Aa for the dominant model) who have the disease, within families in which the disease has already been ascertained. In this case, of course, the individuals through whom the families were ascertained must be excluded from the analysis. This is the approach used in the accompanying paper by Kidd, Ceppellini et al.

In all these cases, as already discussed in relation to approach (3), the estimates of x obtained from family data will most probably be higher, perhaps substantially so, than those that would be obtained from general population data. There are two reasons in addition to the fact that family members are likely to be more intensively studied, why this should be so. The first is simply the ascertainment problem, namely that the probability of detecting a sibship increases with the number of affected individuals it contains. The second is that families containing one or more affected cases will be those that have the appropriate environmental or other genetic factors making susceptible individuals more likely actually to manifest the disease. So these particular families are in fact at higher risk than families who happen to carry the 'disease' gene but do not contain any individuals with the disease.

Following the procedures outlined so far in this paper all the parameters listed in Table 1, except for the recombination fraction R, can be estimated. Thus, for example, in the case of the data on ankylosing spondylitis the antigen genotype frequencies amongst diseased individuals indicate that a dominant mode of inheritance is involved and so the parameter k can be calculated using equation (7). An estimate of the penetrance factor x can next be obtained by considering family data as in the accompanying paper by Kidd, Ceppellini et al. Using this value of x an estimate of the disease gene frequency p_D can then be obtained from the frequency of the disease in the population using equation (10). Finally, the antigen gene frequency can of course be obtained from population data on the antigen phenotype frequency and so, using equations (2), having obtained values for k, p_A and p_D one can obtain estimates of the frequencies of the four haplotypes *AD, Aa, aD* and *ad*.

As already discussed, the biggest problem arises from the differences in the estimates for x and p_D obtained from family as compared to population data. Kidd, Ceppellini *et al.* obtain an approximate answer by using observations on the proportion of a random sample of B27 +ve individuals who have ankylosing spondylitis as diagnosed by the same criteria used in their family studies. Using this value, 0.16, and multiplying by the B27 antigen frequency of approximately 0.1, gives a total population frequency for B27 affected individuals of 0.016. This is then adjusted for the fact that only 0.92 of diseased individuals have B27 to give an approximate disease incidence for ankylosing spondylitis of 0.016/0.92 = 0.017. The rest of their calculations are equivalent to equations (2), (7) and (10) assuming p_A and p_D are small and using an estimate of penetrance x = 0.38 obtained from family data.

So far no affected sib pair data for ankylosing spondylitis has been available for analysis. It will be interesting to see how the estimates obtained from such an analysis compare with those resulting from the above approach.

Discussion

The basis of the methods outlined in this paper for analysing HLA and disease associations assuming an HLA linked disease gene model, is to determine the expected values of various observables such as the antigen frequency amongst diseased individuals, in terms of unknown variables, under the two contrasting assumptions of dominant and recessive 'disease' genes with incomplete penetrance. Using these predictions it should generally be possible to determine whether a given observed set of data fits a dominant or a recessive mode of inheritance, and then to estimate the frequency of the 'disease' gene p_D and the penetrance factor x.

It is, as already discussed, difficult to get good estimates for many of the quantities of interest in studies of disease inheritance. Complications such as variable age of onset of a disease and difficulties in obtaining comparable diagnosis in family and population studies contribute to the problems of estimating the parameters. However, some of the tests outlined above should at least distinguish more clearly between the results expected for dominant as compared to recessive modes of inheritance for the disease gene, even when good estimates of the incidence are not available. For instance, in cases where the frequency of an antigen amongst diseased is high as compared to the population frequency of the antigen, the differences in expected antigen genotype frequencies amongst diseased for the dominant and recessive models are quite striking whatever the values of x and p_D. As more loci within the HLA region are recognised it is likely that stronger associations will be found for some diseases for which the associations are so far weak, thus extending the applicability of this test for the mode of inheritance of the disease gene.

The method of looking at data from affected sib pairs has the advantage that it enables one to get close to the actual disease susceptibility loci by using the HLA haplotypes as markers to trace the inheritance pattern of closely linked disease susceptibility genes. This method is useful even in cases where the population association of the disease with HLA is weak and, of course, allows use to be made of incomplete family data.

The results we have obtained supporting a dominant disease gene model for ankylosing spondylitis and a recessive model for juvenile diabetes, as well as providing some basis for estimating penetrance and disease gene frequencies are at least an indication of the value of these newer approaches to the genetic analysis of HLA and disease associations. Hopefully, a further combination of experimental and statistical analysis of population and family data will help to clarify the nature of these fascinating associations and their implications for understanding the genetics and etiology of the HLA associated diseases.

Acknowledgements

We are grateful to Julia Bodmer and to Hilary and Alan Hill for making available their data on ankylosing spondylitis. This work was supported in part by a grant from the Medical Research Council.

References

1. Bobrow, M., Bodmer, J. G., Bodmer, W. F., McDevitt, H. O., Lorber, J. & Switf, P. (1975) The search for a human equivalent of the mouse T-locus – negative results from a study of HL-A types in spina bifida. *Tissue Antigens* 5, 234–237.
2. Cavalli-Sforza, L. L., & Bodmer, W. F. (1971) *The Genetics of Human Populations*. Freeman & Co. San Francisco, p. 559–561.
3. Cudworth, A. G. & Woodrow, J. C. (1975) Evidence for HLA linked genes in 'juvenile' diabetes mellitus. *Br. Med. J.* 3, 133–135.
4. Day, N. E. & Simons, M. J. (1976) Disease susceptibility genes – their identification by multiple case family studies. *Tissue Antigens* 8, 109–119.
5. Hill, F. H., Hill, A. G. S. & Bodmer, J. G. (1976) The clinical diagnosis of ankylosing spondylitis in Women and relation to presence of HLA-B27. *Annals of Rheumatic Diseases* 35, 267–270.
6. Kidd, K. K. & Cacalli-Sforza, L. L. (1973) An analysis of the genetics of schizophrenia. *Social Biology* 20, 254–265.
7. McDevitt, H. O. & Bodmer, W. F. (1972) Histocompatibility antigens, immune responsiveness and susceptibility to disease. *American J. of Med.* 52, 1–8.
8. McDevitt, H. O. & Bodmer, W. F. (1974) HL-A, immune response genes and disease. *The Lancet*, pp. 1269–1275.
9. Penrose, L. S. (1935) The detection of autosomal linkage in data which consists of pairs of brothers and sisters of unspecified parentage. *Ann. Eugen.* 6, 133–138.
10. Smith, C. (1971) Discriminating between different modes of inheritance in genetic disease. *Clin. Genet.* 2, 303–314.
11. Thomson, G., Bodmer, W. F. & Bodmer, J. G. (1976) The HLA system as a model for studying the interaction between selection migration and linkage. In: *Population Genetics and Ecology*, eds. Karlin, S. & Nevo, E. Academic Press, New York, p. 465–498.
12. Thomson, G. & Bodmer, W. F. (1977) The genetics of HLA and disease association. In: *Measuring Selection in Natural Populations*, eds. Barndorff-Nielsen, O., Christiansen, F. B. & Fenchel, T. Munksgaard, Copenhagen.

93

Rheumatology

D. A. Brewerton[1] & E. Albert[2]

Ankylosing spondylitis is not a simple well-defined disease with clear-cut complications. It is a member of a large group of disorders which overlap and intertwine to produce a wide variety of clinical syndromes. Fortunately, before the current interest in tissue typing, there had been extensive clinical and family studies to clarify the relationships between these disorders and to demonstrate genetic factors in most of them (1–6). The members of the group include: sacro-iliitis and spondylitis, a wide variety of disorders of the peripheral joints and soft tissues, acute anterior uveitis, aortitis, psoriasis, ulcerative colitis, Crohn's disease, reactive arthritis (after sexually transmitted urethritis, or after gut infection with *shigella flexneri, salmonella* or *yersinia enterocolitica),* conjunctival reaction, balanitis, keratoderma blennorrhagica, and Behçet's disease. Closely related in some respect are: rheumatoid disease, amyloidosis, sarcoidosis, and many other disorders.

The discovery of the remarkable association between ankylosing spondylitis and HLA B27 (7, 8) not only provided an excellent human model for studying the relationship between a disease and an inherited antigen, it also

presented clinicians with a thread that could be followed through the labyrinth of diseases that had been so difficult to understand. Now, attention is rightly switching to basic research projects to determine the mechanism by which these diseases are produced.

Ankylosing spondylitis

In most reports of Caucasian populations, B27 has been present in 85–95 % of patients with ankylosing spondylitis. So strong is this association that it has been impossible to determine whether Caucasian patients with certain clinical features, such as peripheral arthritis or uveitis, are more or less likely to have B27. Despite this unprecedented degree of association between an HLA antigen and a disease, it was obvious from the beginning that classical ankylosing spondylitis could develop in the absence of B27. It was also impossible to explain why men were more likely to have a severe form of the disease, why some patients had only trivial symptoms, and why most individuals with B27 had no clinical evidence of the disease. There had to be other factors, probably both genetic and environmental.

Most family studies have shown what should be expected: one parent with B27 (about one third with ankylosing spondylitis, asymptomatic sacro-iliitis, or minor rheumatic symptoms), and B27

[1] Westminster Hospital, Horseferry Road, London SW1P 2AP, England.
[2] Kinderpoliklinik der Universität München, 8 München 2, Germany.

in approximately half the sibs and half the offspring. The occasional exceptions to this familiar pattern have included: two asymptomatic parents with three sons all with severe ankylosing spondylitis and B27; two asymptomatic parents with three sons, one asymptomatic with B27, one with ankylosing spondylitis and B27, and one with ankylosing spondylitis without B27; two parents with ankylosing spondylitis (one with B27 and one without B27) with three sons who have ankylosing spondylitis (two with B27 and one without); identical twins with B27 discordant for ankylosing spondylitis; and families in which homozygosity for B27 led to more frequent or more severe disease.

HLA-A2 and the haplotype A2, B27 have attracted interest, both being moderately increased in most series of patients with ankylosing spondylitis (9, 10). So far, the search for other associations between ankylosing spondylitis and HLA-C or HLA-D has revealed no association greater than that which might be expected in asymptomatic individuals with B27 (11, 12).

There have been several reports of the frequencies of B27 and ankylosing spondylitis in different populations and races. In British Columbia, Gofton et al. (13) found sacro-iliitis in 10 % of adult male Haida Indians, with B27 in 50 % of the Haida population. By contrast, B27 and ankylosing spondylitis are not found in Australian aboriginals or black Africans, and there is a reduced frequency of both antigen and disease in black Americans and in Maoris. In black Americans, patients with ankylosing spondylitis are less likely to have B27, particularly females (14). Calin et al. (15) studied 193 Pima Indians: sacro-iliitis was present in 19.7 %, and B27 in 18 % of the Pima population. Of those with sacro-iliitis, B27 was found in 8 out of 16 males, but only 2 out of 22 females, indicating that the relationship between B27 and sacro-iliitis is weaker than in Caucasians, and in males only. The risk of sacro-iliitis in the Pima without B27 is much greater than in Caucasians. In Israel, Brautbar et al. (16) investigated Ashkenazi Jews, non-Ashkenazi Jews, and Arabs, all with ankylosing spondylitis, and found a comparable frequency of B27 in the three groups, demonstrating a strong association which transcends ethnic differences and varying degrees of geographic isolation for long periods of time. In Japan, although the frequency of B27 in the population is low, there is a high association between B27 and ankylosing spondylitis: Shirakura et al. (17) found B27 in 33 out of 36 patients.

Acute anterior uveitis

Approximately one third of patients with ankylosing spondylitis also suffer acute anterior uveitis. In many respects the uveitis does not appear to be a secondary complication, and so, to test the possibility that the association between the two disorders might be genetically determined, Brewerton et al. investigated patients who had acute anterior uveitis and no evidence of a rheumatic disease. B27 was present in 29 out of 67 patients (43 %), compared with 7 % of controls (18, 19).

Peripheral arthritis

Similarly, one third of patients with ankylosing spondylitis have an arthritis of the peripheral joints, particularly in the lower limbs or shoulders. This peripheral arthritis is unlike rheumatoid arthritis and psoriatic arthritis in that extensive involvement of the hands is uncommon. IgM rheumatoid factor is found in only about 2 % of patients with spondylitic peripheral arthritis.

95

Following the example of the association of B27 with uveitis in the absence of rheumatic disease, it was logical to investigate patients with sero-negative peripheral arthritis who had no evidence of either sacro-iliitis or spondylitis. Cleland et al. (20) found B27 in 30 % out of 73 patients examined; and there were important clinical differences in the groups with and without B27. In those with B27 the sex ratio was equal, the mean age of onset was 24, and the arthritis was predominantly in the lower limbs. By contrast, in the 70 % without B27 the majority were women, the mean age of onset was 40, and almost all had symmetrical upper limb disease. The authors describe the latter group as being exactly like rheumatoid arthritis but without IgM rheumatoid factor or nodules. These findings suggest that sero-negative peripheral arthritis can now be divided into two types, although with clinical overlap between them: a spondylitic type associated with B27 and having a joint distribution similar to the peripheral arthritis of ankylosing spondylitis; and a rheumatoid type with a rheumatoid distribution of joint involvement. Heinrichs et al. (21) studied patients with monarticular arthritis, oligoarthritis, calcaneodynia or tendovaginitis, who had no evidence of rheumatoid arthritis, spondylitis or sacro-iliitis: 42 % had B27. Amor et al. (22) have analysed their results in 115 patients with "unclassified, inflammatory, rheumatic disease": 70 % were male, 83 % had an onset before the age of 40, and 49 of the 115 patients (43 %) had B27. de Ceulaer et al. (23) studied eight patients with non-erosive arthritis of the toes ("sausage toes") occurring without sacro-iliitis, spondylitis or other associated disease: all eight had B27. Bulgen et al. (24) found B27 in 16 out of 38 patients with frozen shoulders.

Aortitis

It might have been expected that aortitis would follow the pattern of uveitis without rheumatic disease and peripheral arthritis without sacro-iliitis, but it does not appear to do so. Calin et al. (25) studied patients with idiopathic aortic insufficiency and found B27 in only one out of the 14 examined.

Polyarthritis in childhood

Ankylosing spondylitis may follow brief episodes of acute polyarthritis in childhood, particularly from the ages of 10–14, which is often misdiagnosed as rheumatic fever. It is also firmly established on clinical grounds that a small proportion of children with juvenile chronic polyarthritis develop sacro-iliitis or ankylosing spondylitis in later life. This occurs particularly in boys with involvement of a few joints in the lower limbs and in children who have acute anterior uveitis. Adults with ankylosing spondylitis who give this history of rheumatic disease in childhood usually have B27, as would be expected; B27 is also found in children with chronic polyarthritis who have clinical features suggesting the later development of ankylosing spondylitis (26). Consequently, B27 may be particularly valuable in the diagnosis and prognosis of children with rheumatic disease. As in adults, a few children with B27 may have chronic polyarthritis in later life without sacro-iliitis or spondylitis.

Chronic inflammatory bowel disease

Spondylitis occurs more frequently in patients with ulcerative colitis and Crohn's disease than in the general population. This spondylitis does not seem to be a secondary complication: it may be diagnosed several years before the onset of bowel symptoms and its clinical course bears little relation to the treatment of the bowel disease. On the basis of clinical family studies there is good evidence of genetic factors in both ulcerative colitis and Crohn's disease, and when Macrae & Wright (3) investigated the first-degree relatives of patients with ulcerative colitis (without rheumatic disease), they found an increased prevalence of sacro-iliitis and spondylitis. In most series of ulcerative colitis and Crohn's disease alone, there has been a normal distribution of HLA antigens, but Van den Berg-Loonen *et al.* (27) now report an increase of A11 in ulcerative colitis and B18 in Crohn's disease. In 39 patients with both chronic inflammatory bowel disease and ankylosing spondylitis, they found B27 in 50 %, and when B27 was absent there was an increase of BW16 (known to be associated with psoriasis). Brewerton *et al.* (28, 29) found B27 in 21 out of 28 patients with chronic inflammatory bowel disease and ankylosing spondylitis, and in 2 out of 6 patients with sacro-iliitis without clinical evidence of spinal involvement. Comparing different series, there appears to be general agreement that the association between spondylitis and B27 is less when chronic inflammatory bowel disease is also present.

Psoriasis and arthritis

Psoriasis without rheumatic disease is well known to be hereditary and it is interesting to note the occasional appearance of psoriasis in family studies of spondylitis, chronic inflammatory bowel disease, or Reiter's disease. It is now accepted that psoriasis alone has modest associations with B13, BW17, and BW16 (BW38), but not B27.

The arthritides associated with psoriasis are complicated and, although they may be divided into arbitrary groups, these do not always behave as would be expected in the absence of psoriasis. Because psoriasis and rheumatoid disease are common diseases, a proportion of patients have a natural combination of the two disorders. Such patients would not be expected to have B27 and have probably been excluded from most studies of HLA antigens. Psoriasis is also associated with spondylitis much more frequently than would be expected and, as with chronic inflammatory bowel disease, the spondylitis does not behave like a complication and may be diagnosed years before the psoriasis appears. Compared with ankylosing spondylitis, patients with psoriatic spondylitis are far more likely to have peripheral arthritis and this usually includes the hands. Furthermore, the spondylitis associated with psoriasis or Reiter's disease has minor radiographic features in common that are not found in other types of spondylitis. HLA results to date (28, 30–32) suggest that the frequency of B27 varies with the severity of spinal involvement, being present in about one third (or less) of patients with sacro-iliitis without clinical evidence of spinal disease, and in 50–90 % of patients with obvious spondylitis. The exclusion of patients with rheumatoid disease, sacro-iliitis and spondylitis leaves a third group of patients with psoriasis and peripheral arthritis, which is itself complicated and may be multifactorial in origin. Moll & Wright (4) studied clinically 181 first-degree relatives of 88 patients with psoriatic peripheral arthritis without sacro-iliitis, and in the relatives found psoriasis and arthritis (or spondylitis) in 13, psoriasis alone in 28, polyarthritis alone in 11, and sacro-iliitis or spondylitis without psoriasis in 10. Hence, a small increase of B27 would be expected in patients with psoriatic peripheral arthritis without sacro-iliitis or spondylitis, but here there is a difference of opinion between British and French results. Brewerton *et al.* (adopting the clinical criteria of Moll & Wright) found B27 in 11 out of 47 patients (28), and now Eastmond & Woodrow (30) report B27 in 7 out of 27 in a similar series. By contrast, Roux *et al.* (31), and Feldmann *et al.* (32) investigated 68 and 44 patients respectively with psoriatic peripheral arthritis without sacro-iliitis, and they reported a normal frequency of B27, or even a decrease. Presumably there was a difference in the method of selection, or in the clinical criteria.

Reiter's disease following urethritis

Reiter's disease following urethritis is particularly interesting because it is assumed to result from sexually transmitted infection. Although it is easy to be puritanical and believe that those who acquire the disease are those who place themselves most at risk, there is good clinical evidence that certain individuals are particularly susceptible to Reiter's disease and that this susceptibility may be hereditary. In Britain, less than 1 % of men with non-specific urethritis develop any evidence of Reiter's disease. Brewerton *et al.* (33) studied 33 matched controls, 33 men with non-specific urethritis, and 33 with Reiter's disease. B27 was present in 2, 3 and 25 (76 %) respectively, indicating that the inherited antigen is not related to the urethritis but to the arthritis and other clinical features that followed a few weeks later. Subsequently, the same authors (34, 29) reported that B27 was present in 19 out of 20 with sacro-iliitis or spondylitis, compared with 29 out of 44 with peripheral arthritis alone. Although the numbers were small, it also appeared that uveitis, keratoderma blennorrhagica and balanitis were more common in patients with Reiter's disease who had B27.

Postdysenteric Reiter's disease

In Finland during the Second World War, there was an epidemic of 150,000 cases of *shigella flexneri* dysentery, followed a few weews later by 350 cases of Reiter's disease, 70 % having the triad of arthritis, urethritis and conjunctivitis. When 100 patients were reviewed 20 years later (35), 32 had spondylitis, 18 peripheral arthritis, and 7 a history of uveitis. In a recent investigation (36), B27 was present in 39 out of 50 of these patients. A different study (37) relates to 602 crew members who developed *shigella* dysentery when on a U.S. naval cruiser in 1963. Nine men developed Reiter's disease; five of them have now been traced and four were found to have B27.

Acute arthritis following specific infections

The term "reactive arthritis" is used to describe arthritis which follows infections of other organs, such as the pharynx, gut, or genito-urinary tract, without direct involvement of the joints by infective agents. Rheumatic fever and Reiter's disease are quoted as examples. After *salmonella* infection, up to 2 % of patients develop acute arthritis in their peripheral joints, and Aho *et al.* (38) found B27 in 15 out of 16 such patients. Similarly, after intestinal infection with *yersinia enterocolitica,* a small proportion of patients may develop an acute arthritis that resembles the acute arthritis of Reiter's disease in adults and may mimic rheumatic fever in childhood. Aho *et al.* (38) found B27 in 43 out of 49 patients with *yersinia* arthritis. In a separate study in Helsinki, Leirisalo *et al.* (39) found B27 in 30 out of 46 patients with *yersinia* arthritis. Of their 46 patients, five had carditis, eight urological symptoms, and five eye complications. Following their *yersinia* infection, five patients developed signs of Reiter's syndrome (three previously asymptomatic, one who had ankylosing spondylitis, and one with sero-negative peripheral arthritis).

Rheumatic fever

Post-streptococcal rheumatic fever is not related to B27, and its possible associations with other HLA antigens are controversial. Falk et al. (40) found an increase of shared antigens in the parents; then came a report of an increase of BW17 in Europeans in New Zealand (41). Joysey et al. (42) have studied 80 patients awaiting cardiac surgery and found an increase of BW15, and Leirisalo et al. report a modest increase of BW35 and a decrease of B5 in recurrent cases. This latter observation is to be studied further in view of the interesting report by Greenberg et al. (43) that individuals with B5 are more likely to have increased in vitro responses to streptococcal antigens.

Vertebral ankylosing hyperostosis

Although the differences between ankylosing spondylitis and vertebral ankylosing hyperostosis have been detailed by Forestier and by others, there has remained a suspicion that the latter condition might be a variant of spondylitis in which the sacro-iliac joints had remained normal. So far there have been three reports, unfortunately reaching different conclusions. Shapiro et al. (44) found B27 in 16 out of 47 patients, while Ercilla et al. (45) reported no increase of B27 in 50 patients, and Graber Duvernay et al. (46) did not find B27 in 20 patients. Rosenthal et al. (47) reported a normal B27 frequency in 50 patients and a significant increase of B8, which was in keeping with the high in-

cidence of diabetes mellitus in their patients.

Osteitis condensans ilii

Like vertebral ankylosing hyperostosis, it seemed possible that osteitis condensans ilii might sometimes be a mild form of sacro-iliitis related to ankylosing spondylitis. In the early stages of disease, sacro-iliac radiographs may occasionally resemble osteitis condensans ilii, and yet the patient has B27 and later proceeds to classical sacro-iliitis or spondylitis. However, this is definitely exceptional. In a careful follow-up study by Singal et al. (48), B27 was present in only 2 out of 25 patients with osteitis condensans ilii.

Behçet's disease

Behçet's disease is reported more frequently in some countries, especially Japan and Turkey, and the distribution of HLA antigens in this disease is not the same in Japan as elsewhere. In Japan, Ohno et al. (49) found B5 in 71 % of patients compared with 30 % of controls. Now Nakagawa et al. (50) report B5 in 30 out of 45 patients, and Hoshino et al. (51) also report B5 in a highly significant proportion of patients. By contrast, in England, Chamberlain (52) found B5 in 18 % compared with 10 % of controls, and B27 in 27 %. In the United States, O'Duffy et al. (53) found B5 in 18 % and B27 in 8 %.

Rheumatoid disease

All the early studies of rheumatoid disease indicated a normal frequency of HLA antigens. In 1974 Stastny (54) reported preliminary evidence of an association with determinants in HLA-D. These findings are now confirmed by Stastny (55) and by several other laboratories, all demonstrating a significant increase of DW4. This clear evidence of HLA-linked susceptibility to rheumatoid arthritis represents one of the most important developments in rheumatology in recent years.

Fallet *et al.* (56) and Good *et al.* (57) report patients who have both rheumatoid arthritis and ankylosing spondylitis. These occasional cases do not seem to indicate an undue association between the two diseases, but they do show that these diseases are not mutually exclusive. It is not yet known whether patients with rheumatoid disease who have B27 (or other HLA antigens) differ in the progress of their disease.

Sjögren's syndrome

In 47 patients with Sjögren's syndrome, Clough *et al.* (58) found B8 in 45 % compared with 22 % of controls. The increase of B8 was significant in patients who also had polymyositis, systemic sclerosis, or both. In patients with rheumatoid disease, B8 was present in 11 out of 31, but this small increase was not significant. The authors conclude that B8 may be more closely related to systemic sclerosis and polymyositis than to Sjögren's syndrome itself.

Polymyalgia rheumatica

In 50 patients with polymyalgia rheumatica, Sany *et al.* (59) reported B5 in 24 % and BW38 in 18 % (compared with 13 % and 5 % respectively in controls). The same antigens were increased in 19 patients with polymyalgia rheumatica who had temporal arteritis, but not in 31 patients with temporal arteritis without polymyalgia rheumatica. This suggests that polymyalgia rheumatica and temporal arteritis are distinct diseases (although commonly associated), or that patients with temporal arteritis who

have B5 or BW38 are likely to develop polymyalgia rheumatica.

Amyloidosis

Pasternack & Tiilikainen (60) compared patients with sero-positive rheumatoid disease, amyloidosis associated with inflammatory peripheral arthritis, and amyloidosis in the absence of rheumatic disease. They found that the majority of patients with amyloidosis and peripheral arthritis were men with an onset of arthritis in early adult life who had B27 but not IgM rheumatoid factor or radiographic sacro-iliitis. They concluded that (in Finland) this type of peripheral arthritis carried a far greater likelihood of being associated with amyloidosis than did classical sero-positive rheumatoid disease.

Disease classification

There is no doubt that in the classification of inflammatory rheumatic disorders rheumatologists have been cutting their cake the wrong way, although most will have had an uncomfortable feeling that this would prove to be so. Previously, the rheumatic disorders associated with ankylosing spondylitis, ulcerative colitis, psoriasis, Reiter's disease and reactive arthritis were usually discussed as if they were separate. Uveitis was described as a complication of spondylitis, ulcerative colitis and Reiter's disease; and radiographic sacro-iliitis was so firmly established as a diagnostic criterion that few physicians would have accepted peripheral arthritis without sacro-iliitis (or uveitis without arthritis) as part of a single disease process linked with ankylosing spondylitis. Now the pieces of the cake must be reassembled, and it might be unwise to cut it again before more facts are available. At present it looks as if there may be a large number of genetic factors, overlapping in various proportions to induce susceptibility to several clinical features, some of which may be found in different members of a family, or occasionally together in a single individual.

Diagnosis

Before considering the value of B27 in diagnosis, it is necessary to define what is to be diagnosed, and for what purpose. In past years the term "ankylosing spondylitis" has concentrated attention on the spine, and in the jungle of chronic backache radiographic sacro-iliitis has been an essential guide. But few physicians who have used tissue typing in studying the outer fringes of spondylitis, unexplained rheumatic syndromes in the limbs, minor symptoms associated with anterior uveitis, or the various clinical features in 'normal' individuals with B27 (in families or in the population), can return to routine clinical practice and be satisfied with current text-book descriptions. To be fair to B27, it is necessary to consider its use in conditions which could not be readily diagnosed before. When examining a young man with typical symptoms of ankylosing spondylitis, radiographic confirmation is wise, but (apart from research) tissue typing is no more than an expensive and time-consuming luxury. Nevertheless, clinicians do encounter patients whose symptoms suggest the possibility of spondylitis, although the physical examination and radiographs are normal or equivocal. In such circumstances does B27 help, or are bone scans more valuable? First, the mathematics: even with classical ankylosing spondylitis in a Caucasian population, at least 5 % with obvious disease will not have B27, and the pro-

portion of "false negatives" will increase (sometimes considerably) in patients with only sacro-iliitis, in the presence of chronic inflammatory bowel disease or psoriasis, and in certain races. Secondly, the "false positives": in adults with B27 there will be no rheumatic symptoms and no evidence of rheumatic disease in 70–80 % of the population, in 60–70 % of first-degree relatives of patients with ankylosing spondylitis, or in 50 % of individuals who have acute anterior uveitis. By definition, B27 cannot be an accurate test, but it can influence appreciably the probability that the individual has spondylitis (or a related disorder). There have been several reports referring to this dilemma. Calin et al. (61) suggest that it is unusual for individuals with B27 to have radiographic sacro-iliitis without symptoms. Bandilla (62) included routine radiographs, bone scans and a search for B27 in a study of 250 patients with backache, and he reports that, although most with sacro-iliitis had B27, there were other patients who had positive bone scans and B27 with normal radiographs. Hedberg & Linberg (63) in a similar study found positive bone scans in 50 % of their spondylitis suspects who had normal sacro-iliac radiographs and, as all of these patients had B27, they suggested that determination of B27 might be used as a screening test to select patients for bone scans.

Knowledge of B27 is probably most valuable when used selectively for particular clinical problems. For instance, the presence of B27 may be helpful in a child with an inflammatory arthritis of a single joint, in a man with arthritis following urethritis (when rheumatoid arthritis or gonococcal arthritis may be suspected), or in a young woman with chronic inflammatory bowel disease who has recently developed backache.

Prognosis

In the future, prognosis may be the strong suit of tissue typing. Unlike rheumatoid factor, which may be absent in the early stages of disease when it is most needed for diagnosis, the HLA antigens may be determined at birth. Little has been worked out in detail so far, except that a child with B27 and chronic polyarthritis is likely to develop spondylitis or sacro-iliitis in later life, and an adult with B27 who has psoriasis, ulcerative colitis or Crohn's disease will probably suffer rheumatic symptoms. This subject is still in its infancy. Much more will be apparent after existing data have been analysed more fully, and particularly when new criteria and markers have been added to the analysis.

Prevention and treatment

With the solitary exception of sexually transmitted Reiter's disease, there is no known method of preventing any of the diseases associated with B27. At this stage, mass screening to identify individuals at risk would cause widespread anxiety with little benefit in terms of disease prevention, and it is unlikely that investigators would wish to tamper with heredity.

In therapy, knowledge of B27 poses more questions than it answers. Are drugs which are particularly helpful in the treatment of spondylitis (such as phenylbutazone and indomethacin) to be used for other rheumatic disorders which are associated with B27 but do not fulfil the present criteria for ankylosing spondylitis? Does the link with acute anterior uveitis add to its value as a model for the study of drugs to be used in the treatment of rheumatic diseases? Do individuals with B27 respond differently to certain drugs, and might the determination of HLA antigens and other constitutional factors join the preliminary assessments before drug trials?

The greatest hope is that knowledge of genetic factors may uncover infective agents or disease processes that can be treated or prevented.

Laboratory resources

So far, tissue typing has been used more for research than for diagnosis. This economical use of resources will not last. Soon clinicians will wish to investigate all rheumatic complaints, including the ubiquitous chronic backache and widespread aches and pains. Unless there is a system of priorities, the demands for tissue typing will become at least as frequent as for the rheumatoid arthritis (RA) latex. That may not be all. The association between rheumatoid disease and DW4 may be the forerunner of genetic markers in many other rheumatic diseases. It is a formidable thought that the advent of an effective method of prevention might necessitate mass screening at birth to identify those individuals most at risk.

Mechanism

Before considering how HLA antigens influence susceptibility to disease and the part that infection might play, it would be wise to emphasise two crucial host factors: age and sex. The prevalence of most inflammatory rheumatic diseases changes on passing from childhood to adolescence, to early adult life, and beyond, and many rheumatic diseases have different clinical features at different ages. It happens that the diseases associated with B27 (ankylosing spondylitis, Reiter's disease, peripheral arthritis and acute anterior uveitis) all have a peak of clinical activity in the age group 20–40. Classically, ankylos-

102

ing spondylitis is a disease of young men, systemic lupus erythematosus of young women, and rheumatoid arthritis of middle-aged women. Reiter's disease is 20 times as common in men as in women. By contrast, after *yersinia* infection, reactive arthritis occurs equally in both sexes, whereas the erythema nodosum and associated arthritis after *yersinia* infection is almost exclusively found in women. Acute anterior uveitis is twice as common in men as in women. Previous explanations for these differences of prevalence have included the influence to hormones, or the effects of pelvic anatomy on responses to genito-urinary infection. These may be correct, but could recent knowledge of the H-Y antigen (64) provide an alternative explanation, with fundamental constitutional factors influencing susceptibility to particular diseases?

The concept of reactive arthritis is intriguing. There is no doubt that individuals with B27 who have sexually transmitted urethritis, or infection of the gut with *shigella flexneri, salmonella* or *yersinia enterocolitica,* are about 40 times as likely to develop acute arthritis as the rest of the population, and at the same time some of them may have involvement of the skin, conjunctivae or mucous membranes. However, it should not be assumed that a similar mechanism applies to other diseases associated with B27. Even the later features of Reiter's disease, such as sacro-iliitis, spondylitis, uveitis and aortitis, could result from different disease mechanisms, possibly more closely related to ankylosing spondylitis. Nevertheless, the presence of B27 in reactive arthritis and in ankylosing spondylitis must strengthen the long-standing belief that ankylosing spondylitis may also follow infection, even though there is no positive evidence that it does. While, as a corrective to excess enthusiasm for the theory of infection, the preliminary evidence (65, 66) should be remembered that asbestos workers with B27 may be more susceptible to lung disease and more likely to suffer severe disease.

Although it is difficult for clinicians to choose between the theories as to how HLA antigens may lead to disease, when considering human rheumatic disease there are clinical facts suggesting that the HLA antigens may not be directly involved in disease processes. Most people with B27 remain symptom-free throughout their lives, and all the diseases associated with B27 can occur with identical clinical features in the absence of the antigen. Moreover, in families, the heredity of ankylosing spondylitis is not always linked to the heredity of B27; and B27 is not associated with susceptibility to a single disease but to a complex array of diseases which appear to be influenced by a number of separate genetic and environmental factors.

The incomplete penetrance of ankylosing spondylitis makes it difficult to study a joint segregation of spondylitis and HLA antigens in families. At present the question whether the antigen B27 itself or the product of a closely linked gene is involved in the pathogenesis of spondylitis cannot be answered with certainty. The critical family study, which would have to show a joint segregation of spondylitis with an HLA antigen other than B27 in three generations, has not been reported so far. The observation by Woodrow (67) of an HLA-identical B27-negative pair of siblings, one with ankylosing spondylitis and the other with Reiter's disease, may favour the hypothesis of a linked gene being responsible for disease susceptibility. Equally inconclusive are the available epidemiologic data. The fact that spondylitis is associated with B27 in widely differing ethnic groups suggests, at least at face value, the direct involvement of the B27 antigen. On the other hand, the association of B27 with spondylitis is clearly weaker in the Pima Indians of Arizona, in whom spondylitis is frequent. This finding fits better with the hypothesis of a closely linked gene with varying degrees of linkage disequilibrium in different ethnic groups. If the antigen itself were involved, one would expect *a priori,* and without further complicating assumptions, that the association of spondylitis with B27 would be equally strong in all populations tested, which is clearly not the case. The finding of a high association of B27 with spondylitis, even in such distant ethnic groups as the Japanese, is of course compatible with the linked-gene hypothesis, if one assumes that spondylitis has arisen a long time ago as a single mutation af a gene very closely linked with HLA-B in a person who happened to be B27 positive. This B27-coupled spondylitis-susceptibility gene would then have spread throughout the world, and, due to the very close linkage of the spondylitis gene with the B locus, recombination between these loci would be very rare, so that B27 remains highly associated with the spondylitis gene, which is particularly impressive in populations where B27 is very rare (e.g. the Japanese). In spite of these speculations, it should be stressed that the argument over the direct involvement of B27 *versus* the action of a closely linked gene remains unresolved, perhaps with a slight advantage for the latter hypothesis.

Since the genetic region between the HLA-B and -D loci is expected to contain immune-response genes, it is appealing to speculate, as is done for a number af HLA-associated diseases, that the disease-susceptibility gene could be a defective immune-response gene which upon confrontation with an environmental factor (e.g. infection with *yersinia)* causes the disease through a pathological immune response. Nikbin *et al.* (68) have studied the one-way mixed-lymphocyte response (MLR) in patients with ankylosing spondylitis, their relatives and controls, and suggest that there may be an hereditary defect in people with B27 (whether or not they have spondylitis). There was also evidence that this defect may be hereditary in individuals who do not have B27.

The heredity of ankylosing spondylitis in families (Ceppellini, this book) and the fact that there is an excess of B27 heterozygotes in the unrelated patients population (Albert 1975 (69)) indicates a dominant heredity of the disease-susceptibility gene. This would suggest that the susceptibility gene is producing an excessive or wrongly directed (auto-) immune reaction rather than a lack of reactivity. Nikbin's data could be reconciled with this finding by the simple assumption that suppressor cells cause the decreased reactivity in the MLR.

The discussion of mechanisms must also include the possibility of cross-reactivity of B27 (or a highly associated antigen) with certain bacteria, which could lead to the inability of the individual to mount an appropriate immune response against these bacteria. This theory of "molecular mimicry" is also compatible with the observed dominant type of heredity. Preliminary evidence suggesting cross-reactivity between Klebsiella Aerogenes and B27 has been reported by Ebringer *et al.* (70).

In conclusion, it must be admitted that the question of the mechanism of HLA-disease associations remains unresolved. In view of the importance of the HLA region for the regulation of the immune response, it seems unlikely that the HLA-disease association is a chance product. It can reasonably be expected that the eventual elucidation of the mechanism of this association will provide new knowledge of pathogenesis. Hopefully, this may lead to fresh approaches to prevention and treatment.

Acknowledgements

We are grateful to Drs. F. Delbarre, B. Amor, and A. O. Carbonara for assisting us during the Rheumatology Workshop of the HLA and Disease Symposium.

References

1. Bremner, J. M., Emery, A. E. H., Kellgreen, J. H., Lawrence, J. S. & Roth, H. (1968) A family study in ankylosing spondylitis. In: *Population Studies of the Rheumatic Diseases,* eds. Bennett, P. H. & Wood, P. H. N., p. 299. Excerpta Medica Foundation, Amsterdam.
2. Wright, V. & Reed, W. B. (1964) The link between Reiter's syndrome and psoriatic arthritis. *Ann. rheum. Dis.* **23**, 12.
3. Macrae, I. & Wright, V. (1973) A family study of ulcerative colitis, with particular reference to ankylosing spondylitis and sacro-iliitis. *Ann. rheum. Dis.* **32**, 16.
4. Moll, J. M. H. & Wright, V. (1973) Familial occurrence of psoriatic arthritis. *Ann. rheum. Dis.* **32**, 181.
5. Haslock, I. (1973) Arthritis and Crohn's disease. A family study. *Ann. rheum. Dis.* **32**, 479.
6. Lawrence, J. S. (1974) Family study of Reiter's disease. *Brit. J. vener. Dis.* **50**, 140.
7. Schlosstein. L., Torasaki, P. I., Bluestone, R. & Pearson, C. M. (1973) High association of an HL-A antigen, W27, with ankylosing spondylitis. *New Eng. J. Med.* **288**, 704.
8. Brewerton, D. A., Caffrey, M., Hart, F. D., James, D. C. O., Nicholls, A. & Sturrock, R. D. (1973) Ankylosing spondylitis and HL-A 27, *Lancet* **i**, 904.
9. Terasaki, P. I. & Mickey, M. R. (1975) HL-A haplotypes of 32 diseases. *Transplant. Rev.* **22**, 105.
10. Kastelan, A., Kerhin-Brkljacic, V., Jalic, kylosing spondylitis and the major histo-

I., Brkljacic, L. & Balog, V. (1976) The frequency of HL-A haplotypes and their segregation in families of patients with ankylosing spondylitis. (Abstract).
11. Dausset, J. & Hors, J. (1975) Some contributions of the HL-A complex to the genetics of human disease. *Transplant. Rev.* **22**, 44.
12. Sachs, J. A., Sterioff, S., Robinette, M., Wolf, E. & Currey, H. L. F. (1974) An compatibility system. *Tissue Antigens.* **5**, 293.
13. Gofton, J. P., Chalmers, A., Price, G. E. & Reeve, C. E. (1975) HL-A 27 and ankylosing spondylitis in B.C. Indians. *J. Rheumatol.* **2**,314.
14. Sewzey, R. L., Zucker, L. M. & Terasaki, P. I. (1974) Reduced prevalence of HL-A antigen W27 in black females with ankylosing spondylitis. *J. Rheumatol.* **1**, 260.
15. Calin, A.. Bennett, P. H., Jupiter, J. & Terakasi, P. I. (1976) HLA B27 and sacroiliitis in Pima Indians. (Abstract).
16. Brautbar, C., Porath, S., Nelken, D. & Cohen, T. (1976) HLA B27 and ankylosing spondylitis in the Israeli population. (Abstract).
17. Shirakura, R., Mori, T., Shichikawa, K., Tsujimoto, M. & Manabe, H. (1976) Genetic significance of HL-A B27 in ankylosing spondylitis. A study of 27 families. (Abstract).
18. Brewerton, D. A., Caffrey, M., Nicholls, A., Walters, D. & James, D. C. O. (1973) Acute anterior uveitis and HL-A 27. *Lancet* **ii**, 994.
19. Brewerton, D. A. (1975) HL-A 27 and acute anterior uveitis. *Ann. rheum. Dis.* **34** (suppl. 1), 33.
20. Cleland, L. G., Hay, J. A. R. & Milazzo, S. C. (1975) The relation of HL-A 27 to disease pattern in sero-negative rheumatoid arthritis. *Scand. J. Rheumatol.* Suppl. 8, Abs. 30, 20.
21. Heinrichs, K., Zeidler, H., Eckert, G. & Wittenborg, A. (1975) HL-A 27 in patients with oligoarthritis and lower back pain. *Scand. J. Rheumatol.* Suppl. 8, Abs. 30, 21.
22. Amor, B., Kahan, A & Delbarre, F. (1976). HLA-B27 in unclassified inflammatory rheumatic disease (URID). (Abstract).
23. de Ceular, Van der Linden, J. M. J. P. & Cats, A. (1976) Sausage-like toes and HLA-B27. (Abstract).
24. Budgen, D. Y., Hazelman, B. L. & Voak, D. (1976) HLA-B27 and frozen shoulder. *Lancet i*, 1042.

25. Calin, A., Fries, J. F.. Stinson, F. B. & Payne, R. (1976) Normal frequency of HLA B27 in aortic insufficiency. (Abstract).
26. Edmonds, J., Morris, R. I., Metzger, A. L., Bluestone, R., Terasaki, P. I., Ansell, B. M. & Bywaters, E. G. L. (1974) Follow-up study of juvenile chronic polyarthritis with particular reference to histocompatibility antigen W27. *Ann. rheum. Dis.* **33**, 289.
27. Van den Berg-Loonen, E. M., Dekker-Saeys, B. J., Meuwissen, S. G. M., Nijenhuis, L. E. & Engelfriet, C. P. (1976) Histocompatibility antigens and other genetic markers in ankylosing spondylitis and inflammatory bowel disease. (Abstract).
28. Brewerton, D. A., Caffrey, M., Nicholls, A., Walters, D. & James, D. C. O. (1974) HL-A 27 and the arthropathies associated with ulcerative colitis and psoriasis. *Lancet* **ii**, 956.
29. Brewerton, D. A. (1976) Joseph J. Bunim Lecture: HLA B27 and the inheritance of susceptibility to rheumatic disease. *Arthr. and Rheum.* **19**, 656.
30. Eastmond, C. J. & Woodrow, J. C. (1976) HLA antigens and arthritis associated with psoriasis. (Abstract).
31. Roux, H., Mercier, P., Maestracci, D., Serratrice, G., Sany, J., Seignalet, J. & Serre, H. (1976) Psoriasis arthritis and HLA antigens. (Abstract).
32. Feldmann, J. L., Amor, B., Cazalis, P., Dryll, A., Hors, J. & Hacquart, B. (1976) Dismemberment of psoriasis arthropathy by HLA antigens. (Abstract).
33. Brewerton, D. A., Caffrey, M., Nicholls, A., Walters, D., Oates, J. K. & James, D. C. O. (1973) Reiter's disease and HL-A 27. *Lancet* **ii**, 996.
34. Nicholls, A. (1975) Reiter's disease and HL-A 27. *Ann rheum. Dis.* **34**, suppl. 1, 27.
35. Sairanen, E. & Paronén, I. (1969) Reiter's syndrome: a follow-up study. *Acta med. Scand.* **185**, 57.
36. Sairanen, E. & Tiilikainen, A. (1975) HL-A 27 in Reiter's disease following shigellosis. *Scand. J. Rheumatol.* suppl. 8. Abs. 30. 11.
37. Calin, A. & Fries, J. F. (1976) An "experimental" epidemic of Reiter's syndrome revisited. *Ann. Int. Med.* **84**, 564.
38. Aho, K., Ahvonen, P., Lassus, A., Sievers, K. & Tiilikainen, A. (1974) HL-A 27 in reactive arthritis: a study of *yersinia* arthritis and Reiter's disease. *Arthr. and Rheum.* **17**, 521.
39. Leirisalo, M., Tiilikainen, A. & Laitinen, O. (1976) HLA phenotypes in rheumatic fever and *yersinia* arthritis. (Abstract).
40. Falk, J. A., Fleischman, J. L., Zabriskie, J. B. & Falk, R. E. (1973) A study of HL-A antigen phenotype in rheumatic fever and rheumatic heart disease patients. *Tissue Antigens* **3**, 173.
41. Caughey, D. E., Douglas, R., Wilson, W. & Hassall, I. B. (1975) HL-A antigens in Europeans and Maoris with rheumatic fever and rheumatic heart disease. *J. Rheumatol.* **2**, 319.
42. Joysey, V. C., Bullman, W. & Roger, J. H. (1976) HLA antigens in patients with rheumatic heart disease. (Abstract).
43. Greenberg, L. J., Gray, E. D. & Yunis E. J. (1975) Association of HL-A 5 and immune responsiveness in vitro to streptococcal antigens. *J. exp. Med.* **141**. 935.
44. Shapiro, R. F., Utsinger, P. D., Wiesner, K. B., Resnick, D., Bryan, B. L. & Castles, J. J. (1976) The association of HLA B27 with Forestier's disease (vertebral ankylosing hyperostosis). *J. Rheumatol.* **3**, 4.
45. Ercilla, G., Brancos, M. A., Breysse, Y., Vives, J., Rotes, J., Castillo, R. & Alonso, G. (1976) Histocompatibility antigens in Forestier's disease, polyarthrosis and ankylosing spondylitis. (Abstract).
46. Graber Duvernay, B., Gras, J. P., Dutertre, P. & Bensa, J. C. (1976) Histocompatibility antigens in Forestier's disease. (Abstract).
47. Rosenthal, M., Bahous, B. & Müller, W. (1976) Increased frequency of HLA-B8 in hyperostotic spondylosis. (Abstract).
48. Singal, D. P., de Bosset, P. & Gordon, D. A. (1976) Comparison of osteitis condensans ilii and ankylosing spondylitis in female patients: clinical, radiological and HLA typing characteristics. (Abstract).
49. Ohno, S., Aoki, K., Sugiura, S., Nakayama, E., Itakura, K. & Aizawa, M. (1973) HL-A5 and Behçet's disease. *Lancet* **ii**, 1383.
50. Nakagawa. J., Ikehara, Y., Ito, K. & Fukase. M. (1976) HLA antigens in various autoimmune and related diseases. (Abstract).
51. Hoshino. K., Inouye, H., Unokuchi, T., Ito, M., Tamaoki, N. & Tsuji, K. (1976) HLA and diseases in Japanese. (Abstract).
52. Chamberlain, M. A. (1975) Behçet's disease. *Ann. rheum. Dis.* **34**, suppl. 1, 53.
53. O'Duffy, J. D., Taswell, H. F. & Elve-

back, L. R. (1976) HL-A antigens in Behçet's disease. *J. Rheumatol.* **3**, 1.

54. Stastny, P. (1974) Mixed lymphocyte culture typing cells from patients with rheumatoid arthritis. *Tissue Antigens* **4**, 571.

55. Stastny, P. (1976) Personal communication.

56. Fallet, G. H., Mason, R. M., Berry, H., Mowat, A. G., Boussina, I. & Gerster, J. C. (1976) Rheumatoid arthritis and ankylosing spondylitis occurring together. (Abstract).

57. Good, A. E., Schultz, J. S. & Kapur, J. J. (1976) Rheumatoid arthritis associated with ankylosing spondylitis. (Abstract).

58. Clough, J. D., Aponte, C. J. & Braun, W. E. (1976) HLA-B8 and clinical features of Sjögren's syndrome. (Abstract).

59. Sany, J., Seignalet, J., Serre, H. & Lapinski, H. (1976) HLA in polymyalgia rheumatica. (Abstract).

60. Pasternack, A. & Tiilikainen, A. (1976) HL-A antigens in rheumatoid arthritis and amyloidosis, (in press).

61. Calin A., Fries, J., Schurman, D. & Payne, R. (1976) The close correlation between symptoms and disease expression in HLA B27 positive subjects. (Abstract).

62. Bandilla, K. (1976) HLA B27 typing in combination with bone scintiscanning for differential diagnosis of back pain. (Abstract).

63. Hedberg, H. & Linberg, S. (1976) HLA, ankylosing spondylitis and scintigraphy of the sacroiliac joints. (Abstract).

64. Gasser, L. L. & Silvers, W. K. (1971) Genetic control of the immune response in man. III An association between H-2 type and reaction to H-Y. *J. Immunol.* **106**, 875.

65. Merchant, J. A., Klouda, P. T., Soutar, C. A., Parkes, W. R., Lawler, S. D. & Turner-Warwick, M. (1975) The HL-A system in asbestos workers. *Brit. Med. J.* **1**, 189.

66. Matej, H. & Lange, A. (1976) HLA antigens in asbestosis. (Abstract).

67. Woodrow, J. C. (1975) Family studies. *Ann. rheum. Dis.* **34**, suppl. 1, 42.

68. Nikbin, B., Brewerton. D. A., James, D. C. O. & Hobbs, J. R. (1976) Diminished mixed lymphocyte reaction in ankylosing spondylitis, relatives, and normal individuals all with HL-A 27. *Ann. rheum. Dis.* **35**, 37.

69. Albert, E. D. (1975) The significance of HLA-disease associations. *Z. Immun. Forsch.* **148**, 382.

70. Ebringer, A., Cowling, P., Ngwa Suh, N., James, D. C. O. & Ebringer, R. W. (1976) Crossreactivity between Klebsiella Aerogenes species and B27 lymphocyte antigens as an aetiological factor in ankylosing spondylitis. (Abstract).

Neurology

T. Fog[1], E. Schuller[2], C. Jersild[3], C. P. Engelfriet[4] & J. Bertrams[5]

Multiple Sclerosis = m. s.

Introduction

M.s. is a chronic disease developing over the years severe and disabling signs and symptoms from the central nervous system (CNS). The course is generally characterized by initial acute episodes, followed some years later by a more even progress, overlapped by acute episodes (11).

The cause is unknown. The pathogenesis is only partially understood, but the pathology is characterized by so called "plaques" which are localized around the venous system, especially around the great subependymal venous complex in the brain, along the cortico-subcortical veins, and in the central white matter along other central veins. Macroscopically the plaque looks like islets when cutting the brain. In the spinal cord these plaques follow the veins, particularly in the posterior and lateral funiculi, and along the anterior vein in the median fissure. In the plaques a demyelination can be demonstrated, the axial cylinders being relatively preserved, the glia (astroglia) proliferates, but little by little the tissue within a plaque will disentegrate totally, and a cystic cavity may ensue result.

Since the end of last century infectious agents have been considered as a possible cause of m.s., both spirochetes and virus. At the beginning of this century measles was in the limelight, based upon neuropathological findings in children dying from measles encephalitis. At the end of the twenties a high incidence of both postvaccinial, post-measles encephalomyelitis, but also cases with unknown etiology occured, and the analogy to m.s. was drawn because of the perivenous inflammatory changes. At this time Pette (51) advocated a virus hypothesis in m.s., and he emphasized the allergic hypothesis, strongly supported by the succes in provoking disseminated encephalomyelitis in animals by injection of homologous brain (57), (24), (23). This was the basis for the autoimmune hypothesis, later so extensively explored after the discovery of the accelerating effect of Freund's adjuvans (5). Over the years discussions have taken place concerning the relationship between the experimental allergic encephalomyelitis (EAE) and the human disease m.s., a discussion which is still going on, not least after the isolation of the active antigen from myelin and the unravelling of the amino-acid-sequence of this antigen (21), (58).

Even in humans an EAE has been provoked, of course accidental: Rabbit

[1] Kommunehospitalet, Department of neurology, DK-1399 Copenhagen,
[2] Laboratorie d'Immunologie du Systeme Nerveux, Hôpital de la Salpetriere, 75013 Paris.
[3] Blood type serological department, Hvidovre hospital, DK-2650 Hvidovre, Denmark.
[4] Centraal Laboratorium Van de Bloedtransfusiedienst, Amsterdam.
[5] Tissue Typing and Central Laboratory, Elisabeth-Krankenhaus, D-43 Essen, Germany.

spinal cord antigen was present in vaccine against rabies, and some Japanese dying from an EAE like disease showed at autospy also EAE like foci and plaques in the brain (64). The well known case described by Jellinger & Seitelberger (31) received several injections of calf brain during an 18 months period of treatment for Parkinson's disease. He developed a rapidly progressing disseminated encephalomyelitis verified by autopsy.

The postmeasles virus infection hypothesis was renewed by the findings of an increase in the measles antibody titer in serum of m.s. cases (1), a finding which was later confirmed in about 25 different laboratories throughout the world. Although the titers vary from patient to patient, and the average titer is not impressively increased, it remains significantly elevated compared with titers in age and sex matched normal controls.

Among healthy family members of m.s. patients, increased antibody titers to measles virus have also been demonstrated, average levels being between those of m.s. patients and normal controls. Of more significance is the finding of elevated antibody titers in cerebro spinal fluid (CSF), which can be found in some m.s. cases. Ratios between antibody titers in CSF and serum were obtained for several viruses by Norrby *et al.* (47) and significantly increased ratios for measles virus were also found in some m.s. cases, indicating antibody production within the CNS, which should then contain the virus antigen, or another cross-reacting antigen.

No direct proof of measles virus in the brain of m.s. patients has been given so far, and in some cases an elevated titer towards other virus can be demonstrated, but generally it seems to be measles. Only very few cases of other CNS diseases have an elevated antibody titer to measles in CSF, and in quantitative studies only measles antibodies were found in high concentrations in m.s. cases compared with other CNS diseases, except Subacute Sclerosing Panencephalitis (SSPE) (16).

Recently Carp *et al.* (12) found a new virus-like substance in homogenates of brain, spleen, and in serum of m.s. patients. The size of the substance range between 25 and 50 nm, and evidence has been presented, of its ability to multiply during repeated passages in cell cultures of mouse fibroblasts, as well as in vivo, when inoculated intracerebraly in different small animals. Antibody to this substance has been detected in the CSF of m.s. cases, as well as in serum of family members and nursing personnel of m.s. patients. The substance has not been demonstrated so far in tissues of patients with other CNS diseases. Antibody towards this substance have been found generally in the population of Uganda, where m.s. does not exist.

The geographic distribution of m.s. follows a pattern which divides the world in high-, intermediate- and low risk zones. The high risk zone in Europe is between 47° and 60°, and in North America north of 40°. The prevalence rate for the high risk zone is from about 60–150 per 100,000, depending on the method used for registrating. The intermediate risk zone shows a rate less than 20 per 100,000. In Africa and India very few cases have been found, except in South Africa and Argentina. The Australian continent belongs to the intermediate zone, with an increase towards the south (Tasmania, South Island of New Zealand). We do not know the prevalence rate in USSR, but it seems to follow the European rate in the western part of the country, declining towards the eastern part. In Japan only a relatively small number has been found, 4 per 100,000 towards the north, and 2 per 100,000 in the south. This is a general map. Some clustering has been demonstrated in different parts of the high-risk zones, especially convincing in Finland (73). The highest prevalence rate has been registered on the Orkney Islands, where m.s. has been named "the Orkney disease" (about 300 per 100,000). M.s. mainly occur among Caucasians, however, in USA the black population also suffers from m.s., although prevalence rates are lower. M.s. does not exist among several million negroes of the Bantu stock in Africa.

The prevalence rates of m.s. must be considered with reservation. The diagnosis of m.s. is clinical, based upon the registration of the course and localization of signs and symptoms. No diagnostic test exists. Abortive and very benign cases of m.s. have been found and verified by autopsy, and the possibility of a much wider distribution of the disease throughout the world must seriously be taken into account. Prevalence rates have most frequently been based on a registration of disabled patients. Various, more sophisticated clinical findings may contribute and increase the probability of a correct diagnosis, but such criterias have so far only been partially used in the geomedical studies. Serious difficulties are to be faced, especially in genetic studies of m.s. Familial m.s. has been found in most studies in about 5 to 8 %. The hereditary risk in a family with m.s. patients is, according to some studies, increased to 30 to 40 fold among sibs, compared with families without m.s., even in the high risk zones. The risk decreases with a more distant relationship to the m.s. patient in these families. M.s. in two generations exists, but m.s. in more than two generations has to the author's knowledge never been proved by autopsy.

M.s. may be very difficult to differentiate from cases of hereditary ataxias, both hereditary spinal ataxia (Edie's definition (20)), different types of spinocerebellar degenerations, and even Mb. Friedreich. No doubt a tendency exists to diagnose a chronic CNS disease even if there are fluctuating symptoms and a progressive course as a hereditary CNS disease, if there is more than one case in the same generation say in more than one generation. Several studies in hereditary ataxia have been published, based upon a few cases in the same generation, demonstrating a recessive type of heredity. Some of these cases may have been m.s.

Very few cases of both m.s. and hereditary CNS disease are verified by autopsy. This is a very general and deplorable fact, even in countries with an advanced medical profession.

There is a tendency to publish family studies in chronic CNS diseases, and this is greatly needed for scientific reasons, but these families should be studied extensively in order to obtain a sufficiently detailed picture to allow differentiation. The analysis of CSF, the search for periphlebitis retinae and an EMI-scan (28) may especially increase the possibilities for a true diagnosis of m.s.

Hauge (29) has provided a critical analysis of the genetic aspects of m.s. He concluded "that classical genetic analysis has not really been of much help in furthering the understanding of the aetiological background of m.s.", but "other areas of research may now be able to produce the proof of the importance of genetic elements and open new perspectives of profound interest to geneticists also. The new observations also seem to suggest the possibility of delineating aetiologically separate subgroups as has been done in psoriasis and diabetes. If HLA types could be used as a tool in subdividing m.s. this might solve some of the riddles which have appeared only too often in the genetic studies of m.s."

Serologic and immunologic studies in m.s. demonstrate an elevation, absolute or relative, of gammaglobulins in the CSF in about 80 % of all m.s. cases. This has been demonstrated in many laboratories throughout the world. Using the agar-gel-electrophoresis, one or more sharp bands in the gamma 3–4–5 areas are found in 60 % of all cases (40), and if the electro-diffusion technique is used (18) such bands can be demonstrated in about 90 % of the cases. According to Link (41) these oligoclonal bands may be demonstrated in 90 % of the cases by agar-gel-electrophoresis alone. This oligoclonal response is not specific for m.s., as it may be found in infectious diseases of the CNS (41), as well as in a few cases of non-inflammatory CNS diseases. In some cases of optic neuritis these oligoclonal bands may be found (60, (42). Sandberg-Wollheim (61) made prospective studies in cases of optic neuritis to find out if cases which later developing m.s. were those showing bands earlier, but it is still too early to draw firm conclusions from these studies. The presence of sharp oligoclonal bands in the CSF gammaglobulin area is an important diagnostic clue towards m.s., and this test should be included in the range of diagnostic techniques; it should, however, be remembered that cases of m.s. without the presence of such oligoclonal bands are known, and also that these bands may occasionally be transitory (41), (77).*)

*) Recently SCHULLER et al. (78 and 79) have demonstrated 1) the elevation of DNA and RNA precipitating antibodies in the serum and 2) presence of these nucleic antibodies in 40 % of the MS–CSF, obviously correlated with oligoclonal aspect.

No major abnormalities have been found in the blood of m.s. patients, except for serum antibodies (vide supra), studies of thrombocytes, and lymphocytes. Discrepancies exist concerning the serum lipids, especially linoleic acid concentrations, which in some studies showed decreased levels. A higher tendency to agglutination of thrombocytes was shown by Fog in 1949 (24), later confirmed by other studies, and recently reviewed by Baker et al. (5). Srivastava et al. (65) found i disturbance in the metabolism of prostaglandins in the thrombocytes of m.s. patients supporting the findings of anomalies in the thrombocytes reactivity.

Using lymphocyte transformation in the study of random m.s. patients. Platz et al. (54) were unable to demonstrate any major abnormalities in the general immune capacity of these patients. The study included lymphocyte transformation with various mitogens (PHA, PWM), different bacterial antigens (PPD, E. Coli, SKSD, Staph. Aur.), as well as fungal antigens (Candida Albicans). Percentage of T- and B-lymphocytes were also determined, using rosette- and fluorescense techniques. Although several of the patients repeatedly were tested, other studies seem to indicate that some patients may show marked changes in the number of T-lymphocytes, since very low levels were occasionally observed in a single patient (Jersild et al. (35)). More impressive are the abnormally low responses in the Migration Inhibition Test when m.s. leucocytes are challanged with measles and parainfluenza virus antigens. This was first demonstrated by Ciongoli et al. (14) in Copenhagen, and simultaneously by Utermohlen et al. (71) in New York. This abnormality has been confirmed by Ciongoli et al. (14) and followed up in further studies, using purified virus antigens, by Sever

111

et al. (63) and others (55). The lymphocytes behave as if the patient has never had measles, even if he did have it years earlier. A normal reactivity of the lymphocytes towards PPD and some other antigens was shown. Utermohlen et al. (71) reported that in vitro addition of Transfer Factor restored the reactivity towards measles, but that injection of T.F. to the patients can normalize this reactivity (26). In our experience (Platz et al. (54)) there is an initial and significant change in reactivity towards measles virus following T.F. injections; after continuous therapy for more than 24 months, these changes are not very significant, although there seems to be a trend indicating a slightly better responsiveness towards measles during treatment (Platz et al. (54)).

Studies of HLA in multiple sclerosis

During 1972 several reports appeared which described an increased frequency of certain HLA antigens in random Caucasian m.s. patients (46), (8), (37). These studies were confirmed during the next years by similar studies in other laboratories (4), (3), (67), and also by more intensive investigations by Bertrams et al. In 1973 HLA-D typing was introduced in several laboratories (19), (69). Grosse-Wilde et al. (38), and it was also applied to the study of m.s. by Jersild et al. (34), (35). These studies indicated for the first time, that susceptibility to a disease could be more strongly associated to the HLA-D antigens, than to antigens of any of the other segregant series, in m.s. to the HLA-DW2 antigen, which were originally called LD-7A. These studies also indicated a correlation between the HLA-DW2 type and the course of m.s. On the following pages the authors will briefly summarize the present status of HLA studies in m.s., as it appeared to them from the meeting and the workshop.

(1) HLA-A, B and C series antigens in m.s.

a. *Caucasian* patients have now been intensively studied and no information further during the meeting to what was already known appeared in terms of ABC antigens. In summary the following deviations have been observed: A increased frequency of HLA-A3 and B7, an insignificant, but consistently found minor increase in A1 and B8, as well as B18. Decreased frequencies of HLA-A2, B12 and B15. Decreased frequency of CW3 has been observed in two studies, but only 100 patients in Bertrams study have been typed for the C series antigens, and these results vary slightly from those reported earlier (33). In the normal population a high frequency of A3 and B7 has been found in North European Caucasians (Scandinavians and Scottish) as weel as in North Americans, whereas lower frequencies are found in other Caucasians, as well as other ethnic groups, especially the Japanese (Table I). The differences in A3 and B7 frequencies in normal populations seem to fit the geographic occurrence of m.s. (see above), however, more firm conclusions can not, of course, be reached, since many other genetic as well as environmental factors differ in these populations, differences which will certainly influence the occurrence of m.s. Of considerable interest in this context is the distribution of the DW2 determinant in various Caucasian populations, as well as other ethnic groups, data which at present are lack-

TABLE I

Frequencies in per cent of some HLA antigens in various normal population groups[1])

Population:	N. Europe	France	Italy	Britain	Amer. Cauc.	Afr. Blacks	Japanese
Number tested:	704	806	762	1003	503	411	416
HLA-A1	29	23	19	32	32	9	3
A2	50	47	45	44	49	22	45
A3	24	25	16	26	22	10	3
A9	22	22	27	18	17	23	58
A10	10	11	10	10	13	15	17
A11	11	13	11	13	8	0	24
A28	10	9	9	10	11	23	6
W19	23	30	38	28	28	62	14
HLA-B5	9	17	20	10	11	4	34
B7	21	17	9	23	23	18	11
B8	21	16	10	25	20	7	1
B12	22	26	16	29	24	16	15
B13	5	6	5	5	6	4	5
B14	6	7	10	7	11	9	2
B18	7	12	19	10	9	10	2
B27	11	8	6	9	8	1	4
BW15	17	11	8	12	7	6	14
BW16	6	9	10	8	12	4	7
BW17	7	8	11	8	7	33	4
BW21	4	8	12	5	4	2	3
BW22	5	6	5	5	5	1	16
BW35	16	20	25	17	17	14	19
BW40	16	11	5	12	12	2	31
HLA-CW1	8	6	7	6	6	0	33
CW2	9	8	13	10	10	24	4
CW3	32	16	13	24	17	15	41
CW4	19	20	26	18	20	22	6
CW5	11	11	11	18	12	6	3
HLA-DW1[2])	19						
DW2	15						
DW3	16						
DW4	16						
DW5	15						
DW6	11						
LD-107	10						
LD-108	8						

[1]) From Histocompatibility Testing 1975, Joint Report, p. 31.

[2]) From Histocompatibility Testing 1975, Joint Report, p. 451. HLA-D typing performed only on 171 random Caucasians. HLA-D data on other ethnic groups are not included in this table since materials are too small, or simply lacking.

ing, or at least insufficient to be conclusive.

b. *Other ethnic groups* suffering from m.s. have been studies. Dupont *et al.* (20) reported on American Black m.s. patients, in whom they could demonstrate the DW2 antigen in 34 % of the m.s. cases, whereas none of the age and sex matched controls carried this antigen. Also interesting was the observation that A3 and B7 do not seem to be increased among the patients. Thus m.s. seems to occur frequently among those rare Black American individuals, who carry the DW2 antigen, which is characteristic for Caucasian m.s. patients. It was also of interest, that A3 and B7 antigens showed no deviations from these frequencies found in healthy controls. The HLA-A'W30' antigens, which are characteristic for the Black Americans, were however found with a consider-

TABLE II

HLA-DW2 in random Caucasian patients with Multiple Sclerosis

Investigator		m.s. patients			Controls			Relative Risk	p value (Fish. exc.)[1]
		N	Pos	%	N	Pos.	%		
Jersild et al. Platz et al.	(33)	88	51	58	157	37	24	4.5	8.8×10^{-8}
Grosse-Wilde Bertrams et al.	(8)	111	60	54	405	84	21	4.5	2.8×10^{-11}
Thorsby et al.	(67)	37	25	68	215	65	30	4.8	2.0×10^{-5}
Möller et al.	(45)	105	49	47	100	30	30	2.0	1.0×10^{-2}
van den Berg-Loonen & Lucas	(72)	46	25	54	49	10	20	4.6	5.9×10^{-4}
Stewart et al.	(66)	40	25	63	28	5	18	7.7	2.5×10^{-4}
Opelz, Terasaki et al.	(50)	350	175	50	136	25	18	4.4	4.8×10^{-11}
Oger et al.	(48)	24	18	75	21	10	48	3.3	5.6×10^{-2}

Combined estimate: Relative risk: 4.0 X^2sign 151.8 X^2het. 7.5 (n.s.)
(1 d.f.)   (7 d.f.)

[1] One sided.

ably lower frequency (50 to 56 % versus 9 %), and thus again indicating that Black Americans m.s. patients are probably more "Caucasian" than the normal Black. It should be remembered that the American Black population does represent a genetically mixed population. Estimates of the genetic admixture of Caucasian genes, based on frequencies of the blood group antigen Duffy Fy (a+), range from 1.06 % in the south to 0.22 % in the northern states (56), and thus seem to fit the north-south gradient observed for both the Black and Caucasian populations in USA.

Studies of the Afro-asian m.s. patients in Israel were recently reported by Alter et al. (2), and decreased frequency of B7 was observed. A3 showed no deviation from normal, whereas B18 occurred in 20 % of the cases, compared with 8 % among normals. The DW2 antigen was not determined. A preliminary report by Saito et al. (60) showed no major deviations of the A and B series antigens among 41 Japanese m.s. patients, compared with nor-

mals. Also in this study DW2 was not reported.

Since the original report of an increased frequency of the DW2 antigen among m.s. patients (Jersild et al. (35)), several studies have now confirmed these findings af which Table II presents a summary.

(2) Ia typing in m.s.

Recent attempts to demonstrate by serological methods the antigens responsible for reactivity in the Mixed Leucocyte Culture (MLC) have opened a new area of extensive research. These antigens have been called I-region associated or Ia, in analogy with the findings in mice, where strong MLC antigens and Immune response genes (Ir) are coded for in the I-region of H-2 (the Major histocompatibility Complex of mice). Although it seems possible to detect these Ia antigens on B-lymphocytes also in humans as well, more extensive studies will have to be made to clarify their relationship with the HLA-

D antigens. Preliminary results obtained by several investigators indicate, however, that a particular DW2 related Ia antigen occur frequently among the m.s. patients. (Winchester *et al.* (75), Thorsby *et al.* (68), Terasaki *et al.* (67), Wernet *et al.* (73)), even when different antibodies and techniques were used. These studies seem to indicate that the DW2 associated Ia antigen occur even more frequently than the DW2 antigen among these patients. If Ia also is closely associated with Ir in humans, these findings may indicate a common characteristic immune response among these patients.

In conclusion, HLA studies at the population level in random m.s. patients indicate that a certain proportion of the Caucasian m.s. patients carries a specific HLA-DW2 determinant, which is 4 to 5 times more frequent in m.s. patients than in controls. In the genetically mixed American Black population this antigen is rare, but still m.s. is occurring in this population more frequently among those individuals who do carry the DW2 determinant. In the study of m.s. in other ethnic groups, DW2 determination has not yet been carried out.

It should be stressed that the HLA-DW2 antigen probably only serves as a genetic marker for a disease susceptibility gene, and if the presence of such a gene is a necessary prerequisite for development of disease, the association between this gene and DW2 is not absolute since approximately 40 % of cases are DW2 negative. However, in the light of experimental models of infectious diseases, genetic control of infection and its outcome with respect to disease is far more complex, and not always linked to MHS (52). If m.s. can be compared to such a model, one would expect a polygenic control of disease susceptibility, where HLA linked genes are only some of several genes working together, probably at different levels in the pathogenic process. Alternatively one would have to postulate different forms of m.s., some with a considerable genetic element which are HLA linked, and other forms which seem mainly to be non-genetic, and thus not HLA linked. These two extremes do not seem to exclude each other, and reality could be somewhere in between.

(3) Linkage studies

If the presence of a gene, linked to HLA, is a major genetic factor determining occurrence of m.s., families in which two or more cases occur will provide an opportunity to evaluate the strength of linkage between this gene, and those controlling HLA. Results obtained in this approach may be influenced by several factors which should be kept in mind:

1) Ascertainment of m.s.: Since diagnosis of m.s. is clinical – (no single laboratory test alone provides the diagnosis) – it is important to exhaustively examine all family members for possible signs and symptoms, as well as to use all relevant laboratory tests, which usually give indications of the presence of m.s.

2) Due to the wide range of the age of onset of m.s., many members of a family studied at one point in time may still be at an age with a considerable risk for developing m.s. Although this can be mathematically corrected in larger studies, such a correction seems of little help in the study of linkage in a single family.

3) HLA antigens are inherited after a simple Mendelian principle as co-dominant characters, and thus among random siblings, the four possible HLA genotypes have been observed equally frequently. Thus the chance for two

HLA identical siblings is 25 %. Compared with what is known about the genetics of m.s., it seems unlikely that classical linkage studies indicate a close linkage between HLA and the hypothetical m.s. susceptibility gene: The frequency of affected siblings of m.s. patients ranges from 0.8 to 5.9 %, and only a low concordance rate in monozygotic twins has been found. For the study of the genetics of a disease it is, however, useful to have a genetic marker which, at the population level showes some degree of association with the disease.

The studies of HLA markers in families with two or more cases of m.s. have not so far provided a clear-cut picture indicating linkage. Thus, if a genetic linkage exists between a single m.s. susceptibility gene and HLA, it would be a rather weak linkage, or alternatively several genes could comprise the susceptibility phenotype.

Alter *et al.* (2) reported on 10 families with two or more cases and could not establish a close linkage, using classical lod score analysis. However, they noted that all affected individuals in these families, as well as in an additional two families reported elsewhere (35), (9) shared one parental haplotype, which only occurred in 7 of 28 unaffected individuals in these families, and this difference was found to be significant, indicating linkage. Similarly, Bertrams *et al.* (6) analyzed HLA markers in a total of 38 families, including 76 parents, 56 m.s. patients and 69 healthy siblings. They used a different approach in analyzing these data: Only informative families were considered, i.e. backcross families where one parent is heterozygous for one HLA gene, the other negative. In such families, the particular antigen under analysis should occur equally frequent in patients and healthy siblings, thus giving a 1:1 segregation.

In these families 17 were informative for A3, and a surplus of A3 positive m.s. patients occurred. Among the normal siblings, a 1:1 ratio of A3 positive to A3 negative was found. Similarly, disturbed segregation could be detected for B7 in 21 families, and also for the A3, B7 haplotype, as observed in 11 families, in all cases the m.s. patients carried the corresponding antigens more frequently.

At this conference further results were presented which did not support HLA linkage to a m.s. susceptibility gene, using classical tests for linkage (75), (30), (65). Only one study included the DW2 determination (48), as well as extensive studies of CSF proteins on diseased members.

It is assumed that a large number of well studied families will be needed in order to detect a linkage by classical lod score techniques. However, by using modified techniques, as shown by Bertrams *et al.* (6), it is possible to show an abnormal segregation ratio of certain HLA antigens in the m.s. patients. However, some observation would be expected in segregation studies of families namely ascertained by HLA-A3, B7-positive children. Nevertheless the increased sharing of haplotypes in affected sibpairs strengthens the influence of HLA.

(4) Other studies

A certain proportion of m.s. patients show abnormally high antibody titers to measles virus (vide supra). Several investigators have shown that high titer antibodies in serum occur predominantly among those patients who carry the HLA antigens associated with this disease, A3, B7 or B18 (32), (50), (44). Other investigators have not, however, been able to confirm these findings (39), (65). Support for a genetic influence on antibody titers to virus has also been provided by Haverkorn *et al.* (29 A), who studies 143 twin pairs, those being HLA identical had more similar titers than the HLA non-identical.

Of particular interest were the studies of complement levels in m.s. patients, since DW2 has been shown to be associated with a *C2°* gene for defective synthesis of C2. It should be noted, however, that the *DW2, C2°* genes are most frequently carried on an *A10, B18* haplotype, and recent evidence also indicates that the *Bf*^{S} allele is included. Bertrams *et al.* (8) presented evidence that low C2 levels were frequent among m.s. patients, but this was not found in a similar study by Day & Jersild (17). Furthermore, none of these studies included a study of families, which is mandatory to claim that the defect is genetically determined. Low levels of C3 and of Factor B were detected in several cases of m.s. by Trouillas *et al.* (68), and in some of these cases these levels were also segregating in healthy family members with particular haplotypes often containing B18. Although these findings suggest abnormalities in the complement sytem, it remains to be shown whether these are not secondary fluctuations reflecting disease activity.

References

1. Adams, J. M. & Imagawa, D. T. (1962): *Proc. Soc. exp. Biol.* (N.Y.) **111**, 562.
2. Alter, M., Harshe, M., Anderson, V. E., Emme, L. & Yunis, E. J. (1976): *Neurology* **26**, 31–36.
3. Arnason, B. G. W., Fuller, T. C., Lehrich, J. R. & Wray, S. H. (1974): *J. Neurol. Sci.* **22**, 419–428.
4. Armstrong, D. & Falk, J. Personal communications (see Jersild *et al. Transplant. Rev.* **22**).
5. Baker, R. W. R., Thompson, R. H. S. &
   Zilkha, K. J. (1966): *J. Neurol. Neurosurgery. Psychiatry* **29**, 95.
6. Bertrams, J. & Kuwert, E. HLA antigen segregation analysis in multiple sclerosis families. *Z. Immunol. Forsch.* (in press).
7. Bertrams, J. & Kuwert, E. (1972): *Europ. Neurol.* **7**, 74–78.
8. Bertrams, J., Opferkuch, W., Grosse-Wilde, H., Netzel, B., Rittner, Ch., Kuwert, E. & Schuppien, W. (1976): C2 levels in m.s. Paris Symposium, September 1976. (No abstract number).
9. Bird, T. D. (1975): *Arch. Neurol.* **32**, 414–416.
10. Brautbar, C., Alter, M. & Kahana, E. (1976): *Neurology* **50**, 50–53.
11. Buchwald, P. I. (1972): Deutsch. Arch. Klin. Med. **2**, 478.
12. Carp, R. I., Merz, G. A. & Licursi, D. C. (1974): *Infection and Immunity* **9**, 1011.
13. Ciongoli, A. K., Platz, P., Dupont, B., Svejgaard, A., Fog, T. & Jersild, C. (1973): *Lancet* ii, 1147.
14. Ciongoli, A. K., Lisak, R. P., Zweiman, B., Koprowski, H. & Waters, D. (1973): *Neurology* **25**, 891–893.
15. Conolly, J. H., Allen, I. V., Hurwitz, L. J. & Millar, J. H. (1967): *Lancet* i, 542.
16. Day, N. K. & Jersild, C. (1976): *C2 functional levels in m.s.* (Unpublished observations).
17. Delmotte, P. 1976): *Proc. Symp. on multiple sclerosis,* p. 113, Melsbroek, April 1976.
18. Dupont, B., Jersild, C., Hansen, G. S., Nielsen, L. S., Thomsen, M. & Svejgaard, A. 1973): *Transplant. Proc.* **5**, 1543–1549.
19. Dupont, B., Lisak, R. P., Jersild, C., Hansen, C., Silberberg, J. A. Whitsett, D. H., Zweiman, B. & Ciongoli, A. K. HLA antigens in Black American patients with multiple sclerosis. *Transplant. Proc.* (in press).
20. Edie, M. J. 1975): In: *Handbook of Clinical Neurology,* eds. Vinken, P. J. & Bruyn, G. W. Vol. 21, p. 365.
21. Eylar, E. H. & Hashim, G. A. (1968): *Proc. nat. Acad. Sci.* (Wash.) **61**, 644.
22. Ferraro, A. & Cazzulo, C. (1948): *J. Neuropathol. exp. Neurol.* **7**, 235.
23. Ferraro, A. & Jervis, G. A. (1940): *Arch. Neurol. & Psychiat.* **43**, 94.
24. Fog, T. (1949): Comp. rend. *IV. Int. Congr. Neurol.,* Paris. Vol. 3, 274. Masson & Cie 1951.
25. Fog, T., Kristensen, I. & Helweg Larsen, H. F. (1955): *Arch. Neurol. Psychiat.* **73**, 267.
26. Fog, T. (1975): Rep. *Int. Symp. on Histo-*

compatibility System. September, Copenhagen (in press).

27. Freund, J., Thomsen, K. J., Hough, H. B., Sommer, H. E. & Pisani, T. M. (1948): *J. Immunol.* **60**, 383.
28. Gyldensted, C. (1976): *Acta Neurol. Scand.* **53**, 386.
29. Hauge, M. (1975): M.S. Symposium, Copenhagen, September. *Acta Neurol. Scand.* (in press).
29a. Haverkorn, M. J., Hofman, B., Masurel, N. & van Rood, J. J. (1975): *Transplant. Rev.* **22**, 120–124.
30. Hens, L., Vlietinck, R. & van de Putte, I. (1976): Symp. HLA and Disease, p. 86. Inserm Paris Abstract II 26.
31. Jellinger, K. & Seitelberger, F. (1958): *Klin. Wchschr.* **36**, 437.
32. Jersild, C., Ammitzbøll, T., Clausen, J. & Fog, T. (1973): *Lancet* i, 151–152.
33. Jersild, C., Dupont, B., Fog, T., Platz, P. & Svejgaard, A. (1975): *Transplant. Rev.* **22**, 148–163.
34. Jersild, C., Dupont, B., Fog, T., Hansen, G. S., Nielsen, L. S., Thomsen, M. & Svejgaard, A. (1973): *Transplant. Proc.* **5**, 1791–1796.
35. Jersild, C., Fog, T., Hansen, G. S., Thomsen, M., Svejgaard, A. & Dupont, B. (1973): *Lancet* ii, 1221–1225.
36. Jersild, C., Platz, P. Thomsen, M., Dupont, B., Svejgaard, A., Ciongoli, A. K., Fog, T. & Grob, P. (1976): *Scand. J. Immunol.* **5**, 141–148.
37. Jersild, C., Svejgaard, A. & Fog, T. (1972): *Lancet* i, 1242–1243.
38. Jørgensen, F. H., Lamm, L. U. & Kissmeyer-Nielsen, F. (1973): *Tissue Antigens* **3**, 323—339.
39. Kuwert, E. K. & Hoher, P. G. (1976): Symp. HLA and Disease, p. 70. Inserm Paris Abstract II 10.
40. Link, H. (1967): *Acta Neurol. Scand.* Suppl. **28**, 1–136.
41. Link, H. (1973): *Ann. Clin. Res.* **5**, 330.
42. Link, H. (1975): Report *Int. Symp. on Histocompatibility System in M.S.* (in press), September, Copenhagen.
43. Mempel, W., Grosse-Wilde, H., Bauman, P., Netzel, B., Steinbauer-Rosenthal, I., Scholz, S., Bertrams, J. & Albert, E. D. (1973): *Transplant. Proc.* **5**, 1529–1534.
44. Myers, L. W., Ellison, G. W., Fewster, M. E., Terasaki, P. I. & Opelz, G. (1976): *Neurology* **26**, 54–55.
45. Möller, E., Link, H., Matell, G., Olhagen, B. & Stendahl, L. (1975): In: *Histocompatibility testing* 1975, Munksgaard, Copenhagen, pp. 778–781.

46. Naito, S., Namerov, N., Mickey, M. R. & Terasaki, P. I (1972): *Tissue Antigens* **2**, 1–4.
47. Norrby, E. & Vandvik, B. (1975): Report Int. Symp. on Histocompatibility System in M.S. *Acta Neurol. Scand.*, September 1975, Copenhagen (in press).
48. Oger, J., Sabouraud, O., Fauchet, R., Genetet, N. & Genetet, B. (1976): Symp. HLA and Disease, p. 74. Inserm. Paris Abstract II 14.
49. Olsson, J. E., Link, H. & Möller, E. (1976): Symp. HLA and Disease, p. 75. Inserm Paris Abstract II 15.
50. Opelz, G., Terasaki, P., Myers, L., Ellison, G., Ebers, G., Zabriskie, J., Kempe, H., Sibley, W. & Sever, J. (1976): Symp. HLA and Disease, p. 76. Inserm. Paris Abstract II–16.
51. Paty, D. W., Cousin, H. K., Stiller, C. R., Furesz, J. & Boucher, D. W. (1976): Symp. HLA and Disease, p. 77. Inserm Paris Abstract II–16.
52. Pette, H. (1928): *Deutsch. Ztsch. f. Nervenh.* **105**, 76.
53. Pincus, T. & Snyder jr., H. W. (1975): In: *Viral Immunology and Immunopathology*, ed. Notkins, A. L., p. 167, Academic Press, N.Y.
54. Platz, P., Fog, T., Morling, N., Svejgaard, A., Sønderstrup, G., Ryder, L. P., Thomsen, M. & Jersild, C. *Acta Pathol. Microbiol. Sect. C.* (in press).
55. Platz, P., Jersild, C., Fog, T. & Raun, N. E. Studies in progress.
56. Platz, P., Jersild, C. Thomsen, M., Svejgaard, A., Fog, T., Midholm, S., Raun, N. E., Hansen, S. K. & Grob, P. (1976): Transfer Factor treatment of patients with multiple sclerosis: II. Immunological parameters in a long-term clinical trial. Proc. II. *Int. Workshop on Transfer factor*, Academic Press, N.Y. (in press).
57. Reed, T. E. (1969): *Science* **165**, 762–768.
58. Rivers, T. & Schwentker, F. (1934): *J. exp. Med.* **60**, 559.
59. Roboz Einstein, E., Nakao, A., Dicaprio, J. & Moore, W. D. (1961): Proc. VII Cong. Neurol., Rome 1961. *Soc. Graf. Romana* **2**, 748.
60. Saito, S., Naito, S., Kawanami, S. & Kuroiwa, Y. (1976): *Neurology* **26**, 49.
61. Sandberg-Wollheim, M. & Bynke, H. (1973): *Acta Neurol. Scand.* **49**, 443.
62. Sandberg-Wollheim, M. (1975): *Acta Neurol. Scand.* **52**, 167.
63. Sever, J. L., Fucillo, D. A., Madden, D. L. & Castellano, G. A. (1976): *Neurology* **26**, 72–74.

64. Shiraki, H. & Otani, S. (1959): In: *"Allergic" encephalomyelitis*, eds. Kies, M. & Alvord, E., Charl. Thomas Publ. Springfield, Illinois.
65. Srivastava, K. C., Fog, T. & Clausen, J. (1974): *Acta Neurol. Scand.* **51**, 193.
66. Stewart, G. J., Basten, A., Guinan, J. & Bashir, H. (1976): Symp. HLA and Disease. Inserm. Paris Abstract II–23.
67. Terasaki, P. I., Ting, A. & Mickey, M. R. B-lymphocyte allo-antigens in Caucasians. *Transplant. Proc.* (in press).
68. Thorsby, E., Helgesen, A., Solheim, B. G. & Vandvik, B. (1976): Symp. HLA and Disease, p. 84. Inserm. Paris Abstract II–24.
69. Trouillas, P., Betuel, H. & Devic, M. (1976): Symp. HLA and Disease. Inserm. Paris Abstract II–25.
70. Tweel, J. G. van den, van Oud Albtass, A. B., Keuning, J. J., Goulmy, E., Termijtelen, B., Bach, M. L. & van Rood, J. J. (1973): Typing for MLC (LD) I. *Transplant. Proc.* 5, 1535–1538.
71. Utermohlen, V. & Zabriskie, J. B. (1973): *Lancet* ii, 1147–1148.
72. van den Berg-Loonen, E. N. & Lucas, K. J. (1975): LD-7a typing in 46 patients with multiple sclerosis. In: *Histocompatibility testing 1975*, pp. 773–777, Munksgaard, Copenhagen.
73. Wernet, P. (1976): Human Ia-type alloantigens. *Transplant. Rev.* **30**, 271–298.
74. Wikström, J. (1975): *Acta Neurol. Scand.* **52**, 207–215.
75. Winchester, R. J., Ebers, G., Fu, S. M., Espinosa, L., Zabriskie, J. & Kunkel, H. G. (1975): *Lancet* ii, 814.
76. Zander, H., Knutz, B., Scholz, S. & Albert, E. D.: Symp. HLA and Disease, p. 91. Inserm. Paris Abstract II–31.
77. Schuller, E., Deloche, G., Delasnerie, G. & Loridan, M. Report Intern. Symposium on Histocompatibility System in Multiple Sclerosis. *Acta. Neurol. Scand.* (In press) September 1975, Copenhagen.
78. Schuller, E., Fournier, C., Reboul, J., Cosson, A., Dry, J. & Bach, J. F. Determination of DNA Antibodies in normal and pathological sera by a new Counterimmunoelectrophoresis Method. *J. Immunol. Methods* (1976) 11–355.
79. Schuller, E., Allinquant, B., Delasnerie, N. & Reboul, J. Determination of RNA Antibodies in Serum and CSF by Counterimmunoelectrophoresis. *J. Immunol. Methods* (in press).

Myasthenia gravis = m. g.

Introduction

M.g. has been known for the last 100 years. It is a disease of neuro-muscular transmission producing muscle weakness and easy fatigability. M.g. must be differentiated from the so called myastehnic syndrome. Herrmann (8) has compared the signs and symptoms between these two completely different diseases, and Table I in his paper ought to be well known by clinicians, trying to determine the association between m.s. and the HLA system. M.g. produces early symptoms and signs of oculobulbar and then extremity weakness with a rapid decline of action potential and contractile strength with repetitive use and nerve-muscle stimulation. Anticholinsterases improve strength. The myasthenic syndrome produces early symptoms and signs in the pelvic girdle, pectoral girdle and proximal limb muscle weakness. This is worst when first starting to use or carry out nerve muscle stimulation in the rested muscles. It improves significantly for a time with use or on rapid stimulation, and then declines. Deep tendon reflexes are sluggish or absent. Small cell carcinoma of the lung is often associated. Guanidine improves strength. The prevalence of m.g. is said to be between 10 and 40 per 100,000. It may be present in men or women at any age, though women have it more often before the age of 40 (8). The ratio of women to men is about 4:3. The so called neonatal myasthenia is persisting for some days or weeks and is transient. It occurs in about 1 out of 6 or 8 infants born to a myasthenic mother. Congenital myasthenia is persistent and occurs in infante born by non-myasthenic mothers. Family cases have been described by Hermann (9). Only a few cases have been published, but it occurs more commonly in families than can be explained by mere chance. Hermann concludes "that the present available information concerning family aggregates and twin studies is inadequate to clearly support genetic mechanisms as determinants though the evidence cannot entirely exclude them. The possibility of exposure to a common factor(s) at an early age in the environment is suggested as a cause for m.g." . . .

Studies in m.g. are especially interesting on account of the possible role of thymus and T-cells in relation to this disease. Thymomata occur in approximately 15 % of patients, but are seldom seen in patients with onset of disease before the age of 19 or after the age of 70. The thymus may be enlarged and show lymphocytic germinal centers on microscopic examination. In skeletal muscle may be found collections of lymphocytes, the so called lymphorrhages, occasional muscle fiber necrosis and atrophy of type II muscle fibers. Supravital staining of neuro-muscular function at times reveals elongated motor-end plates with preterminal branching (for literature see Herrmann (8) cited above).

A circulating blocking agent like curare is an attractive hypothesis. Today two distinct protein entites have been identified as potential candidates for the role of the "autotoxin" mediating neuromuscular blockade: antibody to acetylcholine receptor and thymopoietin (formerly called thymin), and a polypeptide derived from the thymus (for literature, see Vanda Lenon (12)). However, the mechanism of action of these substances and their relevance to m.g. is far from clear.

It is well known that selected patients with m.s. benefit from thymectomy. About 30 % have antibodies in serum which react with striations of skeletal muscles and with similar elements in the thymus, the so called "myoid" cells. The above mentioned germinal centers are the hallmark of antibody production and are not normally present in primary lymphoid organs. M.g. thymuses contain a large proportion of B-lymphocytes and m.g. thymocytes in tissue culture synthesis immunoglobulins, in contrast to normal thymocytes. The autoimmune hypothesis was supported by production of histologic lesions of autoimmune thymitis in animals by immunization with saline extracts of muscle and thymus tissue in adjuvants (Goldstein & Whittingham (7)) but much doubt exist concerning the relation between this experimental disease and the human m.g., like EAE and m.s.

The association of myasthenia gravis with HLA

Six different groups of investigators (1, 4, 5, 13, 14, 19) have studied a possible association of m.g. with HLA in Caucasians. In all these investigations a highly significant increased frequency of HLA-B8 was found with some increase of HLA-A1 which was shown to be secondary to the increase of HLA-B8 and due to linkage disequilibrium between HLA-B8 and HLA-A1. Only Kaakinen et al. (11) have so far studied the frequency of the HLA-D allele associated with HLA-B8, i.e. HLA-DW3. This allele was found to be strongly linked to HLA-B8, but only a little more (not significantly) in myasthenics than in control persons. They conclude that they did not find a specifically myasthenia-associated HLA-D allele

120

and thus that a possible myasthenia susceptibility gene or genes may be situated closer to the HLA-B than to the HLA-D locus.

Pirskanen *et al.* (12) further reported that female myasthenics have a higher frequency of HLA-B8 than males, which was confirmed by Feltkamp *et al.* (4) and Fritze *et al.* (6). Pirskanen *et al* (12) also noted that the presence of HLA-B8 was correlated with early age of onset of the disease. These observations were also confirmed by Feltkamp *et al.* (4) and Fritze *et al.* (6). While the age at onset of m.g. in females was reflected in the age at onset distribution of HLA-B8 positive patients, HLA-B8 negative myasthenics had a later age at onset and a larger percentage of male patients. Feltkamp *et al.* (4) found a significant correlation between HLA-A2 and a later age at onset and the results of Fritze *et al.* (6) suggested that HLA-A3 was more common in myasthenics with an age at onset of over 40 years. These findings however might be fortuitous. They were not confirmed by Pirskanen (15). Fritze *et al.* (6) noticed thymic hyperplasia (an increased number of germinal centers) in HLA-B8 positive patients. HLA-B8 was found to have a normal or low frequency in patients with a thymoma. All these data suggest that two forms of m.g. exist. One with a high frequency of HLA-B8 in which thymic hyperplasia, early age at onset, female sex and a low incidence of antibodies against skeletal muscle are common and another with a normal or even low frequency of HLA-B8, in which thymomata, a later age at onset and antibodies against striated muscle are often found and which occurs predominantly in males. A new development in this disease is the detection of autoantibodies against the protein of the acetylcholine receptor on the postsynoptal membrane. Whether the frequency of HLA-B8 is different in patients with or without such antibodies has not yet been established. A relation was, however, found (17) between the occurrence of antibodies against striated muscle and these antibodies against the protein of the acetylcholine receptor. All patients with muscle antibodies also had the other kind, but 32 out of 57 patients examined in the study only had the antibodies against the acetylcholine receptor. It will be important to establish the frequency of HLA-B8 in the latter kind of patients. Family studies have been carried out by Dick *et al* (3) and by Pirskanen & Tillikainen (16). Dick *et al.* studied a family with identical twin sisters, one of whom had the disease. Another family with identical twins was studied by van den Berg-Loonen *et al.* (2). In this case too only one of the twins had the disease. This clearly indicates that multiple factors are responsible for m.g., some of which must be non-hereditary. Both groups of investigators found that two members of a family that both have myasthenia do not always share an HLA-hyplotype, which indicates that hereditary factors, not linked with HLA must be involved. In any case these family data clearly show that the genetic background of m.g. is not a simple one. It must be borne in mind in this connection that it is difficult to discriminate between multifactorial models of inheritance of clinical disorders and unifactorial models with low penetrance (18). Pirskanen & Tillikainen (16) noticed that in patients with additional immunological and thyroid disorders, which occur more frequently in myasthenics, the frequency of HLA-B8 was lower (44 %) than in myasthenics without these symptoms (66 %). They suggest that this may mean that such disorders may facilitate the outbreak of myasthenia without the "help" of the HLA-B8 associated susceptibility factor. Finally, the possible association of myasthenia with HLA has also been studied in the Japanese population, in which HLA-B8 is virtually absent. It is very interesting that in the Japanese association with other HLA-B alleles was found. Yoshida et al. (20) found the highest association with HLA-B12 (of the same order as the association with B8 in Caucasians) and less

strong association with HLA-A9 and HLA-BW35. They found no difference in the frequency of antigen in patients with or without autoantibodies against striated muscle.

Hoshino et al. (10) also found an increase in HLA-B12 and HLA-BW35 in myasthenic Japanese. Instead of an increase in HLA-A9 an increased frequency of HLA-A10 was noted.

References

1. Behan, P. O., Simpson, J. A. & Dicke, H. (1973): Lancet ii, 1033.
2. van den Berg-Loonen, P. M., Engelfriet, C. P., Nijenhuis, L. E., Feltkamp, T. E. W., Oosterhuis, H. J. G. H., Galama, J. M. D., van Rijn, A. C. M., Verheugt, F.. W. A., Kort-Bakker, M., van Rossum, A. L. & van Loghem, J. J., in preparation.
3. Dick, H. M., Behan, P. O., Simpson, J. A. & Durward, W. F. (1974): J. Immunogenet. 1, 401.
4. Feltkamp, T. E. W., van den Berg-Loonen, P. M., Nijenhuis, L. E., Engelfriet, C. P., van Rossum, A. L., van Loghem, J. J. & Oosterhuis, H. J. G. H. (1974): Brit. med. J. 1, 131.
5. Fritze, D., Hermann, C., Smith, G. S. & Walford, R. L. (1973): Lancet ii, 211.
6. Fritze, D, Hermann, C., Naeim, F., Smith, G. S. & Walford, R. L. (1974): Lancet i, 240.
7. Goldstein, G. & Wittingham, S. (1966): Lancet ii, 215.
8. Hermann, C. (1970): Medical Progress, Calif. Med. 113, 27–3.
9. Hermann, C. (1966): Neurology 1, 15–85.
10. Hoshino, K., Inonye, H., Unokuchi, T.,

Ito, M., Tamaoki, N. & Tsjui, K. (1976): 1st Int. Symp. on HLA and Disease. Inserm. Paris Abstract (no number).
11. Kaakinen, A., Pirskanen, R. & Tillikainen, A. (1975): Tissue Antigens 6, 175.
12. Lenon, V. (1975): Nature (Lond.) 258, 11–12.
13. Mueller-Eckhardt, C., Gross, W., Friedrich, F., Krüger, J. & Kunze, K. (1974): Z. Immun. Forsch. 147, 331.
14. Pirskanen, R., Tillikainen, A. & Kokkanen, E. (1972): Ann. Clin. Res. 4, 304.
15. Pirskanen, R. (1976): J. Neurol. Neurosurg. Psychiat. 39, 23.
16. Pirskanen, R. & Tillikainen, A. (1976): Symp. HLA and Disease. Inserm. Paris Abstract II–19.
17. Ringel, St. P., Bender, A. & Smith, H. (1975): Lancet i, 1388.
18. Smith, Ch. (1974): Lancet i, 450.
19. Säfwenberg, J., Lindblom, J. B. & Osterman, P. O. (1973): Tissue Antigens 3, 465.
20. Yoshida, T., Tsuchinya, M., Shimabukuno, K., Satoyoshi, E., Tamaoki, N. & Tsuji, K. (1976): Symp HLA and Disease. Inserm. Paris Abstract II–29.

Amyrtrophic lateral sclerosis (A.L.S. or motor neuron disease)

Introduction

A.L.S. is characterized by a progressive and fatal degeneration of anterior horn cells in the spinal cord and bulbar centers. Skeletal muscular wasting and weakness are the results, beginning in about 40 % of the classical cases in the upper extremities, in 25 % in the bul-

bar controlled muscles and in 25 % in the legs (Kurland et al. (5)). Three types exist: the classical and sporadic form, with progression of signs and symptoms to alle muscles except the extrinsic eye muscles; the familial and permanently hereditary form (which, according to a series from the Mayo Clinic, was present in 5–10 % of classical cases), considered as an autosomal dominant pattern of heredity with high penetrance (Kurland & Mulder (1955) and Mulder (1957)) cited from Kurland et al. (5) and a third form which was discovered on the Mariana Islands and some other western Pacific Islands. A high incidence and prevalence of this type was registered in these islands. About 1 % of the adult Chamorros were found to be affected and for an adult Chamorro the lifetime risk of dying from ALS was 10 %. Originally a genetical base was suspected but new studies point to a search for an exogenous factor (for details, see Kurland et al. (5)).

The prevalence rate for the classical form seems to be 6 per 100,000. The annual incidence in the USA, age adjusted to be 1950 US-population, is about 1.3 per 100,000 for a forty year period. The male-female ratio is 1.6:1 for the white population. The average life expectancy after onset varies from 1 to 6 years, the age of onset lying in the late fifthties or early of the sixties.

The cause is unknown. ALS may be more than a single disease entity. Different exogenous substances have been described as causative, such as heavy metals, organic intoxications, metabolic, vascular, prior to poliomyelitis or other infectious agents, and as has been mentioned heredity but without any convincing proof.

The neuropathologic alterations are characterized by a fading of the anterior horn cells, without inflammatory reactions and some slight demyelination in the long fiber tracts in the posterior half of the spinal cord. Special changes are added to this in the Mariana form. Histochemical changes observed in the skin have also been described in the sporadic classical form (Fullmor et al. (1960)) (cited from Kurland et al. (5)).

The HLA-system in A.L.S.

Four reports exist concerning HLA antigens in ALS (1, 2, 3, 4). So far 120 cases have been investigated. The S-D antigens were determined by all four groups, but the L-D antigens also by Pedersen et al. (3) Neither Bartfield et al. (2) nor Pedersen et al. (3) found any significant deviation compared with normal controls. An unusually high incidence of HLA-A2 and A28 was found by Behan et al. (4) (27) patients) but this was not found in the two series mentioned although Bartfield et al. noted an increased frequency of the phenotype HLA-A2, BW17. In contrast, Antel et al. (1) found an increased frequency of HLA-A3.

From these studies it may be concluded that no association is demonstrable between A.L.S. and the histocompatibility system. No studies have been published yet concerning the Guam type of A.L.S.

References

1. Antel, J. P., Arnason, B. G. W., Fuller, T. C. & Lehrich, J. R. Arch. Neurol. 33, 423–425.
2. Bartfield, H., Whitsett, C. & Donnenfeld, H. (1971): Symp. HLA and Disease, p. 61. Inserm. Paris Abstract II–1.
3. Pedersen, L. & Platz, P. (1976): Symp.
4. Behan, P. O., Heather, M., Dick, J. A., Simpson, J. A. & Durward, W. F. (1976): Symp. HLA and Disease, p. 62. Inserm. Paris Abstract II–2.
5. Kurland, L. T., Kurtzke, J. & Goldberg, I.

HLA and Disease, p. 78. Inserm. Paris Abstract II–18.

D. (1973): Epidemiology of neurologic and sense organ disorders. In: *Vital and Health Statistics Monographs*. American Public Health Association, Harvard University Press, Cambridge, Massachusetts.

Other diseases

Only a relatively small number of cases of other different neurological and psychiatric diseases have yet been published concerning a possible association with the HLA system. At the Paris conference Lacert et al. (5) compared 68 paralytic poliomyelitis patients with 591 healthy controls. No relationship was found between the localization of the paralytic attack, the disease itself or the frequency of HLA antigens. Nor did Zander et al. (11) find any significant deviation in 53 unrelated Caucasian polio-paralytic patients from normal controls. 33 antigens were typed, and HLA-D typing was performed using 7 different homozygous typing cells for DW 1, to DW5 plus two more recently defined typing cells E1 and RE. Earlier published data concerning an increase of HLA-A3 and B7 were thus not confirmed by these new studies. No significant frequency of antigens was found in 32 patients with SSPE (7), 26 Black and Caucasian patients were studied for 31 HLA-A and B antigens in St. Louis encephalitis (9). A decreased frequency of BW35 among the Black patients when compared with the Black control group was significant. No other differences were demonstrated. HLA-D allele studies were performed in 15 unrelated children with the Lennox-Gastaut syndrome (8). An HLA-D allele may possibly be associated with this disease. 59 American Caucasians and 35 American Black patients suffering from dementia paralytica were typed for 31 HLA antigens of the A and B loci. In the Caucasian patients the frequency of HLA-B18 was significantly increased.

No other significant deviations were demonstrated (19). 16 patients with vitamin B_{12} neuro-myelopathy associated with pernicious anemia were typed for 27 alleles of A and B loci and compared with 53 cases of pernicious anemia without neurological damage and 60 controls. A significantly increased frequency of the HLA phenotype A2, B12 (44 % versus 4 %) was found (3). Thirty patients suffering from ataxia teleangiectasia and their 27 parents and healthy siblings were typed for 19 HLA allele of the A and B loci. An increase of HLA-BW17 and decreased frequency of HLA-A1 and B8 seems to be associated with this immunodeficiency disease (2).

Studies in the major psychoses, schizophrenia and manicdepressive psychosis are still so small, compared with the great number of patients, that it seems premature to draw definite conclusions, especially as the early results are unequivocal. At the Paris conference, only three groups presented studies of patients. Ivanyi et al. (4) tested 200 male patients with schizophrenia and found a significant increase of HLA-A28 and of the haplotype A10, B18. Bennaham et al. (1) were not able to draw definite conclusions from their small sample, but were able to differentiate schizophrenia from manicdepressive psychosis by the method of discriminatory analysis. They also emphasize the importance of the ethnic influence upon the HLA results. Mercier et al. (6) studied 14 hebephrenic and 15 paranoic patients. The data are too sparse to draw conclusions. The authors feel that the strongly increased frequencies of A9 and B5 in the paranoid group open a new biological aspect.

Future studies in patients suffering from the major psychoses are necessary in order to determine a possible association with the histocompatibility system and the diseases.

References

1. Bennaham, D. A., Troup, G. M., Rada, R. T., Kellner, R. T. & Kyner, T. (1976): HLA antigens in schizophrenic and manicdepressive mental disorders. Symp. HLA and Disease, p. 64. Inserm. Paris Abstract II–4.
2. Berkel, A. I. & Ersoy, F. (1976): HLA antigens in ataxia teleangiectasia. Symp. HLA and Disease. Inserm. Paris Abstract (not numbered).
3. Horton, M. A. & Oliver, R. T. D. (1976): HLA phenotype A2, B12 in vitamin B_{12} neuromyelopathy. Symp. HLA and Disease, p. 68. Inserm. Paris Abstract II–8.
4. Ivanyi, D., Zemek, P. & Ivanyi, P. (1976): HLA antigens in schizophrenia. Symp. HL Aand Disease, p. 69. Inserm. Paris Abstract II–9.
5. Lacert, Ph., Durand, J. J., Guardin, M., Grossiord, A., Gony, J. & Hors, J. (1976): HLA and poliomyelitis. Symp. HLA and Disease, p. 71. Inserm. Paris Abstract II–11.
6. Mercier, P., Kieffer, N., Julien, R. & Sutter, J. M. (1976): Schizophrenia: HLA-A9 and B5 antigens. Symp. HLA and Disease, p. 72. Inserm. Paris Abstract II–12.
7. Reinert, Ph., Mannoni, P., Lehon, P. & Ponsot, G. (1976): HLA and subacute sclerosing panencephalitis. Symp. HLA and Disease, p. 80. Inserm. Paris Abstract II–20.
8. Smeraldi, E., Scorza-Smeraldi, K., Guareschi-Cazullo, S., Cazullo, C. L., Rugarli, C. & Canger, R. (1976): Immunogenetics of Lennox-Gastaut Syndrome: Search for LD Determinants as genetic markers of the syndrome. Symp. HLA and Disease, p. 82. Inserm. Paris Abstract II–22.
9. Whitsett, C., Lee, T., Powell, K., Dupont, B. & Lytle, V. (1976): HLA antigens in St. Louis encephalitis. Symp. HLA and Disease, p. 87. Inserm. Paris Abstract II–27.
10. Whitsett, C., Turner, W. J. & Dupont, B. (1976): HLA antigens in paralytic dementia (syphilis). Symp. HLA and Disease, p. 88. Inserm. Paris Abstract II–28.
11. Zander, H., Grosse-Wilde, H., Scholz, S., Knutz, B., Netzel, B. & Albert, E. D. (1976): Poliomyelitis: Analysis of HLA-A1, B and D alleles. Symp. HLA and Disease, p. 90. Inserm. Paris Abstract II–30.

Dermatology

Walter C. Lobitz, Jr.,[1] Jean Civatte,[2]
Jean Thivolet,[3] Hervé Betuel,[4] &
Eric Thorsby.[5]

Introduction

Association of the HLA system with dermatologic diseases presents unique opportunities for the clinicians and for the HLA scientists. Clinical dermatologists are uniquely equipped for these opportunities because they deal directly with the cellular events and mechanisms in understanding the diseases that confront them. Such understanding makes it possible to apply new knowledge, such as the HLA system, directly to clinical problems, to put them in proper perspective, to use the information to aid in diagnosis and management, to ask significant questions about the present information and even to suggest directions for future investigation in the laboratories of the HLA scientists as well as those laboratories which are investigating the diseases.

In this chapter, the authors are trying to do just that. For example, in certain diseases which are known to be familial and are easy to diagnose, the HLA associations may give the laboratory investigators of the disease a perspective on future research for better understanding (e.g. psoriasis). Certain diseases are difficult to diagnose early; here the HLA associations can help the clinician make earlier correct diagnoses and thus institute early or preventive therapy (e.g. Bechet's disease *versus* recurrent oral ulcerations). Certain diseases which are known to run in families may not have HLA associations, so geneticists must look elsewhere (e.g. acne conglobata). Certain diseases are so well understood from the standpoint of pathologic events and mechanisms that they in turn give the HLA scientists clues as to where to search in the future for even more precise genetic controlling loci (e.g. dermatitis herpetiformis). This interrelating by the HLA scientists and their clinical colleagues is just beginning. It is already fruitful, especially in diseases of the skin.

In this chapter, these diseases will be grouped according to their clinical diagnostic similarities, for example, the vesiculo-bullous diseases, the mucous-membrane ulcreative diseases, the so-called autoimmune diseases, the infectious and allergic diseases, and then a miscellaneous group of diseases where single studies may show positive or negative correlations.

[1] Department of Dermatology, School of Medicine, University of Oregon Health Sciences Center, Portland, Oregon.
[2] Clinique des Maladies Cutanées et Syphilitiques, Hôpital Saint-Louis, Paris, France.
[3] Department of Dermatology, Hôpital Edouard Herriot, Lyon, France.
[4] Tissue-Typing Laboratory of the Blood Transfusion Center, Lyon, France.
[5] Tissue-Typing Laboratory, Rikshospitalet, Oslo, Norway.

At the end of this chapter, some of the significant data are summarized in tabular form according to diseases and first authors. This material will also be referred to in the references but will not be included in the text. In order to keep the reference list as brief as possible, references for the older material will be given to review articles or to the report from the HLA and Disease Registry of Copenhagen, 1976. The latest material just presented in abstract form at the 1st International Symposium on HLA and Disease, Paris, June 23–25 1976, will be referred to as such.

Psoriasis

Affecting 1.0–2.8 % of the world's population, with many variations according to climate and ethnic origin, psoriasis is a papulosquamous skin disease which has long been known to be familial. Many factors play a part in its development among which are the genetic factors. The hypothesis of an autosomal dominant mode of transmission with reduced penetrance is the most popular at present. More recent theories on psoriasis try to explain it as a multifactorial affliction transmitted by a single gene wherein environmental factors play an important role.

The uncertainty of the genetic data is explained by the importance of external or metabolic factors to the disease. These obstacles are now being overcome, thanks to the association of psoriasis with the histocompatibility system by Russell et al (1972) and White et al (1972) (1). For psoriasis, two types of HLA studies are utilized. First, as with other diseases, a sample population of unrelated ill people is studied by typing for the histocompatibility antigens and establishing their distribution in relation to a sample of healthy unrelated subjects of the same racial background. Secondly, and more particularly for psoriasis, hereditary forms of the disease are studied in families, grouping those members of the same family when more than one member is afflicted with the disease.

All the early studies agree that the association of HLA-B13, BW17 and perhaps B16 with psoriasis is significant in Caucasoid populations (1, 2, 3, 4). It is interesting that there is a negligible incidence of psoriasis in the pure American Indian (Amerindian) who is mongoloid. The HLA-gene frequency in the Amerindian is 0 % for HLA-B13 and only 1 % for HLA-BW17. On the other hand, the West African negroid also has a low prevalence of psoriasis (Nigeria 0.5 %, Angola 0.3 %) (5) and a low frequency of HLA-B13 (about 1 %), but BW17 occurs in between 15 and 28 % of Nigerians and between 2 8and 47 % of Angolans.

The Japanese (6) could not confirm the early Caucasoid association of B13, BW16 and BW17 with psoriasis vulgaris. Their studies show significant associations with HLA-A1 and BW37. However, more recent work shows a significant BW37 increase to be the strongest among the Caucasian psoriatic population (8, 14).Interestingly, Ohkido et al. found a decrease in HLA-B12, and when they typed for B-cell Ia-like antigens they showed the B-cell-positive reaction (JE5-487 antiserum) in four out of 13 patients with psoriasis (30.8 % compared with 9 % in healthy controls).

Gross-Wilde et al. (7) studied HLA-D allele frequencies in parallel with HLA-A and -B typing. DW2 and E1 were significantly increased in patients with psoriasis. Since E1 is associated with B13 and B17 among healthy individuals, they believe that the E1 increase can be explained by the increase of HLA-B13 and BW17, but the increase of DW2 remains unexplained.

HLA-B13, BW17 and BW37 were most marked in patients whose psoriasis began before 40 years of age (8). The risk of developing psoriasis in a normal Caucasian population is 2 %, but that risk increases to 5 % if the individual carries HLA-B13 or BW17 and to 6 % for BW37. The risk decreases to 0.8 % if the person carries HLA-B12.

It is well known that respiratory streptococcal infections precede exacerbations of psoriasis. Krain et al. (9) reported a significant association between HLA-B13 and a history of severe streptococcal infections. Karvonen (8) recently confirmed this .Bertrams et al. (10) found that HLA-B13-positive psoriatic patients had significantly lower antistreptolysin-O titers than HLA-B13-negative patients.

Family studies are important and increasing in number. Also, loci are being looked at other than the HLA-A and -B antigens. There seems to be a greater frequency of family psoriasis with psoriatics who have the antigen BW17 than with the other groups.

Many authors agreed early that the haplotype HLA-A1 and BW17 is important in familial psoriasis. In the normal Caucasian population, the haplotype HLA-A1-B8 is four times more frequent than A1-B8 in patients with psoriasis. Karvonen (11) and Civatte et al. (12) investigated families with HLA-B13. Civatte also showed that in families with psoriatic siblings, 9 out of 13 pairs of siblings were HLA identical, three were haplo identical and one was HLA different. The genotype distribution differs significantly from the ex-

pected and is in favor of a linkage between genes controlling psoriasis and those coding for HLA antigens. The excess of HLA-identical siblings supports the hypothesis of a possible dose-haplotype effect. Marcusson et al. (13, 14) believe that the controlling psoriatic gene(s) is not the BW17 allele itself, but other genes in close proximity to the B region. They described two haplotypes (A1-BW17Dx and A1-BW37 DW2) which they called the "pso" haplotype. They found six recombinant children, which was much higher than expected.

Early studies could find no HLA-A- or -B-locus associations with pustular psoriasis. Karvonen (15) could not find any significant HLA associations in patients with persistent palmoplantar pustulosis (P.P.P.) but did have two patients with generalized pustular psoriasis (G.P.P.) with HLA-BW17. Ohkido et al. (6) found that HLA1BW15 was significantly increased in 31 patients with P.P.P.. Zachariae (16) divided pustular psoriasis into subgroups: localized pustular psoriasis of the palms and soles (L.P.P.), acrodermatitis chronica of hallopean (A.C.), generalized pustular psoriasis (G.P.P) and P.P.P. Patients with L.P.P. and G.P.P. had no significant HLA associations, but 36 % of the 14 A.C. patients had BW27 (36 % also had arthritis) and 34 % of 35 P.P.P. patients had BW35. Both results were considered significant.

There are several clinical forms of psoriasis. Psoriasis vulgaris is the classical chronic papulosquamos plaque form and is the most common. In the acute eruptive stage, the small new lesions are more inflamed, producing an acute guttate variety. Sometimes the acute disease can progress to a generalized exfoliative erythroderma which can in turn persist in a more chronic state. Here HLA typing may help in the diagnosis. An acute flare of psoriasis can also become pustular with discrete and confluent superficial subcorneal pustules within hot red inflamed areas of skin (von Zumbush type). Pustular psoriasis can also be localized in the palms and soles as persistent palmer plantar psoriasis (P.P.P. or Barber type). All forms of psoriasis can also be associated with several varieties of arthropathy (central, peripheral, ankylosing spondylitis, rheumatoid-like). The psoriatic arthropathies which seem to be associated with B27 will be discussed in the chapter on Rheumatology.

One can appreciate, therefore, that there is more than one pathologic event in the disease process. The dominant event in psoriasis vulgaris is an accelerated rate of growth or turnover of the epidermis which is nine times the normal rate. There is good evidence that there is a defect somewhere in the cyclic AMP system of the psoriatic epidermal cell or in its chalone hormonal control that allows it to divide and reproduce so rapidly. Any topical or systemic treatment that will decrease this accelerated epidermal turnover will clear the skin of psoriasis vulgaris lesions, (e.g. systemic methotrexate inhibits the DNA-cell cycle in its S phase and will slow down the rate of mitosis and improve psoriasis). Also, in all psoriatic lesions there is a migration of polymorphonuclear leukocytes (PMNs) from the papillary capillaries into the stratum corneum producing a so-called microabscess of Munroe.

The exact mechanism for this PMN stratum corneum chemotaxis is yet unknown, although recent antistratum corneum antibodies have been demonstrated by immunofluorescence in psoriasis. When this PMN-migration event is dominant, the clinical picture is one of pustular psoriasis.

Since the pathologic event in pustular psoriasis is so different from that of accelerated epidermal turnover in psoriasis vulgaris, one wonders whether these two events are under separate genetic control. The B13, B16, BW17 and BW37 association might be in charge of only the accelerated epidermopoesis event. This is particularly attractive to think about since the HLA antigens may interfere with or confuse hormonal receptor sites on cell membranes which in the case of psoriasis may be the sites for the cAMP system or for chalone. The genetic control of the pustular event may be on some other chromosome since HLA associations and pustular psoriasis are still in doubt.

In any event, the fact that three or more HLA antigens are associated with psoriasis suggests that these several markers are secondary to the actual controlling gene(s) which may be closer to the D locus. On the other hand, increases in B13, BW17 and BW37 may be secondary to a primary increase of the newly defined C-series antigen, T7, which includes each of these three B antigens (17). More antigens in more loci need to be correlated with psoriasis. Most important, family studies with a high incidence of psoriasis of three generations or more such as in the Faroe Islands, where there is a 93 % incidence of familial psoriasis, should be thoroughly studied for haplotypes which would include all the antigens of all the HLA loci that are available and pertinent.

Dermatitis herpetiformis

Also known as Duhring-Brocq disease, dermatitis herpetiformis (D.H.) is a benign recurring inflammatory vesiculobullous disease. Of rare incidence, it occurs between the ages of 20 and 55; it occurs twice as frequently in males. There is no racial prevalence. The burning or itching eruption consists of small grouped vesicles usually on top of erythematous and urticarial papules which when resolved may leave hyper or hypopigmentation and scarring. In the more severe forms, bullae occur on normal or inflamed skin. The eruption is symmetrically distributed on the trunk and on extensor surfaces of the extremities. Oral mucous membranes are rarely affected. The disease responds well to sulfapyridine, to Dapsone and to a gluten-free diet. Iodides and bromides taken internally may flare the disease.

The frequency of HLA-B8 is significantly increased in patients with D.H. (18, 19, 20). The first study was undertaken by Katz et al. (18) because D.H. is often associated with jejunal villous atrophy similar to that encountered in gluten-sensitive enteropathy (G.S.E.), where a very high correlation was found with B8. For a few years there was argument as to hether B8 was controlling the enteropathy or the dermatitis (19, 20, 21, 22, 23, 27). Then, as the diagnostic criteria for D.H. became more critical and included the early neutrophil microabscess in the dermal papillae, positive immunofluorescences for IgA in normal as well as abnormal skin, factor B of the alternative complement pathway in inflamed skin plus the lymphoyctic infiltrations in small bowel biopsies, the HLA-B8 correlation rose from 57 % to 85 % thus increasing the relative risk from 4.45 to 18.2.

Solheim et al. (24) and Thomson et al. (25) while confirming the increase in B8 have shown that DW3, which is associated to B8 among healthy individuals, reaches the highest frequency in D.H. Later Solheim et al. (26) typed with antiserum (AH) defining an Ia-like alloantigen closely associated to DW3 which is detectable on human B lymphocytes and macrophages. All patients reacted positively compared with 25 % of controls. The results indicate that association of D.H. may be stronger for the "Ia-like" specificity AH than DW3.

A different approach was used by Mann et al. (28) who typed B lymphocytes of patients with G.S.E. and D.H. The originality consisted in using two antisera obtained from women whose children or husbands were afflicted with G.S.E. and/or D.H. Serum "B1" reacted with cells from 13 out of 16 G.S.E. patients and with those from 15 out of 19 D.H. patients (12 B8-positive and three B8-negative). Antiserum "W1" reacted with 15 out of 16 G.S.E. patients and with all of the 15 D.H. patients tested. None of these sera reacted with B cells from normal individuuals whether or not they were B8. These antigens are not determined by the HLA chromosomal complex. One of the hypotheses considered this B-lymphocyte antigen to be a receptor for gluten. The presence of similar receptors on the skin and on the gut epithelial cells would explain the reaction to gluten and subsequent lesions in both diseases.

In summary, dermatitis herpetiformis is an inflammatory subepidermal bullous disease with separation of the epidermis at the epidermal-dermal junction. It is associated with the small bowel changes characteristic of gluten-sensitive enteropathy (G.S.E.) In addition to the subepidermal bullae and the early inflammatory exudate of neutrophils, direct immunofluorescence reveals IgA in uninvolved skin and also with C3 and properdin factor B in the lesions. When the patient is given a gluten-free diet, the cutaneous lesions disappear, thus implicating this protein and the alternative complement pathway as a mechanism for this inflammatory skin disease. The association with HLA-B8 is strong. Most recently a significant association has been shown with HLA-DW3 and DW3-associated Ia-like antigens. Since there is good evidence that the alternative pathway of the complement system is involved in the pathologic events, future studies should look for the properdin factor B marker which lies between the B and the D loci in the HLA supergene.

Bullous pemphigoid (B. P.)

In the past, this disease has been confused with pemphigus vulgaris (P.V.) and dermatitis herpetiformis (D.H.) until it was demonstrated that acantholysis is present in P.V. and absent from the lesions of B.P. and D.H. The association with D.H. is no longer tenable due to the character of the eruption, the absence of response to sulphones, immunoflourescence and the HLA pattern.

Bullous pemphigoid occurs late in life after the age of 60; both sexes are affected and there is no racial prevalence. After a prodromal rash and erythema, blisters appear on the limbs and abdomen. The bullae are large and tense but after resorption leave no pigmentation. The cause is chronic, but many patients respond well to very high doses of corticosteroids. There is no acantholysis of the epidermis. The bullae are subepidermal. However, patients with B.P. have IgG and IgM antibodies specific for the basement membrane zone (BMZ) of the epidermis (peribullous or normal skin) which can be demonstrated by both direct and indirect immunofluorescence, since these are circulating antibodies in the patients' serum. C3 is also present at the BMZ.

In 1976, Thivolet et al. (29) presented a study on 19 patients typed for HLA-A and -B. Though the p value was not significant after correction, B5 and BW 16 were increased. More patients should be typed for this disease until definite conclusions are reached. Recently, Ahmed et al. (30) studied 19 Caucasoid patients. Again, no statistically significant increased frequency of HLA antigens was noted. Interestingly, Ahmed showed that after his patients with B.P. cleared their skin with azathioprene therapy, those patients with recurrent disease had an 83 % incidence of HLA-B12 compared with 35 % in the control. HLA-BW15 was found in 67 % of patients with recurrent B.P. compared with 7 % of the controls. Although the series is very small, this might suggest that B12 and BW15 are associated with more severe and recurring disease.

However, it is important to stress that B8 has not been associated with B.P. Since B8 is strongly associated with dermatitis herpetiformis, this can help in differential diagnosis and in further separation of the two diseases.

Pemphigus vulgaris

The distribution of this disease of unknown etiology is worldwide, but a higher incidence has been confirmed in Jews. It affects both sexes in the middle age of life. The characteristic histological pattern is the separation of the epidermal cells by loss of intercellular bridges, a change known as acanthylosis. The bulla formed is intraepidermal. Its floor is formed by basal cells which remain attached to the dermis. Clinically, the onset consists in mucous-membrane lesions more often in the mouth and in the vulva. The widespread bullae appear in the skin after several months. The blisters break easily leaving denuded areas which extend as the epidermis strips off. Such erosions are painful, bleed, and show no tendency to heal. Lesions which do heal leave hyperpigmentation. Antiepithelial antibodies (IgG, IgM) directed against the material on or around the epithelial cell and C3 are demonstrated by immunofluorescence either directly on skin-bioposy specimens or indirectly in the patients' serum using as a substrate human skin or monkey or rat esophagus. The severity of the disease correlates directly with the level of antiepithelial antibody in the patients' serum. More than two thirds of the patients respond well to immunosuppressive drugs and steroid therapy though the course may be more severe in Jews. Before treatment the autcome was death.

In a study of 18 Caucasian patients (seven of whom were Jews) Katz et al. (30) found an increase in B13. Though the difference was significant, the author did not support this association firmly on account of the small number of patients.

Interesting findings were the presence of antiepithelial antibodies in all the patients' sera; however, there were no cytotoxic antibodies in these sera directed against the patients' own lymphocytes or against a panel of 118 HLA-typed controls. In addition, two anti-HLA sera (B8, BW40) did not react with the pemphigus interepithelial antigen. These results render unlikely the hypothesis that the pemphigus antigen is related to HLA. The racial prevalence of pemphigus was outlined in the study by Krain (32). On 28 Jewish patients of Ashkenazi extraction, 60 % were A10 compared with 20 % of controls of the same origin. This antigen was even higher in females, 71 % (out of 17) compared with 45 % in males (out of 11). Hoshino (33) also demonstrated an association between HLA-A10 in 19 Japanese with the disease (p<0.001).

Behcet's disease

The syndrome described by Behcet in 1937 is associated with buccal mucosal ulcerations, genital ulcerations and iridocyclitis. In 1941 A. Touraine enlarged the concepts of the disease and reported Behcet's disease to be a general illness. In 1955, he included the visceral complications of the syndrome.

Behcet's disease (34) is a chronic and progressive syndrome of unknown cause which is characterized by recurring ulcers of the mouth and genitalia associated with iridocyclitis, conjunctivitis, iritis and uveitis. Skin lesions (papules and pustules) and cutaneous nodules (erythema nodosum) also occur as do arthritis, thrombophlebitis and diverse visceral and central nervous system involvement. Viral infection and autoimmune disease have been postulated as possible causes.

The disease has a large incidence of morbidity in Japan, the Middle East, and in countries bordering the Mediterranean Sea, suggesting a genetic predisposition. The disease is frequent in young adults between the ages of 15 and 40 years, affecting males more than females, and begins in men at a younger age than in women. Since the disease has such a poor prognosis, it is important to study all the possible explanations of its pathogenesis, particularly the role of the HLA-associated antigens. Because of the many manifestations of Behcet's syndrome, strict diagnostic criteria must be adhered to in any studies.

In order to confirm the diagnosis, different authors have proposed lists of major and minor criteria necessary to establish the diagnoses. For the most part, the major criteria include buccal and genital mucous-membrane ulcerations, eye involvement, and skin lesions. The minor criteria include thrombophlebitis, gastrointestinal and cardiovascular and central nervous system involvement, arthritis, and a familial history of the disease.

Ohno *et al.* in 1973 (35) reported a highly significant frequency of HLA-B5 in 21 Japanese with the disease. In 1975, he (36, 37) added 29 new patients and retyped 15 patients from the previous study with a new anti-B5 antiserum. Among these 44 patients, 35 had a complete form of the illness. The frequency of the gene HLA-B5 was again high. Similar findings have been obtained by Dausset & Hors in 1975 (37), and Rosselet in 1976 (39).

Ohno's original findings have been confirmed by presentations at the First International Symposium on HLA and Disease by other Japanese workers and by studiies from Turkey and France (40 –44). Only one discrepancy in the otherwise unanimous agreement (Orientals and Caucasians) on the increased frequency of HLA-B5 patients with Behcet's disease was reported from England. Jung *et al.* (45) found no increase in B5 in ten British patients with the disease.

Only Ohno (1975) has carried out studies on three families, but they are not sufficient to draw any conclusions about the significance of the haplotypes. He could not correlate HLA-B5 with patients who carried the complete forms of disease and those with only a few symptoms. Nor could he associate B5 with the patients with Behcet's disease who had significantly higher levels of complement-fixing antibodies to Chlamydia (46).

All these combined studies at present establish a strong correlation between HLA-B5 and Behcet's disease, even though the populations (Japanese and Caucasian) have differences in their antigenic distributions in each population. Perhaps HLA-B5 can give clues as to the etiology of the disease (a crossreaction between a virus and B5 or linkage disequilibrium between an immune-response gene and HLA-B5). Some of the syndrome's clinical events could be of infectious (e.g. viral) origin; others could fit well with immune-complex disease (e.g. erythema nodosum and vasculitis). More family studies are needed and also studies involving the HLA-D-series antigens and components of the "Ia" and complement-controlling loci.

It is difficult to make the diagnosis of Behcet's disease in the early stages where the only clinical events of the disease are oral and/or genital ulcerations or ocular involvement or vague systemic aspects of the syndrome. In such incomplete forms of the disease, HLA typing can help improve the diagnosis and permit effective treatment as early as possible.

Recurrent oral ulceration (apthous stomatitis)

The etiology of recurrent oral ulcerations (ROU) is unknown, but much of the recent evidence suggests that ROU is associated with autoimmune responses to oral mucosal antigens or to some crossreacting antigens. Dolby (47) and Platz et al. (48) could not find any deviations of HLA-A and -B antigens in patients with RUO. However, Challacombe et al. (49) typed a series of 100 patients with ROU. HLA-B12 was present in 43 % of the patients with ROU compared with 22 % of the 100 controls. Also, the frequency of the HLA haplotype HLA-A2, B12 was 30 % in ROU, and 11 % in controls. Challacombe's preliminary family studies are consistent with the possibility that ROU may group with an HLA haplotype.

This new information of the possible association of HLA-B12 with ROU is of help in diagnosis, since many oral ulcerating diseases may be confused with ROU. This is particularly so with the early stages of Behcet's disease which is associated with HLA-B5 and with pemphigus vulgaris, pemphigoid and oral herpes simplex infections.

Herpes simplex

Herpes simplex is the most widespread of human viral diseases. The two types of viruses which are responsible are well known (HVS Type I and Type II) as are their immunological reactions.

The primary herpetic infections usually occur in childhood and are not recognized clinically in 85 % of the cases. This primary infection produces specific neutralizing and complement-fixing antibodies. Also, intracutaneous tests are positive to the viral antigen. These antibodies found in 90 % of adults persist a long time in the human, but do not prevent the recurring clinical manifestations of the virus. These recurrences produce benign mucocutaneous lesions which, in a person who is ill, will always reappear in the same sites. There are many known precipitating causes for the recurrences including trauma, sunburn, infection and menses, but many recur without any known cause in otherwise healthy individuals.

Between these recurrences, the virus persists in a latent state in the peripheral nerve-root ganglion. Reactivation of the virus may be linked to a cellular immune deficiency. Cell-mediated immune suppression allows widespread infection throughout the body. Cutaneous immune-complex-like vasculitis, sometimes involving complement (Arthus-type) called erythema multiforme frequently complicates recurring infections. Almost all exposed humans will become infected with HSV Type I and there are no clinical clues that there is a hereditary or genetic aspect to those who have recrudescent clinical episodes of virus activation or to those who develop erythema multiforme. Most herpes labialis is of the HSV Type I origin. Type II infection (herpes genitalis) is now the second-most-common venereal disease. Interpretation of HLA studies is difficult because there is epidemiological, serological, and viral study evidence that HSV Type II may play a role in causing uterine cervical cancer. Therefore, any significant HLA correlations with the disease could be explained by any of the theories including molecular mimicry and breakdown of self tolerance (dominant susceptibility to virus-induced autoimmunity), HLA-antigen incorporation in the surface membrane of the infecting virus, HLA cell-surface factors acting as receptors for the virus, as well as Ia- or Ir-genetic association. HLA complement-controlling factors might help explain those patients who always develop the erythema multiforme complication.

HLA research at present has been carried out by Russell & Schlaut on patients with recurring herpes simplex labialis. Their first studies (50) in 1975 included 90 patients with recurrences at least twice a year. In 1976, Russell (51) extended the studies on herpes simplex Type I by adding 170 new patients (total 260 patients). All of the first 90 patients had humoral and cellular immunity vis-à-vis the herpetic virus. Russell found these same patients to have an increased frequency of HLA-A1. Other modifications of antigenic distributions were noted, such as an increase of HLA-A29 and an increase in HLA-B8 which they attributed to linkage disequilibrium between A1 and B8. These re-sults are confirmed in Russell's additional 1976 studies.

These modifications of antigenic distribution pertain only to herpes simplex virus (HSV) Type I. Recent studies on the recurring genital herpes infections (HSV-Type II) by Dostal (52) do not show any significant difference in antigenic distribution between 36 patients and 450 healthy controls. Finally, in studies on 42 patients with cancer of the cervix of the uterus, an increase in HLA-BW15 was found in 29 % of these patients compared with 10 % of the controls. This study does not bring any supplementary information on the encogenicity of the herpetic virus, since the patients with recurrent herpes genitalis, who were seroepidermiologically determined to have a higher risk of developing cervical carcinoma, showed no significant difference in their HLA-serum-determined antigen frequencies in comparison with the controls and the patients with cervical cancer.

Scleroderma: Progressive systemic sclerosis

Scleroderma is a peculiar induration of the skin caused by sclerosis of the dermis and atrophy of the epidermis. Progressive systemic sclerosis (P.S.S.) includes the skin lesions, vascular and visceral disorders. There are two main clinical types of P.S.S. – acroscleroderma (acrosclerosis) which includes 90–95 % of the cases, and diffuse scleroderma which includes about 5–10 %.

It is difficult to estimate its frequency. An average of 2.7 new cases are described per year per million inhabitants. Females in the fourth decade are more often afflicted (70–80 % of the cases). The incidence is the same in all races. Antinuclear antibodies are detected by immunofluorescence in more than 50 % of scleroderma. Their titer is usually low with speckled appearance, but the pathologic mechanism is very imprecise. The alteration of the connective tissue includes on one hand an increase in collagen synthesis very distinctive in the skin, and on the other hand vascular alteration, especially in the viscera. An autoimmune mechanism has been proposed because of the various antibodies detected and particularly because of the aspect of the antinuclear antibodies.

On the basis of clinical, immunological and histological evidence a single entity called "mixed connective-tissue disorders" has been suggested to unite discoid and systemic lupus erythematosus (S.L.E.), systemic sclerosis, morphea, polyarthritis nodosa, dermatomyositis, rheumatoid arthritis and Sjögren's Syndrome. This concept has not met with universal approval. No sign of unity is apparent when the distribution pattern of A- and B-locus are considered in some of these diseases. Also, there is very little evidence that there is any really significant association with any of the forms of scleroderma and the HLA system (53, 54, 55, 56, 57, 58).

Sjögren's syndrome (Ss)

This disorder of unknown etiology and pathogenesis has a variable clinical picture. The most obvious features are dryness and atrophy of the conjunctiva and cornea, a dry mouth caused by the destruction of the lacrymal and the salivary glands, and a dry skin. The onset occurs from the fourth decade on. Ninety-five percent of the patients are female. Many of the patients have rheumatoid arthritis and, less often, connective-tissues disorders.

An autoimmune etiology has been proposed on account of antinuclear factors and precipiating antibodies in the serum, together with the sex predominance and age distribution. Pathological signs are also suggestive. The exocrine glands are infiltrated by lymphocytes (mostly B cells) and plasma cells; the proliferation in connective tissue is followed by fibrosis. The changes in the salivary glands are similar to those of the thyroid in Hashmoto's disease. Finally, an animal model analogous to Sjögren's syndrome (Ss) has been provided by Kessler (59) with New Zealand Black X White F1 hybrid mice.

Two independent studies by Gerschwin et al. (60) and Ivanyi et al. (61) totaling 60 Caucasoid patients have revealed a highly significant correlation with B8. Both authors have developed arguments to emphasize the autoimmune etiology and the role of sex hormones. Rheumatoid factor was found in 33 % of Ivanyi's patients and its presence was not associated with B8.

Patients suffering from Ss with rheumatoid arthritis were HLA-B8-negative, which would indicate a different form of the disease. In contrast to these concordant studies, Sturrock et al. (62) found no altered HLA pattern in 21 patients' which may be explained by less strict criteria of clinical diagnosis. However, when patients had only the Sicca syndrome without arthritis, HLA-B8 and DW3 associations were significant.

Discoid lupus erythematosus (D. L. E.)

Systemis lupus erythematosus (S.L.E.) will be covered in the chapter on Immunopathology. However, the authors present one interesting report on discoid lupus erythematosus (D.L.E.) by Millard et al. (63).

A study of histocompatibility (HLA) antigens in 66 patients with D.L.E. showed an increased incidence of HLA-B7 and HLA-B8 related to the age at onset and sex of the patient. Female patients with S.L.E. at all ages of onset showed a significant association with HLA-B8. Female patients, with onset between 15 and 39 years of age, with either S.L.E. or D.L.E. which has transformed to S.L.E., showed a significant increase in HLA-B8 compared with the

136

group of females with the same age at onset who had only the discoid disease. The presence of HLA-B8 in a young female with D.L.E. may then represent a risk factor for the development of the systemic disease; and HLA-B7 may decrease the risk or protect the patient with D.L.E. from S.L.E.

Leprosy

Leprosy is an infectious, relatively non-contagious disease due to mycobacterium leprae (M.L.) which enters the body through the skin or the respiratory tract.

Immune factors are important to consider in leprosy. Although leprosy is caused by a single agent (M.L.), the host response can vary from good defense with strong cell-mediated immunity (CMI) as in tuberculoid leprosy (T.L.) to very poor defense with suppressed CMI coupled with high serum antibody production to the antigen (M.L.). Also, this end of the spectrum can be further complicated by Type III immune-complex disease including cutaneous vasculitis (erythema nodosum leprosum), glomerulonephritis, arthritis, uveitis, etc.. Cellular defense against the disease is demonstrated by the reaction of Mitsuda. The antigen, Lepromin, is a crushed preparation of lepromatous nodules rich in bacilli. When injected intradermally this antigen gives rise to the reaction of Mitsuda, a delayed reaction appearing after 20 days. In a leprous environment, the reaction is positive in normal individuals and in patients afflicted with T.L. It is negative in lepromatous leprosy (L.L.) and more or less positive in intermediate forms. Only the two polar forms, T.L. and L.L. constitute well-characterized entities on clinical, bacteriological and immunological criteria.

There is no clear picture of HLA-antigen association in leprosy, even when the two clinical forms are separated. For one thing, the studies conducted so far have been run in various ethnic groups often of mixed origin so that for obvious reasons of antigen divergence the conclusions reached in one racial group cannot be applied to another. In many studies the number of patients investigated was small. This material was reduced further when the group was split according to the clinical types.

Escobar-Gutierez (64) reported an increase of A2 in patients of Hispano-indian origin from Mexico. In Amhara patients from Ethiopia, a mixed group of Caucasoid-negroid descent, Thorsby et al. (65) found no difference with the antigen frequencies of a control group. However, BW21 was present only in leprous patients (tuberculoid and lepromatous)and not in the controls. This antigen has a low frequency in African negroid populations. The authors stress that this finding should be interpreted with caution.

Dasgupta (66) in India and Reis (67) in Brazil found no statistical antigenic divergence. The ethnic origin of the patients is not clearly defined. Later Dasgupta (68) typed for the A and B loci in leprosy patients in an area where the disease is endemic. Again, though no statistical differences in the antigen frequencies were noted between the patients and the same ethnic controls, the frequency of HLA-B5 was decreased in both lepromatous (L.L.) and non-L.L. patients. Also, there was a decreased frequency of HLA-A9 in the non-L.L. patients (27 %) compared with the L.L. group (68 %).

In the only study undertaken on Cau-

137

casoids, Kreisler (69) reported a significant increase of B14 frequency in leprosy patients from Spain. The percentage of B14 was higher in the L.L. group.

Interesting findings were reported by Smith (70) in Filipino patients from Cebu. There was an increase in A10 in the lepromatous group compared with normals, and B5 was present in 16 % of tuberculoid patients. The importance of the control population is well outlined in this study where a Filipino population originally from the Luzon area and presently living in San Francisco had a different HLA pattern from the normal population of Cebu.

de Vries *et al.* (71) of the Netherlands studied infected Sumatran families. When two or more siblings had the same type of disease (T.L., L.L., borderline) they also shared an HLA haplotype more often than expected. The results were interpreted by the authors to indicate that at least two genes are involved, one coding for susceptibility to the infection and the other coding for the type of leprosy; the latter may be linked to the HLA complex.

One reason for the lack of association with certain HLA determinants among unrelated individuals with leprosy is that the bacillus may carry many different anitgenic determinants. Several Ir genes may therefore be involved which are non-randomly associated to different HLA genes. The possible influence of HLA-linked genetic fectors, in diseases involving multispecific immune responses, may only be revealed through family studies, which emphasizes the importance of the approach followed by de Vries *et al.*

Atopic dermatitis

Classical studies in clinical allergy have shown atopic diseases in successive generations of families. Atopy and atopic dermatitis, particularly the clinical reactions associated with Type I allergic diseases such as allergic rhinitis (hay fever) and asthma, will be discussed in the chapter on Allergology. Most of the significant studies with the HLA system have been made showing associations with this type of patient responders. Specific IgE-antibody responses to specific allergens are clearly responsible for many of the clinical manifestations of allergic hayfever and asthma. The role of these in atopic dermatitis is not so clearly understood. The pathogenesis of the eczematous or dermatitis component of atopy is more complex and as yet not extensively studied for HLA-system associations. The few studies that have been reported do not agree and as yet give no clues for the etiology, mechanism, diagnosis, treatment, or prognosis of atopic dermatitis.

In a preliminary study of 45 American Caucasian patients with atopic dermatitis, Krain & Terasaki (72, 73) showed an increased frequency of HLA -A3 and -A9. Tsuji *et al.* (74) found an increased frequency of HLA-B5 in 50 Japanese with atopic dermatitis. In France, Goudemand *et al.* (75) typed 27 unrelated children with atopic dermatitis (11 of whom also had asthma). HLA-BW35 was significantly increased. The families of 23 of the children were then studied allowing typing of 44 parents (33 healthy, 8 with atopic dermatitis, 2 with atopic dermatitis and asthma, and 1 with asthma). Only the increased frequency of BW35 remained significant. Segregation analysis of HLA antigens was processed in these 23 families listing separately the 33 patients and 24 of their first-degree relatives.

The distribution of the HLA antigens was not significantly disturbed, although BW35 was more frequent among the patients than would theoretically be expected considering the HLA phenotypes of the parents.

It is noteworthy that results obtained by Krain and coworkers indicate an increased frequency of A-loci determinants (A3 and A9) and not of B- and D-loci determinants. Associations reported with other forms of atopy are to B-locus determinants (e.g. HLA-B7 for the ragweed RA5 allergen and HLA-B8 for the rye grass allergen (76, 77)). The Tsuji and Goudemand studies both show significant increased frequencies of the B-locus determinants (B5 and BW35, respectively). At any rate the Goudemand study, showing a significant increased frequency of BW35 among both the unrelated patients and their parents, helps to confirm the hereditary nature of atopic dermatitis and might indicate an influence of an HLA-linked Ir gene. However, much work needs to be done, particularly associating determinants of the HLA-L locus with flares and remissions of the dermatitis, as well as with specific etiologic allergens, since patients with severe atopic dermatitis have been shown to have *in vivo* and *in vitro* T-cell-activity suppression as well as a decrease in chemotaxis and cell migration of all leukocytes (neutrophils, macrophages and lymphocytes).

Vitiligo

Vitiligo is a leukoderma. Decreased pigmentation of the skin can result from absence of melanocytes, production of abnormal melanosomes, and distrubances in transfer of melanosomes from melanocytes to epidermal cells. In vitiligo the melanocytes are apparently absent (78). Its pathogenicity is controversial. Both sexes are affected. The average age of onset is about 25. The incidence is about 1 % in Caucasoids. The genetic aspects of vitiligo are well established. It is believed to be an autosomal dominant trait with incomplete penetrance. A history of the disease in families of vitiligo patients was found in 35 % of 430 patients (79). Vitiligo occurs in about 6 % of thyrotoxic patients. The occurrence of biological signs of autoimmunity, antithyroid in particular, has been claimed but not uniformly accepted. No specific or constant biological marker is characteristic of this skin disease.

In the study of Retornaz *et al.* on 90 vitiligo patients, there was no correlation between HLA-A- and -B-antigen frequency and various etiological and clinical criteria (78). A non-significant increase of B12 was noted for vitiligo appearing before the age of 25.

In the families investigated, no haplotype appeared to be correlated with the skin disease; however, there was a significant correlation between B13 and vitiligo with antithyroid antibodies in 13 patients. There was no correlation for any antigen in 44 patients without antithyroid antibodies.

Alopecia areata

This type of hair loss is benign though the esthetic prejudice may be important. It represents about 2–3 % of dermatological outpatients in Europe. It may be more common in mongoloids and less common in negroids. The primary patch may start anywhere, but is usually appears on the scalp. It is clearly circumscribed and often rounded. The skin is smooth and devoid of hair. The prognosis is uncertain; relapses are frequent, and complete recovery from total alopecia is unusual. The pathogenesis is uncertain, but alopecia areata is thought to be autoimmune in origin because it is found commonly in association with other similar disorders such as Hashimoto thyroiditis, pernicious anemia, adrenal insufficiency and vitiligo.

Knutz (80) typed 70 patients from Austria and found a non-significant increase of B8. However, in Finland, Kianto et al. (81) observed a significant increase of B12 in 47 patients. The ages of the patients are not mentioned, but some analogy can be made with the increase of B12 in patients afflicted with vitiligo before age 25.

Acne conglobata

Acne conglobata is a chronic suppurative variant of acne vulgaris characterized by burrowing abscesses and irregular scarring. Males are predominantly affected between the ages of 18 and 30. The bacterial flora are not different from those found in acne. The localization of the lesions is characteristic not only on the face but also on the neck, the axillae, the inferior parts of the limbs, the trunk, the perianal region and the perineovulvar region, i.e. in areas not involved in ordinary acne. Inflammatory nodules form, increase in size and break down to discharge oily pus. The condition is persistent. The healing of some abscesses is followed by cheloidal scars, while others may remain active. The etiology and pathogenesis are obscure. The disease may occur in many generations of a family, but the mode of transmission is unknown.

A study by Schackert et al. (82) on 65 patients could not define any association pattern with HLA-A and -B antigens. The author has also typed 156 relatives, but the results were not given.

Lichen planus

Lichen planus is a disease of adults with specific clinical and histopathologic characteristics. Its pathogenesis is unknown. Although it is a common skin disease, very little research has been done between lichen planus and the histocompatibility system because of the rarity of familial forms. The studies carried out so far are those of Lowe et al. (83) in 1975 and Saurat et al. (84). Lowe found an incidence of HLA-B5 in 49 patients. The antigen B5 was also found six times in 15 patients who had diabetes mellitus associated with their lichen planus. Saurat did not find any significant modification of the antigenic distribution in 43 patients with lichen planus.

At this time, no significant correlation has been definitively established between the HLA system and lichen planus. These two studies found an increase in HLA-B5 but are not yet significant. More work needs to be done to confirm these findings in the future. It will also be interesting to study the modifications of the antigenic distribution of patients with lichen nitidus and lichen pigmentogene. In effect, if the autogenic distribution is the same in lichen nitidus as it is in lichen planus, this would permit more confirmation that lichen nitidus is a variant of lichen planus, which is generally agreed. The same holds for lichen pigmentogene whose histology is not always typical.

Mycosis fungoides

Mycosis fungoides (M.F.) is a slowly evolving T-cell neoplasm that is primary in the skin. Dick *et al.* (85) examined 15 patients with histologically proven early stages of M.F. A high frequency of HL-B8 and a surprisingly high frequency of antigens of the W19 complex, in particular of AW31 and AW32 together, comprised 40 % of the A-series antigens in the group.

Keloids and hypertrophic scars

Laurentaci (86) studied 25 patients with keloids and hypertrophic scars and found an increased frequency of HLA-B14. If confirmed, these findings may be of help in predicting those presurgical patients and traumatic and burn-injured patients who may be predisposed to develop keloid and hypertrophic scars. Preventive therapy may be possible.

Miscellaneous diseases

It is always reasonable to study patients or families who have known hereditary diseases for any HLA associations. This has been done. The following list gives those with negative reults (no significant associations):

Epidermolysis bullosus simplex (87)
Xeroderma pigmentosa (88)
Ehlers-Danlos syndrome (89)
Hailey and Hailey disease (90)

Summary

The association of the HLA system with diseases of the skin is a new and exciting aspect of dermatology which already shows promise of being of practical value to clinicians and investigators.

Prognosis and preventive medicine is enchanced by the new HLA information in many instances. Psoriasis itself and psoriasis with or without arthritis are good examples. Also, young women with discoid lupus erythematosus may be protected from the systemic disease (S.L.E.) if they carry HLA-B7, but may be more susceptible to S.L.E. with B-8.

Diseases that may be confused clinically at different stages such as dermatitis herpetiformis, bullous pemphigoid, pemphigus vulgaris, Behcet's disease, recurrent oral ulcerations and even recurring herpes simplex labialis have different HLA associations thus giving the clinician yet another diagnostic tool to help separate the diseases.

There is also increasing evidence that perhaps different events in the same disease are controlled by different genes, one of which is in the HLA supergene and others on some other chromosome. Atopy is a good example where antigen specificity of the IgE antibody may be under HLA control, but the amount of IgE antibody produced must be on another chromosome. The same may hold true for leprosy where the infectiousness of the individual is under one control, but the type of leprosy once the person is affected is under another. Perhaps other examples of this are psoriasis vulgaris and pustular psoriasis.

The laboratory scientists also benefit. For example, the new HLA information may give the psoriasis investigators new ways to approach the control of the abnormal DNA synthesis in that disease; and, the HLA scientists can look more carefully at properdin Factor B antigen (Bf) in dermatitis herpetiformis since the alternative pathway of the complement system is involved in that disease.

And finally, there are diseases which the clinician knows to be familial but have no known HLA associations. Thus, geneticists and dermatologists must look elsewhere: e.g. acne conglobata, epidermolysis bullosa simplex, xeroderma pigmentosa, Ehlers-Danlos syndrome, Hailey and Hailey disease.

This beginning era of "HLA and Disease" is adding new dimensions of understanding and inquisitiveness to the specialty of dermatology. Close interactions with the HLA scientists promises to increase and be rewarding to all investigators, and through them to the patient.

TABLE I

HLA and dermatologic diseases

Disease	No. of studies	HLA	Patients %	(N)	Controls %	(N)	Rel. risk	*Significance
Psoriasis	8 π	B13	5–27	(851)	1–15	(2692)	2.87	<1 E-10
unspecified	8 π	BW17	8–50	(851)	1–26	(2692)	3.62	<1 E-10
	2 π	BW16	11–22	(555)	3–5	(555)	4.24	2, 1 E-06
Psoriasis	6 π	B13	2–33	(466)	2–8	(4849)	4.65	<1 E-10
vulgaris	6 π	BW17	12–36	(466)	4–11	(4849)	4.90	<1 E-10
	3 π	BW37	4–16	(220)	1–3	(1029)	6.35	7, 3 E-08
Psoriasis	2 π	B13	0–6	(47)	4–8	(1867)	.73	p>05
pustulosa	2 π	BW17	3–13	(47)	4–8	(1867)	1.60	p>05

* Significance is given as p value. Most p values are given in floating-point notation; e.g. p = 3.0 E–06 means p = 3.0×10^{-6}. No p values have been multiplied with the number of comparisons.

π HLA and Disease Registry (A. Svejgaard, L. P. Ryder – 1976).

Disease	First author	Racial group	HLA	Patients %	(N)	Controls %	(N)	Rel. risk	*Significanc
Psoriasis vulgaris	Ohkido 1976	Mongoloid (Japan)	A1	16.6	(54)	1.5	(66)	1.3	
			B37	20.4	(54)	4.5	(66)	5.37	
	Hoshino 1976	Mongoloid (Japan)	A1, A10	?	(19)	?	(1733)	?	p<0.0
			B13, BW40	?	(19)	?	(1733)	?	
	Stenszky 1976	Caucasoid (Hungary)	B13	33.7	(157)	8.6	(450)	5.37	5.0E–05
			BW17	28.6	(157)	9.7	(450)	3.71	5.0E–05
	Jajic	Caucasoid (Yugoslavia)	B13	15.8	(51)	7.3	(302)	1.4	
			BW17	42	(51)	8.3	(302)	8.1	
	Grosse-Wilde 1976	Caucasoid (W German)	DW2	31	(68)	14	(150)	2.74	
			E1	23	(68)	8	(150)	3.54	
Dermatitis Herpeti-formis	Katz 1972	Caucasoid (USA	B8	58	(26)	24	(251)		
	White 1973	Caucasoid (Scotland)	B8	60	(35)	33	(175)		
	Gebhard 1973	Caucasoid (USA+GB)	B8	68	(28)	17-30	(?)		
	Gebhard 1974	Caucasoid (USA)	B8	53	(15)	20	(350)		
	Seah 1976	Caucasoid (GB)	B8	79	(38)	26	(180)		
	Reunala 1976	Caucasoid (Finland)	B8	87	(61)	17	(326)		
	Solheim 1976	Caucasoid (Norway)	B8	79	(34)	25	(1628)		
			DW3	75	(20)	19	(136)		
	Thomsen	Caucasoid (GB)		85	(40)	24	(1967)	18.2	1E–10
			DW3	92.5	(40)	20	(157)	50.1	7.5E–18
			LD 12A	25	(40)	8	(157)	3.7	6.2E–3
	Svejgaard WHO Reg	Caucasoid	B8	24-87	(469)	17-58	(3371)	5.92	1E–10
Bullous Pemphigoi	Retornaz 1976	Caucasoid (France)	None		(20)		(341)		
	Ahmed	Caucasoid (USA)	None		(19)		(60)		
Pemphigu vulgaris	Katz 1973	Caucasoid (USA)	B13	28	(18)	4	(251)	9.37	1.49E
	Krain 1973	Jewish (USA)	A10	61	(28)	20	(94)	5.89	8.29E–05
		Non-Jewish	None	(49)	(870)				
	Hoshino	Mongoloid (Japan)	A10	?	(19)	?	(1733)	?	1E–03?

Disease	No. of studies	Racial group	HLA	Patients %	(N)	Controls %	(N)	Rel. risk	*Significanc
Behcet's Disease	3 π	Caucasoid	B5	18–26	(37)	9–17	(1052)	4.29	8.1 E–05
	1 π	Caucasoid	B18	9–9	(22)	1–1	(700)	13.03	4.0 E–04
	1 π	Caucasoid	B27	27–27	(22)	8–8	(700)	4.77	9.1 E–04
	1 π	Mongoloid	B5	75	(44)	30–8	(78)	6.75	2.38 E–06

Disease	Author	Racial group	HLA	Patients %	(N)	Controls %	(N)	Rel. risk	*Significanc
Behcet's	Godeau France	Caucasoid	B5	54	(39)	13	(591)	7.9	1 E–10
	Ersoy 1976	? (Turkey)	B5	85	(26)	25	(138)	16.8	
	Hoshino 1976	Mongoloid (Japan)	B5	?	(158)	?	(1733)		1 E–10
	Nakawaga 1976	Mongoloid (Japan)	B5	67	(45)	?	(114)	3.17	3 E–04
	Tsuji 1976	Mongoloan (Japan)	B5		(158)				<1 E–03
	Jung 1976	None			(10)				
Recurrent Oral Ulcreation	Challa- combe 1976	Caucasoid (England)	B12	43	(100)	22	(100)	2.67	p=0.0015
Recurrent Herpes Simplex Labialis	Russell 1975	Caucasoid (Canada)	A1 B8	55.5 33.3	(90) (90)	25 16.9	(606)		1.31 E–08 3.38 E–04
	Russell 1976		A1	50.1	(170)	25	(606)		p<0.001
Leprosy	Thorsby 1973	Cauc. Negr. (Ethiopia)	BW21 BW21	T.L.25 L.L.26	(90) (19)	0	(36)		1.5 E–03
	Escobar- Guttierez 1973	Hispano- Indians (Mexico)	A2 A3	28 20	(50) (50)	68 44	(200) (200)		
	Dasgupta 1974	? (India)	None	T.L. LL.	(30) (40)		(40)		
	Reis	? (Brazil)	None	T.L. LL.	(13) (13)				
	Kreisler 1974	Caucasoid (Spain)	BW14	T.L.7 L.L.35	(13) (17)	4	(149)	7.2	2 E–03 (T.L. and L.]
	Smith 1975	Mongoloid (Filipino)	None	T.L. L.L.	(44) (38)				
	Krain 1973	Caucasoid (USA)	A3 A9	33 33	(45)	19 21	(870)		p<0.05 p<0.05
Vitiligo	Retornaz	Caucasoid	None		(90)		(341)		
V+Anti- thyroid Antibodies			B13	30.8	(13)	4.1	(341)	10.3	4 E–04
Alopecia Areata	Kuntz 1976	Caucasoid (Austral.)	None		(70)		(1142)		
	Kianto 1976	Caucasoid (Finland)	B12	38	(47)	15	(326)	3.46	8 E–05
Mycosis Fungoides	Dick 1976	Caucasoid (Scotland)	B8 AW31	46.6	(15) (15)				
Keloids & Hypertro- phic Scars	Laurentaci 1976	Caucasoid (Italy)	B14 BW16	25 31	(40)	4 6	(131)	6.30 4.85	p<0.01

References

1. Ryder, L. P. & Svejgaard, A. (1976) Associations between HLA and Disease. Report from the *HLA and Disease Registry of Copenhagen, 1976.* The HLA and Disease Registry of Copenhagen (sponsored by WHO). Tissue-Typing Laboratory of the Blood-grouping Department, Rigshospitalet of Copenhagen, Blegdamsvej 9, DK-2100, Copenhagen Ø.

2. Dausset, J., Degos, L. & Hors, J. (1974) The association of HL-A antigens with diseases. *Clin. Immunol. and Immunopath.* **3**, 127–249.

3. Svejgaard, A., Platz, P., Ryder, L. P. & Nielsen, L. S. (1975) HL-A and Disease Associations. *Transplant. Rev.* **22**, 3–43.

4. Terasaki, P. I. & Mickey, M. R. (1975) HL-A haplotypes of 32 diseases. *Transplant. Rev.* **22**, 105–119.

5. Shrank, A. B. & Harman, R. R. M. (1966) The incidence of skin diseases in a Nigerian teaching hospital. *Brit. J. Dermatol.* **78**, 235.

6. Ohkido, M., Ozawa, A., Matsuo, I., Niizuma, K., Nakano, M., Tsuji, K., Nose, Y., Ito, M., Sugai, T. & Yasuda, T. (1976) HLA and Ia antigens and susceptibility to Psoriasis Vulgaris (abstract and manuscript). *1st Int. Symp. on HLA and Disease,* Paris, June 23–25.

7. Gross-Wilde, H., Wüstner, B., Albert, E. D., Kuntz, B., Netzel, B., Scholz, S. & Braun-Falco, O. (1976) Frequency of seven HLA-D alleles in psoriasis patients (abstract). *1st Int. Symp. on HLA and Disease,* Paris, June 23–25.

8. Karvonen, J. (1975) HLA antigens in psoriasis with special reference to the clinical type, age of onset, exacerbations after respiratory infections and occurrence of arthritis. *Ann. Clin. Res.* **7**, 301.

9. Krain, L. S., Newcomber, V. D. & Terasaki, P. I. (1973) HL-A antigen in psoriasis. *New Eng. J. Med.* **288**, 145.

10. Bertrams, J., Lattke, C. & Kuwert, E. (1974) Correlations of antistreptolysin-O titre to HLA-B13 in psoriasis. *New Eng. J. Med.* **291**, 631.

11. Karvonen, J., Tiilikainen, A. & Lassus, A. (1976) HLA antigens in psoriasis: a family study. *Ann. Clin. Res.,* (in press).

12. Civatte, J., Ganas, P., Lazarovici, C., Leon, S., Schmid, M., Reboul, M., Hors, J. & Dausset, J. (1976) HLA Genotypes in familial psoriasis. *1st Int. Symp. on HLA and Disease,* Paris, June 23–25.

13. Marcusson, J., Möller, E. & Thyresson, H. (1976) Genetic association of skin and/or point manifestations of disease in families with a high incidence of psoriasis (abstract). *1st Int. Symp. on HLA and Disease,* Paris, June 23–25.

14. Marcusson, J., Möller, E. & Thyresson, H. (1976) Penetration of HLA-linked psoriasis predisposing genes: a family investigation. *Acta Dermatovner,* (in press).

15. Karvonen, J., Tiilikainen, A. & Lassus, A. (1975) HLA antigens in patients with persistent palmoplantar pustulosis and pustular psoriasis. *Ann. Clin. Res.* **7**, 112.

16. Zachariae, H. (1976) Significance of the pustular reaction in psoriasis. *2nd Int. Symp. on Psoriasis,* Stanford, California, July 12–15.

17. Svejgaard, A., Hauge, M., Jersild, C., Platz, P., Ryder, L. P., Staub-Nielson, L. & Thomsen, M. (1975) The HLA system. In: *Monographs in human genetics,* No. 7, pp. 64–65, eds. Beckman, L. & Hauge, M., S. Karger, Basel.

18. Katz, S. I., Falchuk, Z. M., Dahl, M. V., Rogentine, G. N. & Strober, W. (1972) HL-A8: a genetic link between dermatitis herpetiformis and gluten sensitive enteropathy. *J. Clin. Invest.* **51**, 11, 2977–2980.

19. White, A. G., Barnetson, R. St. C., Da Costa, Jag. & McClelland, D. B. L. (1973) The incidence of HL-A antigens in dermatitis herpetiformis. *Brit. J. Dermatol.* **89**, 133–136.

20. Gebhard, R. L., Katz, S. I., Marks, J., Shuster, S., Trapani, R. J., Rogentine, G. N. & Strober, W. (1973) HL-A antigen type and small-intestinal disease in dermatitis herpetiformis. *Lancet* **ii**, 760–762.

21. Gebhard, R. L., Falchuk, Z. M., Katz, S. I., Sessoms, C., Rogentine, G. N. & Strober, W. (1974) Dermatitis herpetiformis, immunologic concomitants of small intestinal disease and relationship to histocompatibility antigen HL-A8. *J. Clin. Invest.* **54**, 1, 98–103.

22. Seah, P. P., Fry, L., Kearney, J. W., Campbell, E., Mowbray, J. F., Stewart, J. S. & Hoffbrand, A. V. (1976) A comparison of histocompatibility antigen in dermatitis herpetiformis and adult coeliac disease. *Brit. J. Dermatol.* **94**, 131–138.

23. Reunala, T., Salo, O. P., Tiilikainen, A. & Mattila, M. J. (1976) Histocompatibility antigens and dermatitis herpetiformis with special reference to jejunal abnormalities and acetylator phenotype. *Brit. J. Dermatol.* **94**, 139–143.

24. Solheim, B. G., Ek, J., Thune, P. O., Baklien, K., Bratlie, A., Rankin, B., Thoresen, A. B. & Thorsby, E. (1976) *Tissue Antigens, 7,* 57–59.

25. Thomsen, M., Platz, P., Marks, J., Ryder, L. P., Shuster, S., Svejgaard, A. & Young, S. H. (1976) *Tissue Antigens, 7,* 60–62.

26. Solheim, B. G., Albreditsen, D., Thune, P. O. & Thorsby, E. (1976) HLA determinants in dermatitis herpetiformis (abstract). *1st Int. Symp. on HLA and Disease,* Paris, June 23–25.

27. Scott, B. B., Losowski, M. S. & Rajah, S. M. (1974) HLA 8 and HLA 12 in coeliac disease. *Lancet* **ii,** 171.

28. Mann, D. L., Katz, S. I., Nelson, D. L., Abelson, L. D. & Strober, W. (1976) Specific B-cell antigens associated with gluten-sensitive enteropathy and dermatitis herpetiformis. *Lancet* **i,** 110–111.

29. Retornaz, G., Betuel, H. & Thivolet, J. (1976) HLA antigen in bullous pemphigoid (abstract). *1st Int. Symp. on HLA and Disease,* Paris, June 23–25.

30. Ahmed, A. R., Cohen, E., Blumenson, L. E. & Provost, T. T. (1976) HLA in bullous pemphiboid. *Arch. Dermatol.,* (submitted for publication).

31. Katz, S. I., Dahl, M. V., Penneys, N., Trapani, R. J. & Rogentine, N. (1973) HL-A antigens in pemphigus. *Arch. Dermatol.* **108,** July, 53–55.

32. Krain, L. S., Terasaki, P. I., Newcomer, V. D. & Mickey, M. R. (1973) Increased frequency of HLA 10 in pemphigus vulgaris. *Arch. Dermatol.* **108,** 803–805.

33. Hoshino, K., Inouye, H., Unokuchi, M., Ito, N., Tamoaki, N. & Tsuji, K. (1976) HLA and disease in Japanese (abstract). *1st Int. Symp. on HLA and Disease,* Paris, June 23–25.

34. Shimizu, T. (1971) Clinical and immunological studies in Behcet's Syndrome. *Folia Ophthal.* (Japonica) **22,** 801.

35. Ohno, S., Aoki, K., Sugiura, S., Nakayama, S., Itakura, K. & Aizawa, M. (1973) HL-A5 and Behcet's Disease. *Lancet* **ii,** 1383.

36. Ohno, S. (1974) Study on HL-A antigens in Behcet's disease. *Acta Soc. Ophthal. Japonica.* **10,** 78.

37. Ohno, S., Nakayama, E., Sugiura, S., Itakura, K., Aohi, K. & Aizawa, M. (1975) Specific histocompatibility antigens associated with Behcet's disease. *Amer. J. Ophthal.* **80,** 636.

38. Dausset, J. & Hors, J. (1975) Some contributions of the HL-A complex to the genetics of human diseases. *Transplant. Rev.* **22,** 44.

39. Rosselet, E., Saudan, Y. & Jeannet, M. (1976) Recherche antigens HL-A dans la maladie de Behcet. *Ophthalmol.* **172,** 116.

40. Tsuji, K., Hoshino, K., Inouye, H., Unokuchi, T., Ito, M. & Tamoaki, N. (1976) HLA and disease in Japanese (abstract). *1st Int. Symp. on HLA and Disease,* Paris, June 23–25.

41. Nagawa, J., Ikehara, Y., Ito, K. & Fukaze, M. (1976) HLA antigens in various autoimmune and related diseases (abstract). *1st Int. Symp. on HLA and Disease,* Paris, June 23–25.

42. Hoshino, K., Inoye, H., Unokuchi, T., Ito, M., Tamoaki, N. & Tsuji, K. (1976) HLA and disease in Japan (abstract). *1st Int. Symp. on HLA and Disease,* Paris, June 23–25.

43. Ersoy, F., Berkel, A. I., Firat, T. & Kazokoglu, H. (1976) HLA antigens association with Behcet's disease. *1st Int. Symp. on HLA and Disease,* Paris, June 23–25.

44. Godeau, P., Torre, D., Campinchi, R., Bloch-Michel, E., Schmid, M., Nunez-Roldman, A., Hors, J. & Dausset, J. (1976) HLA-B5 and Behcet's disease (abstract). *1st Int. Symp. on HLA and Disease,* Paris, June 23–25.

45. Jung, R. T., Chalmer, T. M. & Joysey, V. C. (1976) HLA in Behcet's disease. *Lancet* i, 694.

46. Ohno, S., Aoki, K., Sugiura, S., Nakayama, E., Itakura, K. & Aizawa, M. (1975) HL-A5 and Behcet's disease. *Lancet* **ii, 1383.**

47. Dolby, A. E. (1975) HLA in recurrent apthone stomatitis. *HLA & Disease Registry,* Copenhagen, Feb. 24.

48. Platz, P., Ryder, L. P. & Donatsky (1976) No deviations of HLA-A and B antigens in patients with recurrent apthous stomatitis. *Acta Pathol. Microbiol. Scand.* Sect. C (in press).

49. Challacombe, S. J., Batchelor, R., Kennedy, L. & Lehner, T. (1976) HLA antigens in recurrent oral ulcreation (abstract). *1st Int. Symp. on HLA and Disease,* Paris, June 23–25.

50. Russell, A. S. & Schlaut, J. (1975) HL-A transplantation antigens in subjects susceptible to recrudescent herpes labialis. *Tissue Antigens* **6,** 257.

51. Russell, A. S. (1976) HLA and herpes simplex virus, type I (abstract). *1st Int. Symp. on HLA and Disease,* Paris, June 23–25.

52. Dostal, V. & Mayr, W. R. (1976) HLA-

SD antigens in cervix cancer and in re-recurrent herpes genitalis patients (abstract). *1st Int. Symp. on HLA and Disease,* Paris, June 23–25.

53. Crouzet, J., Marbach, M. C., Camus, J. P., Godeau, P., Heereman, G., Richier, D., Hors, J. & Dausset, J. (1975) Recherche d'une association entre antigens HL-A et sclèrodermie systèmique. *Nouvelle Presse mèdicale.* 4, 35, 2489–2492.

54. Rabin, B. S., Rodnan, G. P., Bassion, S. & Gillt, J. (1975) HLA antigens in progressive systemic sclerosis. *Arthr. and Rheum.* 18, 381–382.

55. Retornaz, G., Betuel, H. & Thivolet, J. (1976) HLA antigens in progressive systemic sclerosis (abstract). *1st Int. Symp. on HLA and Disease,* Paris, June 23–25.

56. Birbaum, N. S., Rodnan, G. P., Rabin, B. S. & Bassion, S. (1976) Histocompatibility antigens in progressive systemic sclerosis (abstract). *1st Int. Symp. on HLA and Disease,* Paris, June 23–25.

57. Nakawaga, J., Ikehara, Y., Ito, K. & Furkase, M. (1976) HLA antigens in various autoimmune and related diseases (abstract). *1st Int. Symp. on HLA and Disease,* Paris, June 23–25.

58. Seignalet, J. (1972) HLA antigens in rheumatoid arthritis. *Vox Sang,* 23, 468–471.

59. Kessler, H. S. (1968) A laboratory model for Sjögren's syndrome. *Amer. J. Pathol.* 52, 671–685.

60. Gerschwin, M. E., Terasaki, P. I., Graw, R. & Chused, T. M. (1975) Increased frequency of HLA8 in Sjögren's syndrome. *Tissue Antigens* 6, 342–346.

61. Ivanyi, D., Drizhal, I., Erbendva, E., Horejs, J., Salavec, M., Macurova, H., Dostal, C., Balik, J. & Juran, J. (1976) HLA in Sjögren's syndrome. *Tissue Antigens* 7, 45–51.

62. Sturrock, R. D., Canesi, B. A., Dick, H. M. & Dick, W. C. (1974) HLA antigens and the Sicca syndrome. *Ann. Rheum. Dis.* 33, 165–166

63. Millard, L. G., Rowel, N. R. & Rajah, S. M. (1976) Histocompatibility antigens in discoid and systemic lupus erythematosus. *1st Int. Symp. on HLA and Disease,* Paris, June 23–25.

64. Escobar-Gutierrez, A., Gorodezky, C. & Salazar-Mallen, M. (1973) Distribution of some of the HL-A system lymphocyte antigens in Mexicans. II studies in atopics and in lepers. *Vox Sang* 25, 151–155.

65. Thorsby, E., Godal, T. & Myrvang, B.

(1973) HL-A antigens and susceptibility to disease II leprosy. *Tissue Antigens* 3, 373–377.

66. Dasgupta, A., Mehra, N. K., Ghei, S. K. & Vaidya, M. C. (1975) Histocompatibility antigens (HL-A) in leprosy. *Tissue Antigens* 5, 2, 85–87.

67. Reis, A. P., Maia, F., Reis, V. F., Andrade, I. M. & Campos, A. A. S. (1974) HL-A antigens in leprosy. *Lancet* ii, 1384.

68. Mehra, N. K., Dasgupta, A., Ghei, S. K. & Vaidya, M. C. (1976) Histocompatibility antigens in leprosy (abstract). *1st Int. Symp. on HLA and Disease,* Paris, June 23–25.

69. Kreisler, M., Arnaiz, A., Perez, B., Cruz, E. F. & Bootello, A. (1974) HL-A antigens in leprosy. *Tissue Antigens* 4, 3, 197–201.

70. Smith, G. S., Walford, R. L., Shepard, C. C. & Payne, R. (1975) Histocompatibility antigens in leprosy. *Vox Sang* 28, 42–49.

71. de Vries (1976) HLA in Sumatran families with leprosy (Poster) *1st Int. Symp. on HLA and Disease,* Paris, June 23–25.

72. Krain, L. S. & Terasaki, P. (1973) HL-A antigens in atopic dermatitis. *Lancet* i, 1059.

73. Krain, L. S. (1974) Histocompatibility antigens: a laboratory and epidemiologic tool. *J. Invest. Dermat.* 62, 67.

74. Tsuji, J., Hoshino, K., Inouye, H., Unokuchi, T., Ito, M. & Tamaoki, N. (1976) HLA and disease in Japanese. *1st Int. Symp. on HLA and Disease,* Paris, June 23–25.

75. Goudemand, J., Deffrenne, C. L. & Desmons, F. HLA and atopic dermatitis (1976) *1st Int. Symp. on HLA and Disease,* Paris, June 23–25.

76. Marsh, D. B. (1973) Allergology. *Proc. of 8th Congress of the International Assoc. of Allergology,* Tokyo, Oct. 14–20.

77. Levine, B. B., Stember, R. H. & Fotino, M. (1972) Ragweed hayfever: genetic control and linkage to HLA haplotypes. *Science* 178, 1201.

78. Retornaz, G., Betuel, H., Ortonne, J. P. & Thivolet, J. (1976) HLA antigens and vitiligo. *Brit. J. Dermatol.,* (accepted for publication).

79. Fitzpatrick, T. B. & Mihm, M. C., Jr. (1971) Abnormalities of th emelanin pigmentary system. In: *Dermatology in General Medicine,* eds. Fitzpatrick, T., Ahndt, K. A., Clark, W. H., Jr., Eisen, A. Z., Van Scott, E. J., Vaughan, J. H., p. 1615. McGraw Hill Book Co., New York.

80. Kuntz, B., Selzle, D., Braun-Falco, O., Scholz, S. & Albert, E. D. (1976) HLA antigens in alopecia areata (abstract). *1st Int. Symp. on HLA and Disease,* Paris, June 23–25.

81. Kianto, U., Reunala, T., Karvonen, J., Lassus, A. & Tiilikainen, A. (1976) HLA antigens in alopecia areata (abstract). *1st Int. Symp. on HLA and Disease,* Paris, June 23–25.

82. Schackert, K., Scholz, S., Steinbauer, Rosenthal, I., Albert, E. D., Wank, R. & Plewig, G. HL-A antigens in acne conglobata: a negative study. *Arch. Dermatol.* **110,** 468.

83. Lowe, N. J. & Cudworth, A. G. (1975) Lichen planus: investigation of carbohydrate metabolism and the HL-A system. *Brit. J. Dermatol.* **93,** suppl., 11–18.

84. Saurat, J. H., Cosne, A., Puissant, A., Nunez-Roldan, A. & Hors, J. (1976) HL-A A and B marker in lichen planus (abstract). *1st Int. Symp. on HLA and Disease,* Paris, June 23–25.

85. Dick, H. M., Mackie, R. & De Sousa, M. B. (1976) HLA and mycosis fungoides (abstract). *1st Int. Symp. on HLA and Disease,* Paris, June 23–25.

86. Lauretnaci, G. & Dioguardi, D. (1976) HLA antigens in keloids and hypertrophic scars (abstract). *1st Int. Symp. on HLA and Disease,* Paris, June 23–25.

87. Noble, J. P., Dupré-Dérens, F. & Hewitt, J. (1973) Absence of linkage between simple bullous epidermolysis and serum red cell, white cell and platelet groups. *Ann. de Dermatologie et de Syphilographie* **100,** 275.

88. Degos, L., Beth, E., Garbi, R., Day, N., Dastot, H., Rebont, M., Schmid, M. & Giraldo, G. (1976) HLA antigens in 16 families with xeroderma pigmentosa (abstract). *1st Int. Symp. on HLA and Disease,* Paris, June 23–25.

89. Mercier, P. & Zini, G. (1976) Ehlers-Danlas syndrome and HLA haplotype (abstract). *1st Int. Symp. on HLA and Disease,* Paris, June 23–25.

90. Karvonen, J. & Tiilikainen, A. (1976) HLA antigens in Haily-Haily's disease (abstract). *1st Int. Symp. on HLA and Disease,* Paris, June 23–25.

HLA and Endocrine Diseases

J. Nerup[1], Cr. Cathelineau[2], J. Seignalet[3] & M. Thomsen[4]

The family of organ-specific autoimmune diseases (Table I) consists main-

TABLE I

The organ-specific autoimmune diseases. Pernicious anaemia is described on page 181.

IDIOPATHIC ADDISON's DISEASE
GRAVES' DISEASE
PRIMARY MYXEDEMA
HASHIMOTO's THYROIDITIS
INSULIN-DEPENDENT DIABETES
  MELLITUS
HYPERGONADOTROPIC HYPOGO-
  NADISM
IDIOPATHIC HYPOPARATHYROIDISM
(PERNICIOUS ANAEMIA)

ly of endocrine disorders. These autoimmune endocrinopathies have clinical, pathological and immunological featur-

es in common (1). More often than should be expected by chance alone they occur in clinical combination syndromes. The typical pathological lesion in the endocrine glands is a lymphocytic infiltration together with a selective destruction of the hormone-producing epithelial cells, although in the case of Graves' disease the thyroid hormone-producing epithelium is hypertrophied. Autoantibodies and cell-mediated autoimmunity against organ-specific subcellular antigenic components in the cytoplasm of the secreting cells are often found.

Thus, there was ample reason to look for a common genetic factor for susceptibility for these diseases and it is the purpose of this chapter to review the relevant literature dealing with this question.

Diabetes mellitus

Data to suggest that the term diabetes mellitus should be used rather as a label for a heterogenous group of diseases characterized by hyperglycemia and glucosuria than as a name of a well-defined disease entity have accumulated during recent years (2). On the basis of clinical, biochemical, immunological and pathological findings, and data from family studies, at least five nosologically different types of diabetes mellitus can be distinguished (Table II).

[1] Steno Memorial Hospital, DK - 2820 Gentofte, Denmark.
[2] Hôpital St.-Louis, 2 Place du dr Fournier, 25010 Paris, France.
[3] Centre de Transfusion Sanguine, Montpellier, BP 1213, France.
[4] Tissue-Typing Laboratory, Rigshospitalet, Copenhagen, Denmark

Until recently, there has been considerable disagreement as to whether

TABLE II

The five nosologically distinct types of diabetes mellitus

INSULIN-DEPENDENT (JUVENILE-ONSET) DIABETES MELLITUS

NON-INSULIN DEPENDENT (MATURITY-ONSET) DIABETES MELLITUS

MATURITY-ONSET TYPE OF DIABETES MELLITUS IN THE YOUNG (MODY) A RARE DOMINANTLY INHERITED MILD TYPE OF DIABETES MELLITUS (3)

DIABETES MELLITUS OR CARBOHYDRATE INTOLERANCE ASSOCIATED WITH GENETIC SYNDROMES (4)

SECONDARY DIABETES

or not so-called juvenile-onset and maturity-onset diabetes were separate entites. Part of this controversy was probably due to the fact that the age at onset was not a good criterion to distinguish the two groups. As documented by the HLA studies (see below), insulin dependency *vs.* non-insulin dependency are better criteria.

HLA and insulin-dependent diabetes mellitus

In the beginning of the 1970s there was little doubt that genetic as well as environmental factors were involved in the pathogenesis of juvenile-onset insulin-dependent diabetes mellitus (4, 5). However, neither the mode of inheritance (6) nor the nature of the environmental factor(s) was elucidated. The pathological findings characteristic of insulin-dependent diabetes mellitus (IDDM) were a lymphocytic insulitis together with a selective disappearance of the beta-cells of the islets of Langerhans (7, 8), and in 1971 cell-mediated autoimmunity directed against antigenic determinants in the endocrine pancreas was reported (9).

Furthermore, indirect evidence to support a possible role of virus in the pathogenesis of IDDM was published. Increased titres of antibodies to Coxsackie B virus (type 4 in particular) were found in high frequency in IDDM patients, and this virus was, as well as the encephalomyocarditis virus, found to be diabetogenic in some strains of mice (10, 11, 12). Thus the stage was set to look for an association between HLA factors and IDDM.

Population studies

This idea was apparently fostered almost simultaneously in several laboratories. Finkelstein *et al.* (13), however, reported that no association could be demonstrated between HLA and juvenile diabetes, while Singal & Blajchman (14) found an increase of BW15 in a small group of IDDM patients, but in this series several patients were found to carry three antigens from the B-segregant series indicating technical difficulties. However, in 1974 Nerup *et al.* (15) in Copenhagen confirmed the increase of BW15 and found, moreover, a significant increase at B8 in IDDM irrespective of the age of onset of disease. The relative risk (RR) for B8 and BW15 were 2.4 and 2.5 respectively.

These authors proposed as a hypothesis for the aetiology and pathogenesis of IDDM: "One or more immune-response genes associated with HLA-B8 and/or BW15 might be responsible for an altered T-lymphocyte response. The genetically determined host response could fail to eliminate an infecting virus (Coxsackie B4 and others?) which in turn might destroy the pancreatic beta-cells or trigger an autoimmune reaction against the infected organ".

150

The findings of the Copenhagen group were soon confirmed by Cudworth & Woodrow (16) from Liverpool. Since then quite a few papers

TABLE III

Juvenile and/or insulin-dependent diabetes mellitus – combined material

DISEASE WHO CODE: 250.001

HLA	No. of studies	PATIENTS TOTAL	% POS range	CONTROLS TOTAL	% POS range	R. RISK	SIGNIFICANCE (r. risk)	(heterog.)
A1	12	1110	13–46	6704	9–34	1.32	2.3E–04	>0.05
A2	12	1110	41–70	6704	43–66	1.15	4.1E–02	>0.05
A3	11	962	9–55	6246	6–44	0.85	>0.05	>0.05
A9	10	905	22–39	5254	16–28	1.35	5.8E–04	>0.05
A10	9	757	0–25	4796	8–15	0.78	>0.05	>0.05
A11	10	850	0–18	5246	9–18	0.56	1.1E–04	>0.05
A28	10	850	2–10	5246	5–11	0.79	>0.05	>0.05
A29	6	667	3–15	2156	3–16	1.24	>0.05	>0.05
AW19	5	285	5–21	3567	2–20	0.75	>0.05	2.5E–02
AW23	1	93	6– 6	450	6– 6	1.06	>0.05	–
AW24	1	93	16–16	450	16–16	1.03	>0.05	–
AW25	3	227	0– 8	1023	0– 5	1.48	>0.05	>0.05
AW26	4	375	4–11	1481	5–13	0.88	>0.05	>0.05
AW30	5	468	1–31	1785	1–26	1.87	4.4E–04	>0.05
AW31	4	320	0– 8	929	3– 7	0.71	>0.05	>0.05
AW32	6	667	2–13	2156	5–11	0.51	1.4E–03	>0.05
AW33	3	218	0– 6	1034	2– 8	0.48	>0.05	>0.05
B5	11	998	0–14	5704	9–21	0.59	2.5E–05	>0.05
B7	12	1110	3–29	6704	3–32	0.51	<1E–10	>0.05
B8	13	1200	19–55	6856	2–29	2.42	<1E–10	>0.05
B12	11	998	5–26	5704	11–34	0.80	1.5E–02	4.8E–02
B13	11	998	0– 8	5704	3– 6	1.18	>0.05	>0.05
B14	10	850	0– 9	5246	0–15	0.72	>0.05	>0.05
B18	12	1088	5–59	5856	5–50	1.65	1.3E–06	>0.05
B27	11	998	2–14	5704	4–14	0.98	>0.05	>0.05
BW15	13	1200	4–50	6856	2–26	1.89	<1E–10	2.2E–02
BW16	6	425	6–20	4401	4–14	1.42	4.0E–02	>0.05
BW17	11	998	0–13	5704	2–23	0.78	>0.05	>0.05
BW21	7	484	0–14	4671	0–13	1.57	1.5E–02	>0.05
BW22	10	850	0– 6	5246	1– 6	0.94	>0.05	>0.05
BW35	11	998	6–34	5704	6–27	0.74	8.6E–03	1.8E–02
BW37	4	247	0– 3	1920	2– 4	1.01	>0.05	>0.05
BW38	1	59	5– 5	270	4– 4	1.40	>0.05	–
BW40	11	998	4–29	5704	2–21	1.32	8.8E–03	>0.05
BW41	1	102	0– 0	500	1– 1	0.69	>0.05	–

Data compiled by the HLA and Disease Registry, Copenhagen.

dealing with the HLA-IDDM association have been published (17–39).

Table III shows the results of combined calculations performed by the HLA and Disease Registry on A and B antigen frequencies in Caucasian patients with IDDM. It appears that the following antigens are significantly as-

151

sociated with IDDM and/or juvenile diabetes: HLA-B8, B18, and BW15. The increase of A1 is considered secondary to that of B8.

HLA-D typing of a larger series of patients has been reported only by Thomsen et al. (19), who found DW3 and/or DW4 in more than 80 per cent of the patients compared with only 25 per cent in the background population. The RRs of DW3 and DW4 were calculated to be 6.4 and 3.7 respectively (40).

In table IV the data for DW3 and DW4 from Thomsen et al. (19) have been combined with the data from a recent series from this laboratory.

TABLE IV

HLA-D typing of IDDM (Juvenile) patients and controls. Data from (19) and a recent series of Danish patients (52)

	PATIENTS		CONTROLS		REL. RISK
HLA–DW3	46/100	(46 %)	33/176	(18.8 %)	3.69
HLA–DW4	64/125	(51 %)	31/176	(17.6 %)	4.90

As commented upon by Svejgaard & Ryder (this volume, p. 50) it is difficult statistically to show that the association between IDDM and DW3 and DW4 is stronger than that of B8 and BW15 by comparing relative risks. However, by means of testing the presence vs. the absence of one of the antigens in patients and controls in individuals carrying and lacking the other antigen respectively, this assumption can be tested.

TABLE V

Detection of the strongest association: DW3 vs. B8. Data from (52)

	Group	No. af individuals			Relative Risk	Fisher's p
		DW3-pos.	DW3-neg.	Total		
HLA-B8 pos.	Juvenile diabetes	15 (100 %)	0	15	indef.	0.020
	Controls	26 (72 %)	10	36		
HLA-B8 neg.	Juvenile diabetes	6 (22 %)	21	27	4.7	0.015
	Controls	7 (6 %)	114	121		
		B8-pos.	B8-neg.	Total		
DW3 pos.	Juvenile diabetes	15 (71 %)	6	21	0.67	
	Controls	26 (79 %)	7	33		
DW3 neg.	Juvenile diabetes	0 (0 %)	21	21	0.0	
	Controls	10 (8 %)	114	124		

As shown in Table V, DW3 is more strongly associated with IDDM than is B8, the increase of which is secondary to that of DW3. When the same kind of analysis is applied for DW4 vs. BW15 (Table VI), it appears that DW4 too shows a stronger association with IDDM than the corresponding B allele.

TABLE VI
Detection of the strongest association: DW4 vs. BW15. Data from (52)

	Group	DW4-pos.		DW4-neg.	Total	Relative risk	Fisher's p
HLA-BW15 Pos.	Juvenile diabetes	24	(80 %)	6	30	3.73	0.021
	Controls	15	(52 %)	14	29		
HLA-BW15 Neg.	Juvenile diabetes	9	(18 %)	40	49	2.60	0.044
	Controls	11	(9 %)	127	138		
		BW15-pos.		BW15-neg.	Total		
DW4 pos.	Juvenile diabetes	24	(73 %)	9	33	1.96	0.18
	Controls	15	(58 %)	11	26		
DW4 neg.	Juvenile diabetes	6	(13 %)	40	46	1.36	0.36
	Controls	14	(11 %)	127	141		

Data about the HLA-IDDM association in other races than the Caucasian are scanty. Only two reports, totalling 115 juvenile IDDM patients, have been published, both of them from Japan (36, 37). Both reports show that in the Japanese population, where B8 is virtually absent and BW15 frequent, IDDM is associated with neither of these HLA antigens, but with BW22. Clearly more studies on the HLA-IDDM association in different racial groups should be undertaken.

On the other hand, a detailed analysis of the Caucasian HLA-IDDM data shows differences in different ethnic groups. In all series published, an increase of HLA-B8 was demonstrated, although the increase was found not to be statistically significant in a few reports (13, 14, 35) after correction for the number of antigens tested. BW15 was found with increased frequency in reports from Scandinavia (15, 26, 33), Germany (24, 27), Austria (20, 31), and the UK (16, 25), while in France (22, 23, 30, 32) B18 seemed to be the second B allele associated with IDDM instead of BW15. B18 was also reported to be increased in the UK (25). In the Italian population neither BW15 nor

B18 was associated with IDDM (28, 29, 34), but in two rather small series (28, 29) BW35 was increased. It would be of interest to see if these differences in the B alleles in relation to IDDM persist in migrating European populations, e.g. after settling in USA.

As pointed out elsewhere in this volume (Svejgaard & Ryder, p. 46), one does not get a perfectly true picture when calculating the RR for B8 alone, for example, since this antigen is compared to say BW15 which in itself shows an increased RR. However, by analysing the data from three different series (15, 31, Cudworth & Woodrow personal communication), the RR for carriers of both B8 and BW15 is considerably increased (Figure 1) when compared with other B8- and BW15-positive individuals. Furthermore, it is important to note that the RRs for individuals homozygous for B8 and BW15 are not nearly as high, but rather of the same magnitude, as the RRs of heterozygous carriers of B8 and BW15.

These observations are most readily interpreted as demonstrating that there are two genes conferring increased risk of IDDM: one associated with B8 and one with BW15. When present together

153

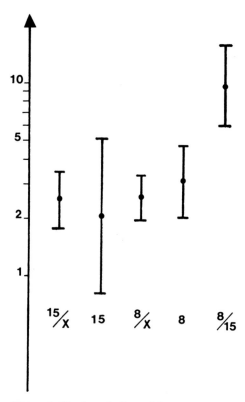

RELATIVE RISK of
JUVENILE DIABETES

Figure 1. The bars indicate 95 per cent confidence limits. X indicates the presence of B-locus antigens other than HLA-B8 or BW15.

the two genes act in concert to further increase susceptibility. This is an example of overdominance (if the genes in question are on the same locus) or epistasis (if they are on different loci), and not an example of recessivity.

Since overdominance or epistasis may simulate recessivity in family studies, this fact is important to note in relation to diabetes mellitus, since it was thought until recently that this condition was inherited as a recessive trait (41).

The data of B8/B18 and BW15/B18 phenotypes in the literature are too small to give useful information about

RRs for such individuals, but Degos et al. (personal communication) have found a similar interaction between B8 and B18 as that described for B8 and BW15.

A decrease of HLA-B7 (Table III) was found by most authors. It was already noted in the first report to appear on the HLA-IDDM association (19). This decrease of B7 has attracted interest and has been claimed (42, 43) to be associated with a gene protective for IDDM. To further support this suggestion, Ludwig et al. (31) reported a lack of B7 in glucose-intolerant young blood relations to IDDM patients.

However, at least 3 other B alleles (Table III) were found to occur with a statistically significant decreased frequency in Caucasian IDDM patients. Thus the evidence in favour of a particular protective role of B7 in relation to IDDM is rather circumstantial and needs confirmation in other test situations (see below).

With regard to the C series of HLA antigens, an increase of CW3 was reported (20, 31) in IDDM patients. A similar observation was made by the Copenhagen group (unpublished). A close linkage disequilibrium exists between BW15 and CW3 and, since the RR for CW3 does not exceed that of BW15 (31, Nerup et al. unpublished), the increase of CW3 is probably secondary to that of BW15.

Family studies

Obviously, further information about the HLA-IDDM association can be obtained from family studies. First of all, such studies have shown that the HLA antigens in diabetics are inherited characters just as they are in normal individuals. Only a limited number of informative families with IDDM in more

154

than one generation have been reported to be HLA typed. A total of 12 families with 37 cases of IDDM distributed over 2 or more generations could be compiled from the literature (17, 19, 28, 35, 44). It is worth noting that in these families, IDDM occurred only in individuals sharing an HLA haplotype with the diabetic proband. Although information from more and hopefully larger families is clearly needed, the available data suggest that the phenotype IDDM – within families – segregates with a certain genotype, i.e. the "Diabetic haplotype" characteristic of that family.

HLA-B8, BW15 or B18 was present in the "diabetic haplotype" of 8 out of the 12 families, a frequency which does not differ significantly from the overall frequency of these three HLA antigens in the Caucasian population studies.

TABLE VII

52 Diabetic probands with 57 diabetic siblings.

	2 haplotypes shared (HLA identity)	1 haplotype shared	No haplotype shared
Observed	61.5 per cent (35/57)	30 per cent (17/57)	8.5 per cent (5/57)
Expected	25 per cent	50 per cent	25 per cent

Data from (28, 29, 31, 35, 63 & Nerup *et al.* unpublished).
Statistics: Data from this table compared to:
A) Normal segregation (25 per cent, 50 per cent, 25 per cent): $\chi^2 = 40.86$, p < 0.001.
B) Hypothesis of dominant susceptibility (33 per cent, 67 per cent, 0 per cent): $\chi^2 = 25.08$, p < 0.01.

The importance of the HLA-IDDM association is further emphasized by typing of sibships comprising two or more diabetics. On the assumption that IDDM was not associated with HLA, 25 % of diabetic sibpairs should be HLA identical, 50 % should share one haplotype, and the remaining 25 % should differ for both parental haplotypes. It appears from Table VII that there are many more HLA-identical sibpairs than expected and the association is very highly significant. If HLA conferred a simple dominant susceptibility to diabetes, one would expect (simply speaking) that 33 % of the sibpairs were HLA identical and that the remaining 67 % shared one haplotype. The values in Table VII are also highly significantly different from this expectation, and this observation (in a smaller series of patients) lead Thomson & Bodmer (this volume) to suggest that IDDM is a recessive disorder. Unfortunately, very few of the siblings in Table VII have been HLA-D typed but it is our prediction that most of the HLA-identical sibpairs are *DW3/DW4* heterozygous. The observations of Suciu-Foca *et al.* (45, 46) that most diabetic sibpairs are MLC identical are compatible with this assumption.

In any case the family studies – although more data are indicated – strongly support the assumption that diabetogenic genes within the HLA region of the sixth chromosome, presumably between the B and the D loci *may be necessary* for IDDM to develop. However, some reservation should be made because families with two affected siblings are probably a biased sample of all families with one or more affected members. There are, however, data to show that the presence of these HLA-associated diabetogenic gene(s) is *not sufficient* for an individual to become an IDDM-patient. The concordance rate of juvenile diabetes mellitus in pairs of identical twins is only about 50 per cent (6), a figure which applies also to the concordance rate of IDDM irrespective of age at onset in this series of identical twins (Pyke 1976, personal communication). Furthermore, only 12–15 per cent of the patients with juvenile IDDM report a positive family history for IDDM in first-degree relatives (47). Lastly, the empirical risk of IDDM is surprisingly low, for example, only about 5 per cent of children of IDDM probands will be IDDM patients themselves at age 30 (48).

Consequently, the twin study implies that non-genetic environmental factors are of importance in producing the disease in the genetically suspectible individuals, and the family studies of the empirical risk of IDDM emphasize this point further, since only about one tenth of the genetically susceptible children of an IDDM patient will ever develop the disease.

On this background, it would be interesting to know if non-diabetic family members sharing haplotypes with the diabetic proband in the family could be earmarked as prediabetics, that is, as having an impaired glucose tolerance or an abnormal insulin response to glucose.

Since the juvenile non-diabetic twins of the discordant identical twin pairs of Pyke & Nelson (49) did not show deterioration of either of these parameters when followed for some years, one would not predict an association between subclinical diabetes and the HLA factors characteristic of IDDM.

The data reported so far are relatively sparse, based on different methods for assessment of glucose tolerance, and do not settle the question entirely. However, only two reports of very limited numbers of persons studied (19, 31) are in favour of an association between subclinical IDDM and HLA, while 5 larger series tend to reject this possibility (21, 27, 29, 30, Nerup et al. unpublished).

Increased recombination frequency

Before leaving the section on the heredity of diabetes, it should be mentioned that a very interesting, but intriguing hypothesis was suggested by Suciu-Foca et al. *(45, 46)* on the basis of their findings of an extraordinarily high (12.5 per cent) recombination frequency in diabetic families. According to these authors, IDDM is inherited as a recessive disorder with the diabetogenic gene closely linked to the HLA-D locus and the high cross-over rate is caused by "a weak spot" on the chromosomes carrying a diabetogenic gene. Another example of B-D recombination has been reported (50). However, in the papers just quoted, no proof of paternity or data from MLC responses between the recombinants were presented, and these findings clearly need confimation. Neither Mayr et al. (51), Cudworth & Woodrow, nor the Copenhagen group found the recombination frequency between the serologically determinable loci to be increased. Furthermore, the Copenhagen group (52), by HLA-D typing 17 IDDM families and performing the above-mentioned controls, was unable to confirm a high recombination frequency to be a feature of IDDM.

Clinical implications

(Seasonal variation, age at onset, severity of disease, insulin antibodies):

In the UK (53) and Denmark (54), seasonal variation in the onset of juvenile IDDM was reported with the highest incidence during autumn and spring. It has been claimed (55, 34) that the B8-positive cases were responsible for the seasonal variation. Others (56) were unable to confirm this observation.

Heterogeneity for age of onset with the B8-positive patients having the lowest age of onset of IDDM was suggested by several groups (31, 33, 34), while Cudworth & Woodrow (25) found no significant evidence to support this.

HLA-DW2 and DW3-positive patients have a more severe type of multiple sclerosis (57) and Graves' disease (58), respectively, than patients without these HLA factors. Severity of IDDM can be assessed in several ways: by measuring preserved endogenous insulin production by means of the C-peptide assay; by the length of the remission period; by calculating the insulin requirement per kilo body weight; and by the degree and time of onset of the late diabetic complications.

Very few reports attempted to elucidate whether any of the IDDM-associated HLA factors showed correlation to the course and severity of the disease. Ludvigsson et al. (26) found no association between B-cell function as estimated by C-peptide analysis and any particular HLA factors with the expectation that the B18-positive patients presented with an increased incidence of detectable C-peptide, and others (59, 21, 60) found that late complications of diabetes, for example retinopathy, prevailed in HLA B8 or BW15-positive individuals.

Obviously, more work is needed in this area of research, especially in relation to the remission period and the late complications of IDDM.

Depending upon the species of insulin used and the form in which it is administered, IDDM patients will develop insulin antibodies during treatment (61). Patients treated with conventionel bovine insulin preparations are most liable to do so, while patients on highly purified porcine insulins rarely do so. Studies of HLA in relation to insulin-antibody formation (24, 26, 62) have shown that genetic factors might influence insulin-antibody forma-

tion since the highest titres were found in HLA BW15-positive IDDM patients and the possession of B7 seemed to protect against insulin-antibody formation.

This observation is of practical interest and should be taken into consideration in assessing the antigeneity of the new highly purified insulin preparations.

Mechanisms

It is still unknown in which way HLA factors confer susceptibility to develop IDDM. Several suggestions have been put forward:

For several decades there have been reports associating IDDM with viral diseases. The viruses most often implicated are mumps, rubella, Coxsackie B4, infectious hepatitis, influenza, and infectious mononucleosis (Review, Gepts (64)). The evidence linking viral infection to IDDM is, however, rather circumstantial and limited to epidemiological data showing a temporal association between outbreaks of viral diseases and onset of IDDM. Naturally, this can be criticized because of the high prevalences of both conditions. But high titres of neutralizing antibodies to Coxsackie-B4 virus have been demonstrated with increased frequency in IDDM patients (53), and a high prevalence of diabetes was found in patients with congenital rubella, predominantly in HLA-B8-positive individuals (65). Furthermore, in newly diagnosed IDDM patients, the high Coxsackie-B4 antibody titres seemed to be associated with the "diabetic" HLA factors (66).

The diabetogenic effect of certain viruses (Coxsackie B4 and the M-strain of encephalomyocarditis virus) has been demonstrated experimentally (67). A genetic influence on the susceptibility

157

is present (68, 69), but in the case of the encephalomyocarditis virus infection, this does not seem to be controlled by the H-2 region (70).

Autoimmunity

Organ-specific anti-pancreatic autoimmunity is a characteristic feature of IDDM (review 71). Insulitis – that is, a lymphocytic infiltration of the islets of Langerhans, together with a selective destruction of the beta-cells – is the typical pathological finding in IDDM patients autopsied within the first year of disease (7, 8).

By means of the leukocyte-migration technique, cell-mediated autoimmunity has been demonstrated in about 30–50 per cent of the IDDM patients (72, 73, 74), and islet-cell antibodies were found by indirect immunofluorescence in 60–85 per cent of the cases at the time of diagnosis (75, 76).

No association between the cell-mediated and humoral autoimmune phenomena could be demonstrated (77). Christy et al. (77) found autoimmunity to be associated with HLA-B8, but others (78) were unable to confirm this.

Interestingly, insulitis as well as both types of autoimmune reactions seem to fade away in the course of IDDM, but it has been demonstrated (39) that persistent autoimmunity, that is, after a duration of IDDM for more than one year, is HLA-B8 dependent.

It might be worth noting that an experimental model bearing most of the characteristics of human IDDM can be produced in mice and that there is ample evidence to suggest a controlling effect of H-2 in this model (70).

Thus, the mechanisms through which genes in the HLA region confer susceptibility to IDDM are still obscure. Much more work, including animal models, is needed, but a suitable working hypothesis could still be the above-mentioned one (15) with minor modifications.

HLA and the other types of diabetes mellitus

Neither non-insulin-dependent (maturity onset) diabetes (15, 25, 28, 36), with one possible exception (79), nor the MODY type of diabetes (80, 81) has been reported to be associated with any particular HLA antigens.

None of the reports available relate HLA to the other types of diabetes mellitus or carbohydrate intolerance listed in Table II.

Summary and conclusions

This literature review can be summarized as follows:

As already suggested from clinical data and stated previously on the basis of HLA data, IDDM is a disease entity in itself and different from non-insulin-dependent diabetes and other types of diabetes mellitus in etiology and pathogenesis (15).

HLA-B8 (RR 2.42) is associated with IDDM in all Caucasian populations studied, irrespective of the age of onset of the disease. HLA-BW15 (RR 1.89) is associated with IDDM in population of Northern European and British origin, while B18 (RR 1.65) seems to replace BW15 in Southern European populations.

IDDM is uncommon in populations where the HLA-B8 frequency is low, and in the Japanese IDDM occurs in association with BW22. The HLA-DW3 and DW4 association with IDDM is stronger than that of the B alleles.

RRs for B8 and BW15 hetero- and homozygous individuals are identical, that is, no gene-dose effect exists. The RR of B8/BW15 carriers is double that of B8 and BW15 alone, i.e. there are two IDDM-associated HLA genes.

In families and sibships, IDDM segregates with the diabetic proband's HLA haplotype. Only a small proportion of family members carrying the "diabetic haplotype" develop IDDM.

On this basis, the following conclusions can be drawn:

Within the HLA region, between the B and D loci, two (or more?) diabetogenic genes are located.

The presence of one or both of these genes is necessary but not sufficient for IDDM to develop, since environmental stimuli are required as triggering mechanisms. It is anticipated that virus and autoimmunity are involved in the pathogenesis of IDDM.

HLA and Graves' disease

In this paper, hyperthyroidism occurring in patients without thyroid nodules was classified under the name of Graves' disease irrespective of whether the patients presented with the classical diffuse goitre and eye symptoms or not.

Graves' disease shows familial aggregation but the pattern of inheritance has not been reported to fit any classical mode. Occasionally Graves' disease occurs in clinical association with other autoimmune endocrinopathies – preferentially with IDDM and idiopathic Addison's disease. Organ-specific autoimmune phenomena are frequent in Graves' disease (82).

A diffuse lymphocytic infiltration of the thyroid gland together with a hypertrophied hormone-producing follicular epithelium and the presence of thyroid antibodies in serum can be demonstrated in about 60 per cent of the cases. Of special interest are the thyroid-stimulating IgG autoantibodies LATS and LATS-protector, demonstrable in about 90 per cent of the patients. These autoantibodies are probably very important in the pathogenesis of the disease. Cell-mediated autoimmunity has been found to be feature of Graves' disease too (83).

These findings served as an impetus to look for a genetic marker for the disease, and in 1973 Grumet et al. (84) reported on the association between HLA-B8 and Graves' disease. This observation was rapidly confirmed by several groups (58, 85–90).

By combining these materials, the RR of Graves' disease in HLA-B8-positive Caucasians was found to be 2.5 ($p < 10^{-10}$).

The frequency of B8 among the patients was about 40 per cent compared with about 20 per cent in the control materials. A slight increase of HLA-A1 was found as well, probably due to linkage disequilibrium with B8. Two reports presented data showing the HLA-Graves' disease association to be stronger for DW3 than for B8 (58, 86), the RR being 5.5 (58).

As previously mentioned, HLA-B8 is virtually absent in the Japanese population, and here Graves' disease was found to be associated not with HLA-B8, but with BW35. The RR being 5 was higher than that for B8 in Caucasian populations (91). No family studies have been published to clarify whether Graves' disease segregates with certain haplotypes like IDDM.

Clinical implications

The studies of the HLA-Graves' disease association might suggest that Graves' disease as defined today is not nosologically uniform. HLA-B8-positive patients were found to have a younger age at onset (89), and furthermore it was shown that the increased frequency of HLA-B8 was found only in patients with ophthalmopathy (92), and that HLA-B8 positivity correlated to a severe course of the disease (88, 89). Bech et al. (58) found a signinficantly higher frequency of DW3 in patients with relapsing Graves' disease than in easily treated patients and suggest that this might be of use in choice of treatment of the disease.

It is, however, difficult to decide whether these findings reflect manifestations of two nosologically distinct disease entities – one associated with DW3 and one not – or merely that the presence of DW3 influences the course of the disease once the patient has contracted it.

Mechanisms

As for IDDM, the concordance rate of Graves' disease is surprisingly low in pairs of identical twins (93), which

points towards the necessity of an external trigger in the aetio-pathogenesis of this condition.

The prevalence of autoimmune manifestations, for example, autoantibodies to thyroglobulin or thyroid microsomes, varied considerably in the different series reported to be HLA typed. However, with two exceptions (85, 86) no association between HLA-B8 positivity and the presence of thyroid antibodies could be demonstrated. Similarly, no association was found between BW35 and thyroid antibodies in the studies of Japanese populations (90).

The lack of an HLA-autoantibody correlation speaks against a causative role for these antibodies in the pathogenesis of Graves' disease.

It should be noted, however, that cell-mediated thyroid autoimmunity as well as the thyroid-stimulating IgGs, which are probably directly involved in the pathogenesis of the condition, have not so far been studied in relation to HLA.

A high frequency of antibodies to *Yersinia enterocolitica* serotype 3 was reported in Graves' disease, especially in relapsing cases (94), but no environmental factor has convincingly been shown related to the onset and cause of the disease.

The difference in HLA-Graves' association in Caucasians and the Japanese is interesting, and suggests that it is not the HLA genes themselves, but rather other genes in the HLA region closely linked to the HLA genes, that play a role in the development of the disease. Such a gene(s) would be anticipated to be located between the B and D loci, probably closer to the latter.

HLA and Addison's disease

Idiopathic Addison's disease – a disease entity of its own, completely distinct from tuberculous Addison's disease – is the autoimmune endocrinopathy *par excellence:* (Review, 95). The prevalence of the other autoimmune endocrinopathies is remarkably high in idiopathic Addison's disease.

Adrenal antibodies and/or cell-mediated autoimmunity to adrenocortical antigens can be demonstrated in about 90 per cent of the cases, and family cases do occur. An association between HLA and this condition was therefore to be anticipated.

Two reports have been published. In one (19) a strong and highly statistically significant association with HLA-B8 (66) per cent) and especially DW3 (70 per cent) was found, the RRs being 7.0 and 10.5 respectively. In the other report (96) no deviations of HLA antigen frequencies were found. Both reports, however, demonstrated a very strong correlation between HLA-B8 and adrenal antibody, which indicates a possible role for this antibody in the pathogenesis of the disease.

The reasons for the different findings in the two materials are not clear. Both materials deal with Caucasians and the diagnostic criteria seem to be the same. Obviously more studies are needed, if possible also in other ethnic groups than Caucasians.

The other autoimmune endocrinopathies

Of the other diseases mentioned in Table I only one has been shown to be associated with HLA. Very recently, Platz et al. (97) found that cases of *hypergonadotropic hypogonadism* with no chromosomal aberrations, but with lymphocytic infiltration of the ovaries and steroid-cell antibodies, were associated with HLA-B8.

Surprisingly, the classical organ-specific autoimmune disease *Hashimoto's thyroiditis* was found not to be associated with any particular HLA antigen (90, 91, 98–100), but the number of patients investigated is still rather small and it might very well be that what is classified Hashimoto's disease comprises more than one disease entity.

No studies of *myxedema* and *idiopathic hypoparathyroidism* have been published so far.

Miscellaneous

Subacute thyroiditis (de Quervain) is a clinical syndrome characterized by a firm, tender goitre, elevated erythrocyte sedimentation rate, fever, and a very low uptake of radioactive tracer in the thyroid gland, but no hyperthyroidism or autoimmune phenomena. The disease is almost exclusively confined to women, and is thought to be of viral origin, This disease is not a member of the group of organ-specific, autoimmune diseases described in Table I. Two reports have dealt with this syndrome. First, Nyulassy et al. 101, 102) demonstrated a strong association with HLA-BW35 ,and this was confirmed by Bech et al. (103).

The relative risk for de Quervain's

thyroiditis for BW35-positive individuals was about 17, and the percentage of BW35-positive patients in the two materials was 87 and 71, respectively, opposed to about 10 per cent in the normal population. This very high frequency makes the HLA investigations almost diagnostic in the individual patient although the number of "false negative" is rather high.

The HLA-DW1, which in the normal population is associated with BW35, was also found to be increased among the patients, but to a much lesser extent, and probably only secondary to the increase of BW35.

These two materials deal only with Caucasians, and it remains to be investigated whether other ethnic groups show the same pattern. It is of interest to note that BW35 is the antigen which in the Japanese population is associated with Graves' disease, but whether this is pure coincidence can only be speculated upon at the present time.

In patients with *adrenocortical hyperfunction (Cushing's syndrome)* there may be a slight increase of HLA-A1 and B8 (104).

No association was found between HLA and *autonomous thyroid adenoma (89)*.

General summary

This review of the present status of HLA in relation to endocrine disorders has shown four out of five autoimmune endocrinopathies studied so far to be associated with HLA-B8 and DW3. Thus, in addition to the previously mentioned clinical, pathological and immunological links between the diseases of this group, there might be a common genetic basis for them. The data suggest, that a gene(s) in the HLA region between the B and D loci – most likely in linkage disequilibrium with D – might be a common genetic denominator for endocrine autoimmunity.

Furthermore, there is strong evidence to suggest that environmental factors are needed to produce these diseases in the genetically susceptible individuals.

More work in this area of research is clearly indicated, and special efforts should be made to try to describe and isolate the environmental triggers. Then, potentially useful clinical information might be obtained as well as important knowledge about the nature of autoimmunity in man.

References

1. Irvine, W. J. (ed.) (1975) Autoimmunity in Endocrine Disease. *Clinics in Endocrinology and metabolism, 4*, no. 2.
2. Creutzfeldt, W., Köbberling, J. & Neel, J. V. (1976) *The Genetics of Diabetes Mellitus,* Springer-Verlag, Berlin, Heidelberg, New York.
3. Tattersall, R. (1976) The Inheritance of Maturity-Onset Type Diabetes in Young People. *Ibid.* p. 88.
4. Harvald, B. (1967) Genetic Perspectives in Diabetes Mellitus. *Acta Med. Scand.* Suppl. **476**, 17.
5. Tattersall, R. & Pyke, D. A. (1972) Diabetes in Identical Twins. *Lancet* **ii, 1120**.
6. Rimoin, D. L. (1976) Genetic Syndromes Associated with Glucose Intolerance. *Ibid.* p. 43.
7. Gepts, W. (1965) Pathologic Anatomy of the Pancreas in Juvenile Diabetes Mellitus. *Diabetes* **14**, 619.
8. Egeberg, J., Junker, K., Kromann, H. &

Nerup, J. (1976) Autoimmune Insulitis. Pathological Findings in Experimental Animal Models and Juvenile Diabetes Mellitus. *Acta Endocrin. (Kbh.)* Suppl. **205**, 129.

9. Nerup, J., Ortved Andersen, O., Bendixen, G., Egeberg, J. & Poulsen, J. E. (1971) Antipancreatic Cellular Hypersensitivity in Diabetes Mellitus. *Diabetes* **20**, 424.

10. Gamble, D. R., Kinsley, M. L., Fitzgerald, M. G., Bolton, R. & Taylor, K. W. (1969) Viral Antibodies in Diabetes Mellitus. *Brit. Med. J.* **3**, 627.

11. Craighead, J. E. & McLane, M. F. (1968) Diabetes Mellitus: Induction in Mice by Encephalomyocarditis Virus. *Science* **162**, 913.

12. Coleman, T. J., Gamble, D. R. & Taylor, K. W. (1973) Diabetes in Mice after Coxsackie B4 Virus Infection. *Brit. Med. J.* **3**, 25.

13. Finkelstein, S., Zeller, E. & Walford, R. L. (1972) No Relation between HL-A and Juvenile Diabetes. *Tissue Antigens* **2**, 74.

14. Singal, D. P. & Blajchmann, M. A. (1973) Histocompatibility (HL-A) antigens, lymphocytotoxic antibodies and tissue antibodies in patients with diabetes mellitus. *Diabetes* **22**, 429.

15. Nerup, J., Platz, P., Ortved Andersen, O., Christy, M., Lyngsøe, J., Poulsen, J. E., Ryder, L. P., Staub Nielsen, L., Thomsen, M. & Svejgaard, A. (1974) HL-A antigens and diabetes mellitus. *Lancet* **ii**, 864.

16. Cudworth, A. G. & Woodrow, J. C. (1974) HL-A antigens and diabetes mellitus. *Lancet* **ii**, 1153.

17. Cudworth, A. G. & Woodrow, J. C. (1975a) HL-A system and diabetes mellitus. *Diabetes* **24**, 345.

18. Cudworth, A. G. & Woodrow, J. C. (1975b) Evidence for HL-A-linked genes in "Juvenile" diabetes mellitus. *Brit. Med. J.* **3**, 133.

19. Thomsen, M., Platz, P., Ortved Andersen, O., Christy, M., Lyngsøe, J., Nerup, J., Rasmussen, K., Ryder, L. P., Staub Nielsen, L. & Svejgaard, A. (1975) MLC typing in juvenile diabetes mellitus and Idiopathic Addison's disease. *Transplant. Rev.* **22**, 120.

20. Scherntaner, G., Mayr, W. R., Pacher, M., Ludwig, H., Erd, W. & Eibl. M. (1975) HL-A8, W15 and T3 in juvenile diabetes mellitus. *Horm. Metabol. Res.* **7**, 521.

21. Barbosa, J., Noreen, H., Goetz, F., Simmons, R., de Leiva, A., Najarian, J. & Yunis, E. J. (1975) Histocompatibility (HLA) antigens and diabetic microangiopathy. *Clin. Res.* **23**, 534 A.

22. Seignalet, J., Mirouze, J., Jaffiol, C., Selam, J. L. & Lapinski, H. (1975) HLA in Graves' disease and in diabetes mellitus insulin-dependent. *Tissue Antigens* **6**, 272.

23. Cathelineau, G., Cathelineau, L., Hors, J., Schmid, M. & Dausset, J. (1976) Les groupes HLA dans le diabete à début précoce. *NOUV. Presse Med.* **5**, 586.

24. Bertrams, J., Jansen, F. K., Grüneklee, D., Reis, H. E., Drost, H., Beyer, J. Gries, F. A. & Kuwert, E. (1976) HLA-antigens and immune-responsiveness to insulin in insulin-dependent diabetes mellitus. *Tissue Antigens* **8**, 13.

25. Cudworth, A. G. & Woodrow, J. C. (1976) Genetic susceptibility in diabetes mellitus: Antlysis of the HLA assiciation. *Brit. Med. J.* **2**, 846.

26. Ludvigsson, J., Säfwenberg, J. & Heding, L. G. (1976) HLA-types, C-peptide and insulin antibodies in juvenile diabetes. *Diabetologia* (in press).

27. Landgraf, R., Landgraf-Leurs, M. M. C., Lander, T., Scholtz, S., Kuntz, B. & Albert, E. D. (1976) HLA haplotypes and glucose tolerance in families of patients with juveninle-onset diabetes mellitus. *Lancet* **ii**, 1084.

28. Contu, L., Puligheddu, A., Mura, C. & Gabbas, A. (1976) HLA antigens in Sardinian patients with diabetes mellitus. *The First International Symposium on HLA and disease*, Inserm, Paris, June 1976. Abstr. no. IV – 4, p. 124.

29. Savi, M., Neri, T. M., Zavaroni, I. & Coselli, C. (1976) HLA antigens and insulin dependent diabetes mellitus. A family study. *Ibid.* abstr. no. IV – 22, p. 142.

30. Vialettes, B., Vague, P. & Mercier, P. (1976) Diabetiques insulino-dépendants, non diabetiques faibles secreteurs d'insuline: deux populations HLA distinctes. *Ibid.* abstr. no. IV – 27, p. 147.

31. Ludwig, H., Scherntaner, G. & Mayr, W. R. (1976) The importance of HLA genes to suspectibility in the development of juvenile diabetes mellitus. *Ibid.* abstr. no. IV – 14, p. 134.

32. Pointel, J. P., Raffoux, C., Janot, C., Sauvanet, J. P., Drouin, R., Streiff, F. & Debry, G. (1976) Antigens HL-A et diabete sucre insulino-dependant. *Ibid.* abstr. no. IV – 19, p. 139.

33. Koivisto, V. A., Kuitunen, P., Tiilikainen,

A. & Åkerblom, H. K. (1976) HLA antigens in patients with juvenile diabetes mellitus, coeliac disease and both of the diseases. *Ibid.* abstr. no. IV – 8, p. 128.

34. Illeni, M. T., Pellegris, G., Del Guercio, M. J., Tarantino, A., Busetto, F., Di Pietro, C., Clerici, E., Garotta, G. & Chiumello, G. (1976) Autoimmunity and histocompatibility antigens in diabetes mellitus of childhood. *Ibid.* abstr. no. IV – 7, p. 127.

35. Gazit, E., Sartani, A., Mizrachi, Y. & Ravid, M. (1976) HLA antigens in jewish patients with juvenile diabetes mellitus. *Ibid.* abstr. no. IV – 6, p. 126.

36. Nakazawa, M., Sakaguchi, S., Nakamura, S., Kono, Y., Hazeki, H. & Kawa, A. (1976). Human leukocyte antigen (HLA) in japanese diabetics. *V International Congress of endocrinology.* Hamburg. Abstr. p. 222.

37. Wakisaka, A., Aizawa, M., Matsuura, N., Nakagawa, S,, Nakayama, E., Itakura, K., Okuno, A. & Wagatsuma, Y. (1976) HLA and juvenile diabetes mellitus in the japanese. *Lancet* **ii**, 970.

38. Garovsoy, M. R., Carpenter, C. B., Myrberg, S. M., Gleason, R. E., Funk, I. B., Flood, T. M. & Craighead, J. E. (1976) Inreased incidence of HLA-B8 in juvenile onset diabetes mellitus. In: *Histocompatibility testing in the Americans.* Grune & Stratton (in press).

39. Morris, P. J., Vaughan, H., Irvine, W. J., Gray, R. S., McCallum, C. J., Campbell, C. J., Duncan, L. J. & Farguha, J. W. (1976) HLA and pancreatic islet cell antibodies in diabetes. *Lancet* **ii**, 652.

40. Nerup, J., Platz, P., Ortved Andersen, O., Christy, M., Egeberg, J., Lyngsøe, J., Poulsen, J. E., Ryder, L. P., Thomsen, M. & Svejgaard, A. (1976) HLA autoimmunity and insulin-dependent diabetes mellitus. In: *The Genetics of diabetes mellitus,* p. 106, Springer-Verlag, Berlin, Heidelberg, New York.

41. Simpson, N. E. (1976) The genetics of diabetes mellitus – a review of family data. In: *The Genetics of Diabetes Mellitus,* p. 12, Springer-Verlag, Berlin, Heidelberg, New York.

42. Ludwig, H., Scherntaner, G. & Mayr, W. R. (1976) Is HLA-B7 a marker associated with a protective gene in juvenile onset diabetes mellitus? *New Eng. J. Med.* **294**, 1066.

43. Van de Putte, I., Vermylen, C., Decraene, P., Vlietinck, R. & van den Berghe, H. (1976) Segregation of HLA-B7 in juvenile onset diabetes mellitus. *Lancet* **ii**, 251.

44. Lestradet, H., Baron, D., Schmid, M., Kolevski, P. & Hors, J. (1976) HLA genotypes in familial insulin dependent diabetes mellitus. *First International Symposium on HLA and disease.* Inserm, Paris, June 1976, abstr. no. IV – 12, p. 132.

45. Suciu-Foca, N., Rubinstein, P. & Nicholson, J. (1976) HLA studies on families with juvenile diabetes. *First International Symposium on HLA and disease.* Inserm, Paris, June 1976, abstr. no. IV – 25, p. 145.

46. Rubinstein, P., Suciu-Foca, N. & Nicholson, J. (1976) Intra-HLA recombinations in juvenile diabetes mellitus. *First International Symposium on HLA and disease.* Inserm, Paris, June 1976, abstr. no. IV – 20, p. 140.

47. Bloom, A., Hayes, T. M. & Gamble, D. R. (1975) Register of newly diagnosed diabetic children. *Brit. Med. J.* **3**, 580.

48. Green-Hansen, A. & Degnbol, B. (1976) Prevalence of diabetes mellitus among relatives of 187 patients with juvenile diabetes. *Diabetologia* **12**, 396.

49. Pyke, D. A. & Nelson, P. G. (1976) Diabetes mellitus in identical twins. In: *The Genetics of Diabetes Mellitus,* p. 194, Springer-Verlag, Berlin, Heidelberg, New York.

50. Shaw, J. F., Kansal, P. C. & Gatti, R. A. (1976) Diabetes mellitus, chromosomal aberration and malignancy. *Lancet* **ii**, 315.

51. Mayr, W. R., Scherntaner, G. & Ludwig, H. (1976) Intra-HLA recombination frequency in juvenile diabetes. *Lancet* **i**, 865.

52. Thomsen, M., Platz, P., Ryder, L. P., Svejgaard, A., Ortved Andersen, O., Christy, M., Buschard, K., Christau, B., Kromann, H. & Nerup, J. (1977) (to be published).

53. Gamble, D. R. (1976) A possible virus etiology for juvenile diabetes. In: *The Genetics of Diabetes Mellitus,* p. 95, Springer-Verlag, Berlin, Heidelberg, New York.

54. Christau, B., Kromann, H., Kristensen, I. H., Steinrud, J. & Nerup, J. (1976) Incidence, sex and seasonal patterns of juvenile diabetes mellitus. *Diabetologia* **12**, 384.

55. Rolles, C. J., Rayner, P. H. W. & Mackintosh, P. (1975) Etiology of juvenile diabetes. *Lancet* **ii**, 230.

56. Barbosa, J., Noreen, H., Goetz, F., Simmons, R., Najarian, J. & Yunis, E. J.

(1976) Juvenile diabetes and viruses. *Lancet* **i**, 371.

57. Platz, P., Dupont, B., Fog, T., Ryder, L. P., Thomsen, M. & Svejgaard, A. (1974) MLC determinants, measles infection and multiple sclerosis. *Proc. Roy. Soc. Med.* **67**, 133.

58. Bech, K., Lumholz, B., Nerup, J., Thomsen, M., Platz, P., Ryder, L. P., Svejgaard, A., Siersbæk-Nielsen, K. & Mølholm-Hansen, J. (1977) HLA antigens in Graves' disease. *Acta endocrin. (Kbh.)* (in press).

59. Ortved Andersen, O., Vejtrup, L., Christy, M., Platz, P., Svejgaard, A., Thomsen, M., Reersted, P. & Nerup, J. (1975) HLA factors in insulin dependent diabetes mellitus: Clinical significance. *Diabetologia* **11**, 329.

60. Bertrams, J., Reis, H. E., Jansen, F. K., Grüneklee, D., Drost, H., Beyer, J. & Griess, F. A. (1976) Diabetic retinopathy and HLA antigen B8. Presented at the *First International Symposium on HLA and Disease*. Inserm, Paris, June 1976.

61. Ortved Andersen, O. (1973) Insulin antibody formation. II The influence of Species difference and method of administration. *Acta Endocr. (Kbh.)* **72**, 33.

62. Scherntaner, G., Ludwig, H., Mayr, W. R. & Willvinseder, R. (1976) Humoral antiinsulin immunity and HLA factors in juvenile onset diabetes mellitus. *First International Symopsium on HLA and disease*. Inserm, Paris, June 1976, abstr. no. IV – 23, p. 143.

63. Woodrow, J. C. & Cudworth, A. G. (1976) The sibship study of HLA and diabetes. *First International Symposium on HLA and disease*. Inserm, Paris, June 1976, abstr. no. IV – 29, p. 149.

64. Gepts, W. (1976) Islet changes suggesting a possible immune aetiology of human diabetes mellitus. *Acta endocr. (Khb.)* Suppl. **205**, 95.

65. Menser, M., Forrest, J. M. & Honeyman, M. C. (1974) Diabetes, HL-A antigens and congenital rubella. *Lancet* **ii**, 1509.

66. Ortved Andersen, O., Christy, M., Arnung, K., Buschard, K., Christau, B., Kroman, H., Nerup, J., Platz, P., Ryder, L. P., Svejgaard, A. & Thomsen, M. (1977) Viruses and diabetes. *Proceedings, The IXX International Diabetes Federation Congress, New Delhi,* (in press).

67. Craighead, J. E. (1975) The role of viruses in the pathogenesis of pancreatic disease and diabetes mellitus. *Prog. Med. Virol* **19**, 161.

68. Craighead, J. E. & Higgins, D. A. (1974) Genetic influences affecting the occurrence of diabetes mellitus-like disease in mice infected with the encephalomyocarditis virus. *J. exp. Med.* **139**, 414.

69. von Yoon, J., Maxine, A. Lesniak, Fussganger, R., Notkins, A. L. (1976) Genetic differences in susceptibility of pancreatic beta-cells to virus-induced diabetes mellitus. *Nature (Lond.)* **264**, 178.

70. Kromann, H., Lernmark, Å., Vestergaard, B. F., Egeberg, J. & Nerup, J. (1977) H-2 influence on experimental diabetes induced by heterologous and homologous immunization and by diabetogenic virus. (To be published).

71. Nerup, J., Christy, M. & Egeberg, J. (1977) Diabetes Mellitus. In: *Immunological Diseases. Third ed.,* ed. Sant, M., Little, Brown & Co., (in press).

72. Nerup, J., Andersen, O. O., Bendixen, G., Egeberg, J. & Poulsen, J. E. (1973) Antipancreatic cellular hypersensitivity in diabetes mellitus. Antigenic activity of fetal calf pancreas and correlation with clinical type of diabetes. *Acta allergol. (Khb.)* **28**, 223.

73. MacCuish, A. C., Jordan, J., Campbell, C. J., Duncan, L. J. P. & Irvine, W. J. (1974) Cell-mediated immunity to human pancreas in diabetes mellitus. *Diabetes* **23**, 693.

74. Richens, E., Ancill, R. J. & Hartog, M. 1976) Autoimmunity and viral infection in diabetes mellitus. *Clin. exp. Immunol* **23**, 40.

75. Botazzo, G. F., Florin-Christensen, A. & Doniach, D. (1974) Islet-cell antibodies in diabetes mellitus with autoimmune polyendocrine deficiences. *Lancet* **ii**, 1279.

76. Lendrum, R., Walker, G., Cudworth, A. G., Theophanides, C., Pyke, D. A,, Bloom, A. & Gamble, D. R. (1976) Islet-cell antibodies in diabetes mellitus. *Lancet* **ii**, 1273.

77. Christy, M., Nerup, J., Botazzo, G. F., Doniach, D., Platz, P., Svejgaard, A., Ryder, L. P. & Thomsen, M. (1976) Association between HLA-B8 and autoimmunity in juvenile diabetes mellitus. *Lancet* **ii**, 142.

78. Lendrum, R., Walker, G., Cudworth, A. G., Woodrow, J. C. & Gamble, D. R. (1975) HLA-linked genes and islet-cell antibodies in diabetes mellitus. *Brit. Med. J.* **1**, 1565.

79. Sakurami, T., Nabaya, N., Nagaoka, K., Kurahachi, H., Kuno, S., Nose, Y., Sumitomo, K. & Tsuji, K. (1976) HLA in

maturity-onset diabetes. *First International Symposium on HLA and disease.* Inserm, Paris, June 1976, abstr. no. IV – 21, p. 141.

80. Nelson, P. G. & Pyke, D. A. (1976) Genetic diabetes not linked to the HLA-locus. *Brit. Med. J.* **1**, 196.

81. Faber, O., Thomsen, M., Binder, C., Platz, P. & Svejgaard, A. (1977) Glucose tolerance and HLA antigens in a family with dominantly inherited non-insulin dependent diabetes mellitus. (To be published).

82. Kendall-Taylor, P. (1975) Lats and Human-specific thyroid stimulator: their relation to Graves' disease. *Clinics in Endocrinology and metabolism* **4**, 319.

83. Calder, E. A. & Irvine, W. J. (1975) Cell-mediated immunity and immune complexes in thyroid disease. *Clinics in Endocrinology and metabolism* **4**, 287.

84. Grumet, F. C., Konoshi, J., Payne, R. & Kriss, J. P. (1973) Association of Graves' disease with HL-A8. *Clin. Res.* **21**, 493.

85. Grumet, F. C., Payne, R. O., Konoshi, J. & Kriss, J. P. (1974) HL-A antigens as markers for disease susceptibility and autoimmunity in Graves' disease. *J. Clin. Endocrinol. metabol.* **39**, 1115.

86. Thorsby, E., Segaard, E., Solera, J. H. & Kornstad, L. (1975) The frequency of major histocompatibility antigens (SD & LD) in thyroxicosis. *Tissue Antigens* **6**, 54.

87. Whittingham, S., Morris, P. J. & Martin, F. I. R. (1975) HL-A8: A genetic link with thyrotixicosis. *Tissue Antigens* **6**, 23.

88. Seignalet, J., Jaffiol, C., Baldet, L., Robin, M. & Lapinski (1975) HL-A et maladie de Basedow. *Rev. Franc. Transf.* **17**, 305.

89. Weise, W. & Wenzel, K. W. (1976) Distribution of HLA-antigens in Graves' disease and in autonomous adenoma of the thyroid. *First International Symposium on HLA and disease.* Inserm, Paris, June 1976, abstr. no. IV – 28, p. 148.

90. Farid, N. R., Barnard, J. M. & Marshall, W. H. (1976) The association of HLA with autoimmune thyroid disease in Newfoundland – The influence of HLA homozygosity in Graves' disease. *Tissue Antigens* **8**, 181.

91. Konishi, J., Grumet, F. C., Payne, R. O., Mori, T. & Kriss, J. P. (1976) HLA antigens in japanese patients with Graves' disease. *First International Symposium on HLA and disease.* Inserm, Paris, June 1976, abstr. no. IV – 9, p. 129.

92. Ludwig, H., Scherntaner, G., Mayr, W. R. & Mehdi, S. Q. (1976) Increased susceptibility to endocrine opthalmopathy in HLA-CW3 positive thyrotoxicosis patients. *First International Symposium on HLA and disease.* Inserm, Paris, June 1976, abstr. no. IV – 15, p. 135.

93. Volpè, R., Edmonds, M., Lamki, L., Clarke, P. V. & Row, V. V. (1972) The pathogenesis of Graves' disease. A disorder of delayed hypersensitivity. *Mayo clin. proc.* **47**, 824.

94. Bech, K., Nerup, J. & Hannover Larsen, J. (1977) Yersinia enterocolitica infection and thyroid disease. *Acta endocr. (Kbh.)*, (in press).

95. Nerup, J. (1974) Addison's disease. A review of some clinical pathological and immunological features. Thesis, University of Copenhagen.

96. Ludwig, H., Mayr, W. R., Pacher, M., Scherntaner, G., Koller, K., Eibl, M. & Erd, W. (1975) HL-A antigens in idiopathic Addison's disease. *Z. Immun. Forsch.* **149**, 423.

97. Platz, P., Thyme, S., Starup, J., Thomsen, M., Ryder, L. P., Svejgaard, A. & Nerup, J. (1977) HLA-antigens in hypergonadotropic hypogonadism. (To be published).

98. Bode, H. H., Dorf, M. E. & Forbes, A. D. (1975) Familial lymphocytic thyroiditis: Analysis of linkage with histocompatibility and blood groups. *J. Clin. endocrinol. metab.* **37**, 692.

99. van Rood, J. J., van Hoff, J. P. & Keuning, J. J. (1975) Disease predisposition, immune responsiveness and the fine structure of the HL-A supergene. *Transplant. rev.* **22**, 75.

100. Mayr, W. R., Scherntaner, G., Ludwig, H., Mehdi, S. Q. & Höfer, R. (1976) Missing evidence of a correlation between Hashimoto-thyroiditis and HLA antigens. *First International Symposium on HLA and disease.* Inserm, Paris, June 1976, abstr. no. IV – 17, p. 137.

101. Nyulassy, S., Hnilica, P. & Stefanovic, J. (1975) HL-A system and subacute thyroiditis – a preliminary report. *Tissue Antigens* **6**, 105.

102. Buc, M., Nyulassy, S., Hnilica, P. & Stefanovic, J. (1976) HLA-BW35 and subacute de Quervain's thyroiditis. A definitive report. *First International Symposium on HLA and disease.* Inserm, Paris, June 1976, abstr. no. IV – 2, p. 122.

103. Bech, K., Nerup, J., Thomsen, M.,

Platz, P., Ryder, L. P., Svejgaard, A., Siersbæk-Nielsen, K. & Mølholm-Hansen, J. (1977) HLA antigens in subacute thyroiditis de Quervain. *Acta endocr. (Kbh.),* (in press).

104. Lada, G., Gyodi, E. & Glaz, E. (1976) HLA antigens in patients with adrenocortical hyperfunction. *First International Symposium on HLA and disease.* Inserm, Paris, June 1976, abstr. no. IV – 10, p. 130.

Abnormalities of the HLA System and Gastrointestinal Disease

Warren Strober

Introduction

The gastrointestinal diseases so far found to be associated with HLA abnormalities are disorders in which the immunologic system is somehow involved, either as a primary factor important to the affector limb of the disease, or as a secondary factor important to the effector limb of the disease. In the review of the association between gastrointestinal disease and HLA abnormalities to follow, it will therefore be of particular interest to try to place the HLA abnormalities found in each disease within the context of our current understanding of the nature of the immunologic defect present.

We shall be concerned with three diseases: gluten-sensitive enteropathy or celiac sprue, where a very tangible and important association with HLA antigens has been found, as well as inflammatory bowel disease and pernicious anemia, where HLA abnormalities are statistically less important but nevertheless present. Chronic active hepatitis is another gastrointestinal disease associated with an HLA frequence disturbance and this abnormality will be covered elsewhere in this volume. If one were to seek other associations between gastrointestinal disease and HLA antigens, one would reasonably investigate other possible immunologic disorders of gastrointestinal function such as Whipple's disease (intestinal lipodystrophy) or Mediterranean lymphoma (with or without associated alpha-chain disease); in both of these cases an underlying immunologic defect may have an important pathophysiologic role (1, 2). One would also study hereditary abnormalities of gastrointestinal function such as familial polyposis and familial gastrointestinal carcinoma. Here again, immunologic phenomena may play a part in disease pathogenesis.

Gluten-sensitive enteropathy (celiac sprue)

Gluten-sensitive enteropathy (GSE) is a disease of the small intestinal mucosa which is due to wheat (gluten) protein

Head, Immunophysiology Section, Metabolism Branch, National Cancer Institute, National Institutes of Health, Bethesda, Maryland 20014.

toxicity (3). The active fraction of gluten responsible for the toxicity is not precisely defined as yet, but it is known that it is associated with the gliadin fraction of gluten, most probably the α-gliadin subfraction of this protein group. The main histological feature of GSE is intestinal villous atrophy or flattening which means that there is a physical loss of absorptive surface in this disease. The villous flattening leads in turn to a complex array of digestive derangements involving abnormalities of intestinal fluid balance, hormonal balance, and bile-salt secretion. The loss of absorptive surface and the consequent physiologic derangements account for the chief clinical abnormality encountered in this disease, malabsorption. From a variety of evidence it is clear that the mature epithelial cell lining the small intestine is the target of the disease process and it is the destruction of mature epithelial cells at a rate in excess of the epithelial-cell replacement rate which results in villous flattening. It is also clear that the disease mechanism mediating epithelial-cell destruction is not a direct cellular cytotoxicity mediated by gluten protein itself, but rather a cytotoxicity mediated by the immune system. The factors responsible for the initiation of gluten sensitivity are, at present, imperfectly discerned. A consideration of such factors will be made following the discussion of the relationship between GSE and the HLA system, since this relationship holds the key to the understanding of the disease.

The study of genetic fectors operating in GSE has its origin in family studies of the incidence of this disease (4–10). These family studies indicate that GSE occurs more frequently in relatives of GSE patients than in the general population. For instance, using intestinal biopsy criteria for diagnosis, an incidence of approximately 10–20 % is found in siblings of patients, whereas a somewhat lower incidence, perhaps 5–10 %, is found in parents of patients. These incidence estimates, even if somewhat imprecise, are clearly more than the incidence estimates of GSE in the population as a whole (one in about 3,000 in western European and North American populations) and thus the presence of genetic factors in GSE is strongly suggested. Analysis of families containing GSE patients has not led to a clear definition of the mode of inheritance of GSE and from such studies it cannot be said whether one or several genes are involved in the pathogenesis of this disease. Similarly, analysis of families has not led to conlusions on whether or not the gene (or genes) involved is dominant or recessive.

In 1972, it was discovered that a genetically determined surface-protein, histocompatibility antigen HLA-B8 was associated with GSE (11). This finding has greatly strengthened the contention that genetic factors play an important role in the cause of GSE and has opened the way to a precise identification of the abnormal genes involved in this disease. In one of the two initial studies, the HLA-antigen distribution in GSE was determined in a group of 24 patients with GSE followed at the National Institutes of Health (NIH). It was found that 21 patients (88 %) of the group had HLA-B8, a B-locus antigen, whereas only 22 % of a large group of normal individuals carried this antigen. This difference was statistically significant and has since been confirmed in a variety of subsequent studies originating in Great Britain, Holland, Australia, and Germany (Table I) (12–24). The combined data, involving close to 600 patients, show that the incidence of HLA-B8 in studies of populations composed mostly of adults ($\sim$300 individuals) is approximately 81 %, and in studies of populations composed mostly of children ($\sim$300 individuals) the incidence is approximately 62 %. These HLA-B8 incidences in adults and in children are far higher than the incidence of this antigen in the control populations studies (which varied between

TABLE I
HLA-B8 Frequency in GSE*

A. *Studies of Adult Patients*	No. B8 Positive/ No. Studied		HLA-B8 Frequency in GSE %	Normals %
Strober & Falchuk (USA) (12)	35/47		75	22
Stokes *et al.* (England) (13)	94/117		80	16
Price Evans (England) (14)	16/21		76	
Seah *et al.* (England) (15)	32/36		89	
van Rood *et al.* (Holland) (16)	33/40		83	
Solheim *et al.* (Finland) (17)	9/10		90	
Overall frequency in adults	219/271		81	
B. *Studies of Pediatric Patients*				
Harms *et al.* (Germany) (18)	80/143		56	18
Falchuk *et al.* (USA) (19)	22/31		71	
McNeish *et al.* (England) (20)	23/30		77	
Rolles & Macintosh (England) (21)	27/37		73	
Solheim *et al.* (Finland) (17)	8/12		66	
Mougenot *et al.* (France) (22)	22/38	European	58	17
	5/15	N. African	33	
Overall frequency in children	182/291		62	
C. *Additional Studies – Age of Patients Unknown*				
Murtagh *et al.* (Ireland) (23)	30/40		75	35
Koivisto *et al.* (Finland) (24)	14/20		70	18

* References in parentheses following country of origin.

16 and 35 %), and it may be concluded that GSE is definitely associated with an abnormally high incidence of HLA-B8. In this regard, it has been calculated using Wolf's method that the risk of having GSE for HLA-B8-positive individuals is 8.8 times greater than for HLA-B8-negative individuals (25).

In addition to the HLA-B8, HLA-A1 is increased in GSE patients, but it seemed clear from the beginning that this was due to the fact that HLA-B8 and HLA-A1 are normally in linkage disequilibrium, i.e., these antigens occur together quite frequently in normal populations. That linkage disequilibrium explains the increased frequency of HLA-A1 in GSE which has been formally proven by Harms *et al.* who have shown that HLA-A1 is not increased in GSE patients who lacked HLA-B8, whereas HLA-B8 is increased in patients who lack HLA-A1 (18).

Other HLA-antigen abnormalities found in GSE include a reduced incidence of HLA-B7 and a possible increase in HLA-B12 in non-HLA-B8-positive patients. The reduction in frequency of HLA-B7 is on the order of one third to one half of normal, and the relative risk of GSE in HLA-B7 individuals can be calculated to be 0.41 (25). This decreased frequency of HLA-B7 requires additional confirmation but, if true, it cannot be attributed solely to an increase in HLA-B8 since one would expect all B-locus alleles to be equally affected by the increase and this is clearly not the case; HLA-B12, for instance, occurs in GSE at a normal frequency. Harms *et al.* have suggested that HLA-B7 may be associated with a gene which confers protection against the occurrence of GSE; this would fit with the observation that the frequency of HLA-B7 is decreased in other disease states where HLA-B8 is increased (e.g., diabetes mellitus, myasthenia gravis) and which suggests that the HLA-B7 gene itself or genes associated with HLA-B7 have reciprocal functions to those of the HLA-B8 gene and/or its associated genes.

As for the possible HLA-B12 abnormality, it was found in studies of 25 adult HLA-B8-negative patients in England, Holland, and the United States that 68 % of HLA-B8-negative patients were positive for HLA-B12, a frequency substantially higher than the normal frequency of HLA-B12 in the general population (12). On the other hand, in studies of children with GSE in Germany and Austria, HLA-B12 is not significantly more frequent in HLA-B8-negative patients than in normals (33 % vs 26.4 %) (26). This difference in HLA-B12 incidence in HLA-B8-negative patients may be related to differences in the ethnic background of the groups studies or may reflect more fundamental differences in patients with early and late onset disease.

The difference in HLA-B8 frequency between populations of adult GSE patients and pediatric GSE patients may be more apparent than real in that the combined frequencies are dominated by studies originating from different geographic areas. The adult populations studied are composed mainly of individuals living in Great Britain, whereas the pediatric populations are largely composed of individuals living in Austria and Germany. This difference in the geographic distribution in the adult and pediatric groups introduces the possibility that the differences between HLA-B8 frequency in adults and children may reflect racial and ethnic differences more than inherent differences between HLA-B8-positive and HLA-B8-negative patients. This possibility finds support in the observation of Mougenot et al. that children in Paris of European origin with GSE have a 58 % frequency of HLA-B8, whereas children in Paris of African origin with GSE have a 33 % incidence of this antigen (22). Mougenot et al. suggest that the differing frequency of HLA-B8 in GSE patients belonging to different ethnic groups reflects the fact that the HLA-B8 gene is linked to another more fundamental gene responsible for GSE and this linkage varies with the different groups (see below). In studies in England and the United States where sizable adult and pediatric groups have been studied utilizing populations comprised of more or less homogeneous ethnic backgrounds (12), small differences between HLA-B8 frequency in adults and children are seen. It therefore remains possible that HLA-B8-positive patients do in fact differ from HLA-B8-negative individuals in that the time of onset of disease differs between these patient groups. It should be noted at this point that this possible difference between HLA-B8-positive and HLA-B8-negative GSE patients is the only one that has been found and that otherwise the patients are clinically indistinguishable.

Family studies of GSE in relation to HLA-B8 have been used to show that this antigen is an hereditary characteristic and is not present in GSE merely as an acquired and secondary effect of the disease. In addition, family studies have allowed the analysis of the distribution of GSE in families in which one parent is negative and one parent is heterozygous for a given HLA antigen (18). In this situation, one would expect that if there is no association between GSE and the HLA antigen in question, it would appear at a 50 % frequency in the GSE-negative and the GSE-positive offspring. Thus, if the antigen in question is associated with GSE, it will be overrepresented in the GSE-positive offspring. In such analyses it was found that only HLA-B8 was overrepresented in children with GSE of appropriate parental pairs, whereas nonaffected sibs of these children had a 50 % incidence of HLA-B8. On the other hand, HLA-B7, which was found to be lower in GSE patients in general, tended to be less frequent in affected children of appropriate parental pairs, whereas it again occurred at a 50 % frequency in unaffected siblings. These analyses provide additional proof that the HLA-B8 gene is associated with GSE.

On the basis of the data reviewed so far, only safely may conclude that HLA-B8 is somehow associated with GSE and the question must now be asked whether the HLA-B8 gene is itself wholly or partly responsible for GSE or whether a gene usually, but not always, linked to HLA-B8 is responsible for this disease. The latter possibility can occur in outbred human populations because of linkage disequilibrium, a genetic mechanism already mentioned whereby two genes on the same chromosome are found associated in normal populations because of cross-over suppression, selection or other unknown factors. The available data are strongly in favor of the linked-gene concept. To begin with, there is the fact that GSE occurs in individuals who do not carry HLA-B8 and GSE does not occur in the vast majority of HLA-B8-positive individuals. Then there is the fact that, while GSE usually groups with HLA-B8 within families, there is at least one family in which GSE segregates with another HLA type (18). Finally there is evidence from the family analyzed by Sasporte et al. (27). In this family, peripheral lymphocytes obtained from two siblings with GSE, one with HLA-B8 and one without HLA-B8, gave a negative mixed-leukocyte reaction. This could be explained by a paternal crossover which resulted in the HLA-B8-negative sibling receiving the paternal D-locus antigen,

as did the HLA-B8-positive sibling. Thus, the siblings were A- and B-locus non-identical, but D-locus identical, suggesting that the latter locus is more important than the former in the causation of the disease. Taken together, the foregoing facts are compatible with the concept that the HLA-B8 gene is mainly a marker gene, usually associated with another gene more closely related to the disease. However, before this idea can be unequivocally accepted, there are two observations to be explained that suggest that the HLA-B8 gene is something more than a marker gene. First, there is the observation, alluded to above, that HLA-B8-positive patients may differ clinically from HLA-B8-negative patients with respect to the time of onset of the disease. Secondly and more important, there is the observation that the sensitivity of GSE jejunal tissue to α-gliadin in organ culture differs among GSE patients depending on the HLA-B8 status of the patient: HLA-B8-positive patients react to α-gliadin in culture where HLA-B8-negative patients do not (28). These data can be interpreted to mean that the HLA-B8-gene product itself can somehow affect the quality of the disease in GSE patients even if it cannot play a primary role.

Accepting now that a gene linked to HLA-B8 (and not HLA-B8 itself) is solely or partly responsible for GSE, the question of the nature of this linked gene can be considered. Here the possibility that the linked gene is an HLA-D-locus gene must be considered first and indeed Solheim et al. and van Hoof et al. found, in studies of mixed-leukocyte cultures composed of cell populations obtained from GSE patients, that GSE may be associated with particular D-locus antigens (29, 30). More recently, the possibility that a D-locus antigen is associated with GSE was put

172

on much firmer ground by Keuning *et al.* who used typing cells as well as antisera reacting with D-locus determinants (but not HLA-A or HLA-B locus determinants) to type GSE patients (31). These authors found that 27 out of 28 patients with GSE carried the HLA-DW3 antigen, an antigen previously found to be in linkage disequilibrium with HLA-B8. The frequency of the HLA-DW3 specificity exceeded the frequency of HLA-B8 (22 out of 28 patients) and statistical analysis showed that the HLA-DW3 antigen occurred in patients whether HLA-B8 was present or absent, whereas HLA-B8 occurred only in patients where HLA-DW3 was present. In parallel studies, Solheim *et al.*, using typing cells, observed that HLA-DW3 is found in 61.5 % GSE patients which compared with a 67.4 % incidence of HLA-B8 (32). In this case the HLA-DW3 antigen was not more frequent than HLA-B8 in GSE patients, so that no conclusion regarding the relative importance of HLA-B8 and HLA-DW3 could be drawn. Although additional studies of the relative frequency of D-locus and B-locus antigens in GSE are necessary, on the basis of parallel studies in other diseases in which HLA abnormalities have been found it seems increasingly likely that the D-locus antigen (HLA-DW3) will be more highly correlated with GSE than the B-locus antigen (HLA-B8). This is not to say that either of the genes responsible for these antigens is the primary gene operating GSE, but only that the D-locus gene is more closely linked to the primary gene than the B-locus gene.

Whereas it can scarcely be denied at this point that an H-complex gene is important in the pathogenesis of GSE, it must not be concluded that this gene is the sole genetic factor involved. This observation comes from several pieces of information: first, particular H-complex genes found in most patients with GSE are also found in considerable numbers of normal individuals; secondly, within families several members may share the D-locus antigen yet may be discordant for disease; in this regard, many family members of GSE patients may be HLA identical or haplotype identical with patients, yet may be free of disease even when examined with intestinal biopsy and organ-culture techniques (19); and finally, one family has been found in which the transmittance of GSE does not follow that of HLA; this is a family in which a grandmother and two grandchildren have GSE and the grandmother is totally HLA nonidentical to the grandchildren (19). These facts point inexorably to the conclusion that a gene or set of genes not associated with the H complex must also be present for GSE to occur.

In searching for such an antigen at the National Institutes of Health, the serum of mothers of children with GSE was examined for the presence of antibodies to cell-surface proteins developed during pregnancy with the child destined to have GSE (33). This approach had its origin with the discovery by Mann *et al.* that maternal serum may contain antibodies specific for B-lymphocyte surface proteins (34). In fact, two serums from mothers of GSE patients proved to be active. The first was present in a mother of two young patients with GSE and the second was present in the wife of a man with dermatitis herpetiformis;* in the latter case the couple had a young child who was free of disease, but who nevertheless had lymphocytes bearing GSE-specific antigens.

Using these maternal antisera in a cytotoxicity test specifically designed to

* Dermatitis herpetiformis is a skin disease associated with covert or overt gluten-sensitive enteropathy (see fuller description later).

173

detect B-lymphocyte antigens, it was found that 29 out of 30 patients with GSE and dermatitis herpetiformis (DH) bore B-lymphocyte surface antigens whereas none of approximately 40 control individuals bore such antigens. Thus, the antigen detected, termed the GSE-associated B-cell antigen, appears to be highly correlated with GSE and more or less specific for this disease.

Family studies of the gene controlling GSE-associated B-cell antigen indicated that it is not linked to HLA genes (35). Thus, in several of the families studies, the B-cell antigen was inherited in a manner separate from the HLA antigens and in the remaining families the data were indeterminate. In addition, in at least one instance, HLA-D-locus-identical siblings as determined by nonreactivity in mixed-leukocyte cultures, were GSE B-cell antigen discordant. This indicates that the GSE-associated B-cell antigen is also not part of, or linked to, the HLA-D locus.

On the basis of the new genetic data just mentioned one can hypothesize that GSE is caused by at least two genes acting together: one gene is in the H complex, is associated with HLA-B8, and may be an HLA-D-locus gene; this gene is associated with GSE but is not specific for GSE; the other gene is not part of the H complex, yet its product is found on the surface of B cells; this gene does appear to be specific for GSE. This "two-gene construct" gives rise to the expectation that within GSE families, affected members carry both genes whereas unaffected members do not have either gene or only one of them. This expectation is, of course, testable and is currently under investigation.

The genetic data summarized here can be utilized to propose several mechanisms which may serve as a framework for current thinking and future work on the pathogenesis of gluten-sensitive enteropathy. From a variety of studies, particularly those involving organ culture, it can be shown that gluten is not directly toxic to epithelial cells in patients with GSE but instead activates an endogenous mechanism of toxicity. All indications are that this endogenous mechanism is the immunologic system, but this point requires additional proof. Be this as it may, it can be shown that a number of immunologic effector mechanisms are indeed present in the intestinal mucosa of active GSE patients (having been activated by gluten challenge) and any of these mechanisms can well serve as the endogenous mechanism of toxicity.

Carrying on from these considerations and assuming now that the immune system does mediate gluten toxicity in patients with GSE, an answer must still be provided to the question why the immune system is activated in such patients and not in normal individuals. The answer to this question must surely lie in the explanation of the association of GSE with the genetically determined cell-surface markers discussed above and, in this regard, several broad hypotheses deserve consideration.

In the first hypothesis, the immune system is considered to be activated in GSE by virtue of the fact that there exists in such patients a binding site for gluten protein (or some breakdown product resulting from gluten ingestion). This binding site could be the product of the HLA-B8 gene or the product of the HLA-B8 gene acting together with an associated H-complex gene such as the D-locus gene, HLA-DW3; alternatively, it could consist of the GSE-associated B-cell antigen described above. In any case, such binding would change the physical form with which gluten protein is presented to lymphoid cells in those areas of the GI tract (such as the organized gut-associated lymphoid tissue) where immunological responses are ordinarily induced. Here one touches on a fundamental enigma of GI function: the ability of the GI tract to respond immunologically to certain antigens and to respond poorly (if at all) to other antigens. The secret of this discriminative power could be that immunogenicity in the GI tract is heavily dependent on the physical form of the antigen and that only those antigens presented to GI-tract lymphoid cells in a specifically ordered form are immunogenic. Alternatively, only those antigens in a certain physical form are able to avoid activation of immunologic suppressor mechanisms normally dominating immune response in the gut. Thus, the mere binding of ingested protein to gastrointestinal cell structures may allow protein which is ordinarily nonimmunogenic to become immunogenic and thereby to activate an endogenous mechanism of toxicity.

This binding theory has the advantage that it provides an explanation of the cytotoxicity for epithelial cells characteristic of GSE in that the theory not only allows for the formation of immunogenic signal, but it also allows for the formation of a target of the immunocompetent cells induced as a result of the immunogenic signal. More specifically, epithelial cells with bound gliadin become the target cells of cytotoxic immune-effector cells or their products. It follows that the binding theory would also find important confirmation if one were demonstrate the binding of gliadin to epithelial cells. However, this has not been unequivocally demonstrated, perhaps because of the fact that appropriate and relevant gliadin subfractions have not been available.

A second important possibility for the pathogenesis of GSE is that this disease is due to the presence of an abnormal immune-response gene. In this view, gliadin activates an immunologic and endogenous mechanism of toxicity because patients with GSE possess an abnormal immune-response gene which dictates anti-gliadin antibody production in all individuals who harbor the gene and who are exposed to gluten. Direct support for this idea is limited at the moment and relies heavily on the analogy between GSE and inbred animal models in which it has been shown that response to many antigens are controlled by histocompatibility-linked genes, termed Ir genes (36). The discovery that GSE is associated with a specific B-cell antigen also offers some support for the immune-response gene theory; in this regard it is possible that the B-cell antigen may be a specific receptor for gliadin on the surface of immunocompetent cells and, therefore, that the B-cell antigen could be the Ir-gene product. The fact that the gene controlling the B-cell antigen is not linked to the H complex is not an insuperable barrier to this explanation inasmuch as non-HLA-linked Ir genes have been described in animals. It is, however, more difficult to postulate that the B-cell antigen is a receptor for gliadin in the knowledge that this antigen is not clonally distributed, i.e., found on only a small population of B cells. The resolution of this difficulty may lie in the observation that at least certain kinds of Ir-gene products (such as the Ia antigens of mice) are not clonally distributed either.

One final mechanism to consider is that the H-complex genes associated with GSE and indeed with other diseases involved with immunological abnormalities may be a nonspecific facilitative gene for immune responses generally. In this view, when such genes are present, the organism has a generally heightened ability to respond immunologically, but the response is relatively nondirected and autoimmune in nature. In GSE, on the contrary, such a gene is coupled with a specific gene for anti-gliadin responses and the result is that a heightened ability to respond is channeled toward anti-gliadin antibody production.

In considering which of these hypotheses is more likely, it is fair to point out that these hypotheses are not mutually exclusive. Thus, in stating that a surface antigen associated with GSE leads to binding and, thereby, to an antibody response in GSE, one may in fact be describing the mechanism through which immune-response genes initiate immunologic reactions.

Dermatitis herpetiformis and HLA antigens

An important and still unexplained disease association is that between GSE and the skin disease dermatitis herpetiformis (DH). The latter is a pruritic vesicular skin disease occurring usually, but not exclusively, on extensor surfaces. Histologically, the skin lesions are characterized by an epithelial blister surrounded by a local granulocytic infiltration. Immunologically, these lesions are characterized by the deposition of IgA immunoglobulin in the fibrous tissue just below the epithelial basement membrane (37). In recent years it has become apparent that the great majority of DH patients also have GI lesions similar to that seen in GSE and, as in the case of GSE, this gut lesion is responsive to gluten exclusion (38, 39). It was originally felt that only about two thirds of GH patients have a GI lesion; later with the use of more sophisticated biopsy techniques and by challenging DH patients with large amounts of gluten, it became apparent that most, if not all, DH patients have gluten sensitivity and some degree of villous flattening (40, 41).

As the above facts indicate, GSE and DH are clinically associated. In addition, these disease can be linked together at a genetic level by virtue of the fact that dermatitis herpetiformis patients have a very high frequency of HLA-B8 as well as the D-locus antigen DW3 (32, 42, 43). In addition, the B-cell antigen specific for GSE mentioned above and detected with antisera obtained from mothers of GSE patients can also be detected on the cells of DH patients (33). On the basis of these facts, dermatitis herpetiformis may be visualized as the disease which is essentially similar to ordinary gluten-sensitive enteropathy in that both diseases are fundamentally brought about by a common disease mechanism centering in the gut and resulting in the production of anti-gliadin antibodies. Furthermore, it may be speculated that the consequences of this immune reaction differ in the two diseases. In ordinary GSE the main consequence of the abnormal production of anti-gliadin is felt in the GI tract itself and the focus of the cytotoxicity reaction is the mature gut epithelial cell. On the contrary, in DH the main consequence of the abnormal antibody production is in the skin and is brought about by the deposition of antibody-antigen complexes (gliadin-anti-gliadin) which binds to a skin-receptor site specific for gliadin.

This speculation is presently unsupported by direct demonstration of the presence of gliadin in the skin of DH patients. However, it is supported by the clinical observation that gluten exclusion is efficacious in the treatment of the skin in at least some patients

176

(44). Moreover, circulating immune complexes have been detected in the blood of DH patients and the histological nature of the skin lesion in DH is consistent with that caused by immune-complex deposition and complement activation (45). Finally, the concept that DH skin contains a receptor for gluten protein is a logical supposition in that DH (as well as GSE) is associated with a variety of genes that code for surface antigens.

The inflammatory bowel diseases

The imflammatory bowel diseases (IBD) are a spectrum of disorders comprising the various forms of ulcerative colitis and Crohn's disease (regional ileitis). A variety of evidence supports the view that these diseases are closely related etiologically in spite of the fact that they usually involve different parts of the gastrointestinal tract and have distinctive (but overlapping) histologic features. Recently, evidence has accumulated that both forms of inflammatory bowel disease may be caused by a transmissible agent (a virus) (46, 47). This evidence consists of the observation that inflammatory bowel disease can be produced in both rabbits and mice injected with homogenates of diseased human tissue, but not homogenates of normal tissue. Furthermore, unidentified RNA viruses are recovered from affected tissue of most inflammatory bowel disease patients but generaliy not from normal gastrointestinal tissue. These findings suggest that inflammatory bowel disease is an infectious disease, but it is likely that, if indeed that is so, only individuals with preexistent immunologic and/or genetic abnormalities will be susceptible to the infection.

As far as a possible underlying immune defect is concerned, a number of immunologic abnormalities have been quite definitely identified. Some of these are almost certainly secondary elements in the disease, but others are quite possibly primary elements. Chief among these immunologic abnormalities are 1) the presence in many patients of anti-colon antibodies which crossreact with widely distributed bacterial antigens (common enterobacterial antigen) but which are not active in complement-mediated lysis of colon epithelial cells and are not correlated with disease activity (48, 49); 2) the local infiltration of diseased mucosa by lymphoid cells, particularly IgG-containing plasma cells (50); 3) the presence of circulating effector cells with cytotoxicity for colonic epithelial cells, effector cells which are probably a type of K-cell (Fc-receptor positive, surface-immunoglobulin negative) (51); 4) the presence of circulating antibodies capable of mediating antibody-dependent cellular cytotoxicity involving normal lymphoid effector cells and colonic epithelial cell targets (52); 5) the presence of minimally depressed cell-mediated immunity as assessed by peripheral-lymphocyte response to nonspecific mitogens in vitro (53); and 6) increased reactivity of peripheral cells to colon antigens and enterobacterial common antigen as assessed by ability of such cells to produce migration inhibition factor (MIF) (54). In summary, a spectrum of immunologic abnormalities is seen in IBD which gives rise to the suggestion that immunologic defects play some role in the causation of disease. On the one hand such defects may lead to an increased susceptibility to a harmful virus infection which is ordinarily nonvirulent. On the other hand, such defects may in fact be caused by a viral infection and the immunologic system may then directly mediate the disease. In any case, both of these views provide wide latitude for the operation of pathogenic genetic factors, including the operation of abnormal genes in the histocompatibility region of the genome.

Turning specifically to the genetic factors there is first the fact, derived from epidemiologic data, that inflammatory bowel disease is at least in part an hereditary condition (55). Thus, approximately 15 % of cases occur in individuals with affected relatives, particularly close (first degree) relatives, whereas affected spouses and environmentally clustered cases have only rarely been reported. In addition, identical twins have usually been concordant for disease, especially in the case of Crohn's disease. Additional evidence in support of genetic influences are the facts that anti-colon antigen specificity occurs in higher-than-expected frequency in (female) unaffected relatives of patients and that inflammatory bowel disease is associated with another disease of undoubted genetic background, ankylosing spondylitis (56–58).

The foregoing considerations suggest but do not prove that hereditary factors play a role in the pathogenesis of inflammatory bowel disease. To approach this question more directly, considerable effort has been directed toward discovering a set of genetic markers unique to this disease. In the late 1950s and early 1960s blood-group antigens were studied as possible genetic markers, but no special association between inflammatory bowel diseases and any particular blood type was found (55). In recent years many studies have focused on finding a link between histocompatibility antigens and inflammatory bowel disease. These studies seemed particularly promising since there was already considerable evidence, such as that presented above, that IBD is associated with immunologic abnormalities. Nevertheless, the composite result of HLA studies in IBD has been generally negative in that no single HLA-antigenic specificity has been found which occurs in unequivocally greater-than-normal frequency. This conclusion can be drawn from the results of some 14 studies emanating from Western Europe, Japan and the United States

TABLE II

*HLA Antigens in Ulcerative Colitis**

Reference	No. of Patients Studied	HLA Abnormalities	Comments
Asquith *et al.* (59) ⎫ same patient Mallas *et al.* (60) ⎭ group	100	No HLA abnormalities	B27 associated with total colitis
Berger *et al.* (61)	51	No HLA abnormalities	
Gleeson *et al.* (62)	16	No HLA abnormalities	? B27 typed
Lewkonia *et al.* (63)	37	No HLA abnormalities	B27 not typed
Morris *et al.* (64)	11	B27 may be increased (no statistical analysis)	? Patients selected for presence of arthritides
Murtagh *et al.* (23)	30	No HLA abnormalities	
Tsuchiya *et al.* (65)	40	HLA-B5 ↑	Japanese patients
Vachon *et al.* (66)	42	No HLA abnormalities	
Van den Berg-Loonen *et al* (67)	58	HLA-A11 ↑	

* Reference numbers in parentheses.

TABLE III

TABLE III
HLA Antigens in Crohn's Disease*

Reference	No. of Patients Studied	HLA Abnormalities	Comments
Asquith et al. (59) } same patient Mallas et al. (60) } group	100	No HLA abnormalities	
Bergman et al. (61)	62	HLA-BW17 ↑ (not significantly)	
de Deuxchaisnes et al. (68)	21	No HLA abnormalities	
Gleeson et al. (62)	18	HLA-A3 ↑ but anti-A3 not specific	
Jacoby & Jayson (69)	74	HLA-B13 ↑ (not significantly)	
Lewkonia et al. (63)	30	No HLA abnormalities	B27 not typed
Morris et al. (64)	18	B27 may be increased (no statistical analysis)	? Patients selected for presence of arthritides
Russell et al. (70)	77	B27 (not significantly)	
Thorsby & Lie (71)	19	HLA-BW17 ↑ (not significantly)	
Vachon et al. (66)	24	HLA-A10 ↑ (not significantly)	B-locus blank increased
Van den Berg-Loonen et al. (67)	51	HLA-B18 ↑	Increased incidence of blood-group Kell

* Reference numbers in parenthesis.

and including approximately 400 patients with ulcerative colitis and approximately 500 patients with Crohn's disease (Tables II and III) (23, 59–71). Thus, whereas some studies report an increased frequency of a particular antigen, these increases were not consistently found, and, in one large series, deviations seen initially were not observed as the study group was expanded (59, 60). In one recent study, HLA-BW17 was increased in patients with Crohn's disease, but not to a significant degree (61). If these data are combined with another study in which HLA-BW17 was also investigated (71), the risk of Crohn's disease in A17-positive individuals is 3.3 times greater than the normal risk. The significance of this finding is tempered by the fact that in other studies HLA-BW17 is found in normal frequency; in addition, even in the studies where it is found to be increased, HLA-BW17 was found in only 10–11 % of the patients (vs 3–5 % of controls) and therefore the proposed excess of HLA-BW17 is not impressive.

The evidence of normal and nearly normal HLA frequency in inflammatory bowel disease is somewhat at variance with the fact that IBD (both ulcerative colitis and Crohn's disease) is associated with ankylosing spondylitis and the latter disease is highly correlated with HLA-B27 (approximately 75 % incidence in patients vs 6 % in the normal population) (57, 58, 72). However, since the occurrence of ankylosing spondylitis in IBD is relatively infrequent (7 %), this apparent discrepancy could be explained if HLA-B27 in IBD patients is found exclusively or mainly among those IBD patients with associated ankylosing spondylitis. In fact, this appears to be true: Morris et al. analyzed 31 patients with IBD and found that of the eight with associated ankylosing spondylitis, six (75 %) had HLA-B27, whereas none of the IBD patients without ankylosing spondylitis had HLA-B27 (73); similarly, HLA-B27 was more frequent in IBD patients with ankylosing spondylitis than without ankylosing spondylitis in studies by Brewerton *et al.*, Mallas *et al.*, and Van den Berg-Lonnen *et al.*, although in the latter studies the incidence of this antigen in IBD and ankylosing spondylitis patients (50 %) was significantly lower than in patients with ankylosing spondylitis alone (60, 67, 74). The lowest incidence of HLA-B27 in IBD patients with associated ankylosing spondylitis is reported by de Deuxchaisnes *et al.* (about 30 %), yet even here the incidence is clearly higher than in the IBD population as a whole or in the general population (68).

The interpretation of the HLA data with respect to HLA-B27 and ankylosing spondylitis is unclear. On the one hand, the data seem to indicate that despite the association with ankylosing spondylitis, HLA-B27 is not a genetic factor in IBD since the incidence of this antigen in IBD patients with ankylosing spondylitis is no higher than that in normals. Rather it may be that IBD is a predisposing "environmental" influence which results in the occurrence of ankylosing spondylitis in B27-positive patients in the same way that yersinia and salmonella infections of the gastrointestinal tract can lead to arthritides in otherwise normal B27-positive individuals (75). Stated differently, it is as if the presence of a chronic intestinal inflammation occurring for diverse environmental and genetic reasons is, in turn, a precipitating "environmental" factor for the development of another disease, ankylosing spondylitis, in individuals with the appropriate genetic background (including HLA-B27).

On the other hand, HLA-B27 may indeed be part of the genetic beckground of IBD even though it is not increased among IBD patients. This may be inferred from the facts that: 1) the incidence of ankylosing spondylitis is vastly increased among the relatives of both ulcerative colitis and Crohn's disease patients, including those patients with associated ankylosing spondylitis and patients without associated ankylosing spondylitis; and 2) ankylosing spondylitis may precede IBD temporally and seems to progress independently of the bowel disease, thereby shedding doubt proposition that IBD is an "environmental" influence precipitating ankylosing spondylitis. These observations are best explained if one assumes that both IBD and ankylosing spondylitis are determined by multiple genetic factors, some of which are shared; in this context, HLA-B27 is one of such shared genetic factors.

In any case, the fact that IBD patients developing ankylosing spondylitis are usually HLA-B27 positive is clinically important because it helps one to predict which IBD patient is likely to develop ankylosing spondylitis even before it develops. In this regard, Mallas *et al.* propose that HLA-B27-positive IBD patients may be subject to a more severe form of disease (ankylosing spondylitis or inflammatory bowel disease) so that HLA status may help to predict the clinical course (60). Finally, the association of HLA-B27 in IBD and ankylosing spondylitis is important becasue of the fact that another form of arthritis associated with IBD, namely peripheral "enteropathic" arthritis, is not associated with an increased incidence of HLA-B27, whereas iritis associated with IBD does appear to be associated with HLA-B27 (73). Thus the HLA status of a particular patient may help to predict the nature of the complications that can be expected in IBD.

To conclude, while the HLA antigens have not emerged as a key genetic-marker system in IBD, genes determining HLA antigens may be linked to (or act together with) other genes more directly relevant to the disease. Additionally, HLA genes may be part of a complex array of genes forming the multigenic background necessary for disease development. Finally. knowledge of HLA in IBD may help predict the particular form of inflammatory bowel disease manifested in any given patient.

Pernicious anemia

A third distinct gastrointestinal disease associated with HLA abnormalities is pernicious anemia. This condition occurs as a result of gastric atrophy associated with achlorhydria and reduced intrinsic-factor secretion. It appears to be the end stage of a chronic inflammatory process involving the gastric mucosa which starts as an atrophic gastritis with reduced acid secretion and which ends as a severe gastric atrophy and intrinsic-factor deficiency (76). Patients with pernicious anemia have serum and gastric juice antibodies to intrinsic factor which are more or less specific for the disease as well as anti-gastric parietal cell antibodies which are less specific but are detected earlier. There is considerable evidence that the antiperietal cell antibodies play a role in destruction of parietal cells and, as a result, gastric atrophy and pernicious anemia may be considered an organ-specific autoimmune disease (77).

In view of the foregoing, it is not suprising that pernicious anemia frequently occurs in association with other organ-specific autoimmune endocrine diseases including Graves' disease, diabetes mellitus, and idiopathic Addison's disease. As in the case of these diseases, it has now been established that pernicious anemia is associated with a relatively minor but definite abnormality in HLA frequency. This consists of an increased incidence of HLA-B7 which occurs at about twice the rate in patients as in controls (37–52 % in patients vs 19–26 % in controls) and it can be calculated that the risk of pernicious anemia in B7-positive individuals is twice as great as in normals (78–80 %). HLA-A3 is also increased in all studies, but this is attributable to linkage disequilibrium: HLA-A3 and HLA-B7 are frequently found together in the normal population. It is of interest that the occurrence af HLA-B7 is not correlated with the presence of autoantibodies (anti-intrinsic factor or anti-parietal cell antibodies), clinical features of the disease or blood group states (blood group A is associated with pernicious anemia; 62 % in patients vs 44 % in controls) (80). Furthermore, in one study HLA-B7 was not increased in patients with "simple" atrophic gastritis (although HLA-A3 was marginally increased), in spite of the fact that this condition, as indicated above, is felt to be antecedent to pernicious anemia (78).

The significance of the HLA abnormality in pernicious anemia is far from clear. In other autoimmune endocrine diseases, even those which are in fact associated with pernicious anemia, the HLA antigen present at an increased frequency is HLA-B8 (Graves' disease, Addison's disease and diabetes mellitus). This, taken with the observations that other abnormalities of HLA-A3 and HLA-B7 involve not the endocrine system but rather the nervous system (multiple sclerosis and poliomyelitis)

(81) lead one to the conclusion that one cannot postulate a unifying theory which involves a specific HLA gene and various organ-specific autoimmune abnormalities. Instead, one must assume that HLA-B7 and HLA-A3 antigens influence the development of pernicious anemia in a more specific but as yet completely unknown manner.

Conclusion

The gastrointestinal diseases associated with HLA abnormalities are mediated by a diverse group of pathologic mechanisms. These mechanisms may be characterized in one way as disorders of the immune system and in another way as abnormalities of cell-surface interactions. This leads one to suspect that the number and type of GI diseases associated with HLA abnormalities are by no means exhausted, particularly when one begins to examine associations with D-locus genes and other non-HLA genes which may interact with HLA genes. Certainly, the search for such genes can and should be pursued in an effort to shed new light on the genetic basis of gastrointestinal disease.

Acknowledgements

We are grateful to Drs. B. Genetet, W. Mayr, J. Rey and J. Benhamou for assistance during the Gastroenterology Workshop of the HLA and Disease Symposium.

References

1. Groll, A., Valberg, L. & Simon, J. B. (1972) Immunological defect in Whipple's disease. *Gastroenterology* **63**, 943.
2. Rambaud, J. C. & Matuchansky, C. (1973) Alpha-chain disease. Pathogenesis and relation to Mediterranean lymphoma. *Lancet* ii, 1430–1432.
3. Strober, W. (1976) Gluten-sensitive enteropathy. *Clinics in Gastroenterology* **5**, 429–452.
4. Boyer, P. H. & Anderson, D. H. (1956) A genetic study of coeliac disease. *Amer. J. Dis. Child.* **91**, 131–137.
5. Carter, C., Sheldon, W. & Walker, C. (1959) The inheritance of coeliac disease. *Ann. Human Genetics* **23**, 266–278.
6. MacDonald, W. C., Dobbins, W. O. & Rubin, C. E. (1965) Studies of the familial nature of coeliac sprue using biopsy of the small intestine. *New. Eng. J. Med.* **272**, 448–456.
7. McCrea, W. M. (1969) Inheritance of coeliac disease. *J. Med. Genetics* **6**, 129–131.
8. Robinson, D. C., Watson, A. J., Wyatt, E. H., Marks, J. M. & Roberts, D. F. (1971) Incidence of small intestinal mucosal abnormalities and of clinical coeliac disease in the relatives of children with coeliac disease. *Gut* **12**, 789–793.
9. Mylotte, M. J., Egon-Mitchell, B., Fottrell, P. F., McNicholl, B. & McCarthy, C. F. (1972) Familial coeliac disease. *Quart. J. Med.* **41**, 527–528.
10. Stokes, P. L., Asquith, P. & Coke, W. T. (1973) Genetics of coeliac disease. *Clinics in Gastroenterology* **2**, 547–556.
11. Falchuk, Z. M., Rogentine, G. N. & Strober, W. (1972) Predominance of histocompatibility antigen HL-A8 in patients with gluten-sensitive enteropathy. *J. Clin. Invest.* **51**, 1602–1606.
12. Strober, W. & Falchuk, Z. M. Unpublished observations.
13. Stokes, P. L., Asquith, P., Holmes, G. K. T., Macintosh, P. & Cook, W. T. (1973) Inheritance and influence of histocompatibility (HL-A) antigens in adult coeliac disease. *Gut* **14**, 627–630.
14. Price Evans, D. A. (1973) Coeliac disease and HL-A8. *Lancet* ii, 1096.
15. Seah, P. P., Fry, L., Kearney, J. W., Campbell, E., Mowbray, J. F., Stewart, J. S. & Hoffbrand, A. V. (1974) Lymphocyte infiltration of the small intestine in dermatitis herpetiformis and adult coeliac disease. In: *Proc. 2nd Int.*

Coeliac Symp., eds. Hekkens, W. Th. J. M. & Peña, A. S., pp. 138–140, Stenfert-Kroese, Leiden.

16. van Rood, J. J., van Hooff, J. P. & Keuning, J. J. (1975) Disease predisposition, immune responsiveness and the fine structure of the HL-A supergene. *Transplant. Rev.* **22,** 75–104.

17. Solheim, B. G., Baklien, K. & Ek, J. (1974) Association of coeliac disease with HL-A antigens and MLC antigens. In: *Proc. 2nd Int. Coeliac Symp.*, eds. Hekkens, W. Th. J. M. & Peña, A. S., p. 232, Stenfert-Kroese, Leiden.

18. Harms, K., Granditsch, G., Rossipal, E., Ludwig, H., Polymenidis, Z., Wank, R., Scholz, S., Steinbauer-Rosenthal, I. & Albert, E. D. (1974) HL-A in patients with coeliac disease and their families. In. *Proc. 2nd Int. Coeliac Symp.*, eds. Hekkens, W. Th. J. M. & Peña, A. S., pp. 215–226, Stenfert-Kroese, Leiden.

19. Falchuk, Z. M., Katz, A. J., Schwachman, H., Rogentine, G. N. & Strober, W. (1976) Evidence that at least two genes are necessary for the pathogenesis of gluten-sensitive enteropathy. (Submitted for publication.)

20. McNeish, A. S., Nelson, R., & Macintosh, P. (1973) HL-A1 and 8 in childhood coeliac disease. *Lancet* **i,** 668.

21. Rolles, C. J. & Macintosh, P. (1974) Concordance for HL-A antigens in the parents of children with coeliac disease. *Gut* **12,** 789–793.

22. Mougenot, J. F., Polonovski, C., Sasportes, M. L., Schmid, M. & Hors, J. (1976) HLA and digestive intolerance to gluten and cow's milk proteins. In: *1st Int. Symp. on HLA and Disease,* Paris, France. (Abstract.)

23. Murtagh, T. J., Reen, D. J. & Gerally, J. (1976) HL-A A1 and B8 in coeliac disease. *1st Int. Symp. on HLA and Disease,* Paris, France. (Abstract.)

24. Koivisto, V. A., Kuitunen, P., Tiilikainen, A. & Åkerblom, H. K. (1976) HLA antigens, especially B8 and BW15, in patients with juvenile diabetes mellitus, coeliac disease, and both of these diseases. In: *1st Int. Symp. on HLA and Disease,* Paris, France. (Abstract.)

25. Ryder, L. P. & Svejgaard, A. (1976) Associations between HLA and disease. *Report from the HLA and Disease Registry of Copenhagen, 1976,* p. 2.

26. Ludwig, H. & Granditsch, G. (1974) HL-A antigens in coeliac disease. *Lancet* **ii,** 459.

27. Sasportes, M., Mawas, C., Buc, M., Charmot, D., Mougenot, J. F. & Dausset, J. (1975) LD typing in coeliac disease. *10th Leukocyte Culture Conference,* abstracts II: 85.

28. Nelson, D. L., Falchuk, Z. M., Kasarda, D. & Strober, W. (1975) Gluten-sensitive enteropathy: correlation of organ culture behavior with HL-A status. *Clin. Res.* **23,** 254 (abstract).

29. Solheim, B. G., Baklien, K. & Ek, J. (1974) Association of coeliac disease with HL-A antigens and MLC antigens. In: *Proc. 2nd Int. Coeliac Symp.*, eds. Hekkens, W. Th. J. M. & Peña, A. S., p. 232. Stenfert-Kroese, Leiden.

30. van Hooff, J. P., Peña, A. S., Keuning, J. J., Termiptelen, A., Hekkens, W. Th. J. M., Haex, A. J. Ch. & van Rood, J. J. (1974) In: *Proc. of the 2nd Int. Coeliac Symp.*, eds. Hekkens, W. Th. J. M. & Peña, A. S., p. 233, Stenfert-Kroese, Leiden.

31. Keuning, J. J., Peña, A. S., van Leeuwen, A., van Hooff, J. P. & van Rood, J. J. (1976) HLA-DW3 association with coeliac disease. *Lancet* **i,** 506–511.

32. Solheim, B. G., Ek, J., Thune, P. O., Baklien, K., Bratlie, A., Rankin, B., Thoresen, A. B. & Thorsby, E. (1976) HLA antigens in dermatitis herpetiformis and coeliac disease. *Tissue Antigens* **7,** 57–59.

33. Mann, D. L., Katz, S. I., Nelson, D. L., Abelson, L. D. & Strober, W. (1976) Specific B-cell antigens associated with gluten-sensitive enteropathy and dermatitis herpetiformis. *Lancet* **i,** 110–111.

34. Mann, D. L., Abelson, L. D., Henkart, P., Harris, S. D. & Amos, D. B. (1975) Specific human B lymphocyte alloantigens (L-B) linked to HL-A. *Proc. nat. Acad. Sci. (Wash.)* **72,** 5103–5106.

35. Katz, S. I., Mann, D. L., Nelson, D. L., Abelson, L. D. & Strober, W. (1976) Non-H-complex-linked B-lymphocyte antigens in gluten-sensitive enteropathy and dermatitis herpetiformis. *Clin. Res.* **24,** 447 (abstract).

36. McDevitt, H. O. & Benaceraff, B. (1969) Genetic control of specific immune responses. *Adv. Immunol.* **11,** 31–74.

37. Seah, P. P., Stewart, J. S., Fry, L., Chapman, B. L., Hoffbrand, A. V. & Holborow, E. J. (1972) Immunoglobulins in the skin in dermatitis herpetiformis and coeliac disease. *Lancet* **i,** 611–614.

38. Marks, J., Shuster, S. & Watson, A. J. (1966) Small-bowel changes in dermatitis herpetiformis. *Lancet* **ii,** 1280–1282.

39. Fry, L., McMinn, R. H. M., Cowan, J. D. & Hoffbrand, A. V. (1968) Effect of gluten-free diet on dermatological, intestinal, and haematological manifestations of dermatitis herpetiformis. *Lancet* i, 557–561.
40. Brow, J. R., Parker, F., Weinstein, W. M. & Rubin, C. E. (1971) The small intestinal mucosa in dermatitis herpetiformis. I. Severity and distribution of the small intestinal lesion and associated malabsorption. *Gastroenterology* 60, 355–361
41. Weinstein, W. M. (1974) Latent celiac sprue. *Gastroenterology* 66, 48–493.
42. Katz, S. I., Falchuk, Z. M., Dahl, M. V., Rogentine, G. N. & Strober, W. (1972) HL-A8: a genetic link between dermatitis herpetiformis and gluten-sensitive enteropathy. *J. Clin. Invest.* 51, 2977–2979.
43. Thomsen, M., Platz, P., Marks, J., Ryder, L. P., Shuster, S., Svejgaard, A. & Young, S. H. (1976) Association of LD-8a and LD-12a with dermatits herpetiformis. *Tissue Antigens* 7, 60–62.
44. Fry, L., McMinn, R. M. H., Cowan, J. D. & Hoffbrand, A. V. (1968) Effect of gluten-free diet on dermatological, intestinal, and haematological manifestation of dermatitis herpetiformis. *Lancet* i, 557–561.
45. Seah, P. P., Mazaheri, M. R., Fry, L., Mowbray, J. F., Hoffbrand, A. V. & Holborow, E. J. (1973) Alternate-pathway complement fixation by IgA in the skin in dermatitis herpetiformis. *Lancet* ii, 175–177.
46. Beeken, W. L., Mitchell, D. N. & Cave, D. R. (1976) Evidence for a transmissible agent in Crohn's disease. *Clinics in Gastroenterology* 5, 289–302.
47. Forsyth, B. (1975) Isolation and characterization of a viral agent from intestinal tissue of patients with Crohn's disease and other chronic intestinal disorders. *Prog. Med. Virol.* 21, 165–176.
48. Broberger, O. & Perlmann, P. (1963) In vitro studies of ulcerative colitis. I. Reactions of patients' serum with human fetal colon cells in tissue culture. *J. exp. Med.* 117, 705–715.
49. Perlmann, P., Hammerstrom, S., Lagercrantz, R. & Campbell, D. (1967) Autoantibodies to colon in rats and human ulcreative colitis; crossreactivity, with Escherichia coli 014 antigen. *Proc. Soc. exp. Biol. Med.* 125, 975–980.
50. Brandtzaeg, P., Baklien, K., Fausa, O. & Hoel, P. S. (1974) Immunohistochemical characterization of local immunoglobulin formation in ulcerative colitis. *Gastroenterology* 66, 1123–1136
51. Stobo, J. D., Tomasi, T. B., Huizenga, K. A., Spencer, R. J. & Shorter R. G. (1975) In vitro studies of inflammatory bowel disease. Surface receptors of the mononuclear cells required to lyse allogeneic colonic epithelial cells. *Gastroenterology* 70, 171–176.
52. Shorter, R. G., Huizenga, K. A., Spencer, R. J., Aas, J. & Guy, S. K. (1971) Cytophilic antibody: The responsible factor in the cytotoxicity of lymphocytes in inflammatory bowel disease. *Gastroenterology* 60, 802.
53. Whorwell, P. J. & Wright, R. (1976) Immunological aspects of inflammatory bowel disease. *Clinics in Gastroenterology* 5, 303–321.
54. Bull, D. M. & Ignaczak, T. F. (1973) Enterobacterial common antigen induced lymphocyte reactivity in inflammatory bowel disease. *Gastroenterology* 64, 43–50.
55. Kirsner, J. B. (1973) Genetic aspects of inflammatory bowel disease. *Clinics in Gastroenterology* 2, 557–575.
56. Lagerkrantz, R., Perlmann, P. & Hammerstrom, S. (1971) Immunological studies in ulcreatve colitis. V. Family studies *Gastroenterology* 60, 391–389.
57. Haslock, I. & Wright, V. (1973) The musculo-skeletal complications of Crohn's disease. *Medicine* 52, 217–225.
58. Jayson, M. I. V., Salmon, P. R. & Harrison, W. J. (1970) Inflammatory bowel disease in ankylosing spondylitis. *Gut* 11, 506–511.
59. Asquith, P. Stokes, P. L., Macintosh, P., Holmes, G. K. T. & Cooke, W. T. (1974) Histocompatibility antigens in patients with inflammatory bowel disease. *Lancet* i, 113–115.
60. Mallas, E., Macintosh, P., Asquith, P. & Cooke, W. T. (1976) Transplantation antigens in inflammatory bowel disease. Their clinical significance and their association with arthropathy with special reference to HLA-B27 (W27). In: *1st Int. Symp. on HLA and Disease,* Paris, France. (Abstract.)
61. Bergman, L., Lindblom, J. B., Syfwenberg, J. & Krause, U. (1976) HL-A frequencies in Crohn's disease and ulcerative colitis. *Tissue Antigens* 7, 145–150.
62. Gleeson, M. H., Walker, J. S., Wentzel, J., Chapman, J. A. & Harris, R. (1972) Human leukocyte antigens in Crohn's disease and ulcerative colitis. *Gut* 13, 438–440.
63. Lewkonia, R. W., J. C., McConnell, R. B.

& Price Evans, D. A. (1974) HL-A antigens in inflammatory bowel disease. *Lancet* i, 574–575.

64. Morris, R. I., Metzger, A. L., Bluestone, R. & Terasaki, P. I. (1974) HL-A-W27, a useful discriminator in the arthropathies of inflammatory bowel disease. *New. Eng. J. Med.* **290**, 1117–1119.

65. Tsuchiya, M., Yushida, T., Mizuno, Y., Kurita, K., Hibi, T. & Tsuji, K. (1976) HL-A antigens and ulcreative colitis in Japan. In: *1st Int. Symp. on HLA and Disease*, Paris, France. (Abstract.)

66. Vachon, A., Gebuhrer, L. & Betuel, H. (1976) HL-A antigens in ulcreative colitis and Crohn's disease. In: *1st Int. Symp. on HLA and Disease*, Paris, France. (Abstract.)

67. van den Berg-Loonen, E. M., Dekker-Saeys, B. J., Meuwissen, S. G. M., Nijenhuis, L. E. & Engelfret, C. P. (1976) Histocompatibility antigens and other genetic markers in ankylosing spondylitis and inflammatory bowel diseases. In: *1st Int. Symp. on HLA and Disease,* Paris, France. (Abstract.)

68. de Deuxchaisnes, C. N., Huaux, J. P., Fiarre, P. & de Brugere, M. (1974) Ankylosing spondylitis, sacroileitis, regional enteritis and HLA-27. *Lancet* i, 1238.

69. Jacoby, R. K. & Jayson, M. I. V. (1974) HL-A-27 in Crohn's disease. *Ann. Rheum. Dis.* **33**, 422–424.

70. Russell, A. S., Percy, J. S., Schlaut, J., Sartor, V. E., Goodhart, J. M., Sherbaniuk, R. W. & Kidd, E. G. (1975) Transplantation antigens in Crohn's disease. Linkage of associated ankylosing spondylitis with HL-AW27. *Am. J. Dig. Dis.* **20**, 359–361.

71. Thorsby, E. & Lie, S. O. (1971) Relationship between HL-A system and susceptibility to diseases. *Transplant. Proc.* **3**, 1305–1307.

72. Brewerton, D. A., Hart, F. D., Nicholls, A., Caffrey, M., James, D. C. O. & Sturrock, R. D. (1973) Ankylosing spondylitis and HL-A27. *Lancet* i, 904–907.

73. Morris, R. I., Metzger, A. L., Bluestone, R. & Terasaki, P. I. (1974) HL-A-W27 - A useful discriminator in the arthropathies of inflammatory bowel disease. *New Eng. J. Med.* **290**, 1117–1119.

74. Brewerton, D. A., Caffrey, M., Nicholls, A., Walters, D. & James, D. C. O. (1974) HL-A27 and arthropathies associated with ulcerative colitis and psoriasis. *Lancet* i, 956–958.

75. Aho, K., Ahvonen, P. & Alkio, P. (1975) HL-A27 in reactive arthritis following infection. *Ann. Rheum. Dis.* (suppl.) **34**, 29–30.

76. Irvine, W. J., Cullen, D. R. & Mawhinney, H. (1974) Natural history of autoimmune achlorhydric atrophic gastritis. A 1–15 year follow-up study. *Lancet* ii, 482–484.

77. Irvine, W. J. (1965) Immunological aspects of pernicious anemia. *New Eng. J. Med.* **273**, 432–438.

78. Mawhinney, H., Lawton, J. W. M., White, A. C. & Irvine, W. J. (1975) HL-A3 and HL-A7 in pernicious anemia and autoimmune atrophic gastritis. *Clin. exp. Immul.* **22**, 47–53.

79. Whittingham, S., Youngchaiyud, U., Mackay, I. R., Buckley, J. D. & Marris, P. J. (1975) Thyrogastric autoimmune disease. Studies on the cell-mediated immune response and histocompatibility antigens. *Clin. exp. Immunol.* **19**, 289–299.

80. Zittoun, R., Zittoun, J., Seignalet, J. & Dausset, J. (1975) HL-A and pernicious anemia. *New Eng. J. Med.* **293**, 1324.

81. Pietsch, M. C. & Morris, P. J. (1974) An association of HL-A3 and HL-A7 with paralytic poliomyelitis. *Tissue Antigens* **4**, 50–55.

HLA and Liver Disease

Ian R. Mackay

Introduction

There are certain liver diseases which, because of associations with autoimmune antibodies as in chronic active hepatitis, or with chronic virus infection, as in hepatitis B carrier states, might be expected to show associations with histocompatibility antigens. The liver disease in which HLA antigens have been studied will be considered from the standpoint of: (i) definition, (ii) genetic and familial predisposition, (iii) racial predisposition, and (iv) histocompatibility-antigen associations.

Chronic active hepatitis (CAH): definition and subgroups

CAH began to be recognized around 1950 (1) as a progressive and usually fatal liver disease predominantly found in young women and characterized by hypergammaglobulinaemia. Needle biopsy of the liver from the 1950s led to wide application of non-formalized histological criteria for diagnosis. Hypergammaglobulinaemia and serological reactions for auto-antibodies raised the possibility of an auto-immune cause, but this was not wholly accepted because of lack of fulfilment of two important criteria, namely presence of liver-specific auto-antibody and a valid experimental model in animals. Latterly these requirements have to some extent been met as a result of work with a liver-specific lipoprotein extracted and characterized by Meyer zum Büschenfelde (2, 3). From 1960–1970 corticosteroid drugs were found to inhibit biochemical indices of activity and modify the otherwise progressive course of the disease (4).

However, problems of definition and nomenclature were augmented with recognition that the hepatitis B surface antigen (HBsAg), a marker of acute Type-B viral hepatitis (5), was demonstrable in some cases of histologically typical CAH. There were also recognized cases of CAH with typical histological and auto-immune serological features, in which a laxative drug, oxyphenisatin, could be implicated, and activity of this varied according to whether the drug was withdrawn or readministered (6); other drugs, particularly alpha methyldopa, likewise appeared to cause CAH (7). From 1968–1970, a

The Clinical Research Unit of The Walter and Eliza Hall Institute of Medical Research and The Royal Melbourne Hospital, Post Office, Royal Melbourne Hospital, Victoria 3050, Australia.

186

group of histopathologists defined and characterized CAH on morphological criteria (8, 9): non-destructive chronic liver disease, called "chronic persisting hepatitis", was differentiated from progressively destructive types which were histologically called "chronic aggressive hepatitis".

There would by now be agreement on this broad definition of chronic active hepatitis: a six-month duration of symptoms with over four-fold elevation from normal of transaminase enzymes in blood, and histological appearances fulfilling criteria for "chronic aggressive hepatitis" (8, 9). However, there is not general agreement as to whether chronic active hepatitis, also known as "chronic active liver disease" (10), should be further subclassified into groups which differ according to a presumed causal agent and/or pattern of host response. However, because HLA phenotypes do appear to differ among subgroups of CAH, the following classification has been proposed (11): (i) a type associated with anti-nuclear and smooth-muscle antibodies in blood – auto-antibody-associated ("classical" or "lupoid") type of CAH (CAH-A); (ii) a type with HBsAg in blood – hepatitis B-virus-associated CAH (CAH-B) (with differences from CAH-A being shown in Table I, adapted from Hadziyannis (12)); (iii) a type with no identifying characteristics, being negative for auto-antibodies and HBsAg – cryptogenic CAH (CAH-C); and (iv) a type dependent on exposure to a medicinal drug – drug-associated CAH (CAH-D). Differentiating features for Types A, B and D were described by Mackay (13). In future studies on HLA and chronic hepatitis, the subtype should be designated prospectively before results of HLA typing are available.

Auto-immune chronic active hepatitis – CAH-A.

Genetic and familial associations

Although CAH has aroused considerable clinical interest over the past 20 years, published observations on familial associations are so few that it may be inferred that direct genetic influences are relatively weak; the available reports concern serological abnormalities in first-degree relatives (14, 15) and multiple cases within families (16, 17).

Racial predisposition

CAH-A has been reported mostly from Caucasian populations and, according to personal communications from colleagues, is rarely seen in those Asian, Oriental and African populations where HLA-A1 and B8 exist in low frequency (18). Moreover, the impression exists that the disease could be more frequent among Caucasians originating from higher than from lower Northern latitudes. In a combined Australian-Asian study of patients with chronic liver disease, prevalences of auto-immune serological reactions to nuclei, smooth muscle and mitochondria were present in marked excess

TABLE I

Differences: CAH-A and CAH-B

	CAH-A	CAH-B
Female sex	>80 %	<10 %
Age < 30	50 %	20 %
Extra-hepatic features	>50 %	<10 %
Mean λ globulin	>30 g/L	<20 g/L
ANA and/or % + SMA	70–100	22
HLA-B8	62-69 %	{ 0 (UK) { 31 (Sweden)
Steroid response	+	?

Adapted from Hadziyannis (12).

among Australian cases (55% of 18) than among Asian cases (0–14 % of 149) originating from Ceylon, India, Singapore and Thailand (18); it was noted that haplotype A1, B8 occurs more frequently among Australians (9 %) than among Indians (0.9 %) and Chinese (0.6 %) (18).

Histocompatibility-antigen associations

Up to 1975 there were reports, some shown in Table II, from various parts of the world on HLA frequencies in which the index group can be taken to have CAH-A, with controls comprising healthy Caucasian subjects. Five studies (19–23) were consistent in showing an increased frequency of HLA-B8 from 61–68 %, as against 17–23 % in the controls, and HLA-A1 was similarly increased; one study (23) reported on haplotypes and of the 21 cases studied, the A1, B8 haplotype was represented in 8 out of the 13 cases carrying HLA-B8. In one report on a normal frequency of HLA-B8 in CAH (24), the data were presented in the course of another study (on coeliac disease), the cases numbered only 17 and, although 16 were female, only five were aged below 40 years. Cumulation of some of the earlier studies, representing 233 subjects with HLA-B8, gave a relative risk for CAH in carriers of B8 of 3.04 (25).

More recent data have further corroborated the association of CAH with HLA-B8. In Melbourne, the earlier series (19) has been extended, with 69 % of 48 cases carrying HLA-B8 (26). In West Germany, in a more detailed analysis of earlier data (20), Freudenberg et al. (27) studied 34 adults and 8 children with CAH-A and found frequencies of HLA-B8 of 82 % and 64 % respectively as against 19.2 % of 5,046 controls, yielding a relative risk for HLA-B8 of 15.4. Also, there was for CAH-A an insignificant decrease in frequency (12 %) of HLA-B7. From the United States, Opelz et al. (28) reported on 38 patients with chronic active liver disease with 32 appearing to be CAH-A; the 34 % frequency of HLA-B8 was higher than in controls (24 %), but not significantly so, although the frequency of DW3 was considerably higher (vide infra). In Finland, Salaspuro et al. (29) found a significantly higher frequency (54 %) for 26 cases of CAH-A, compared with 20 % for controls.

There are three reports relating to D-locus antigens in CAH. Page et al. (23), in a genotype analysis of 21 cases, found an increased frequency of homozygosity for HLA-B8 in patients (6 out of 21) over controls (2.8 %), and three of these homozygous patients were homozygous for a mixed-lymphocyte culture (MLC) determinant called 8a; however, 8a was equally frequent in the patient and control populations (23). Dumble & Mackay (30), in a family study of MLC reactions among a patient with CAH, her parents, and four siblings identical at the A and B loci, found evidence that the patient's lymphocytes carried a different MLC determinant which, however, was apparently not linked to HLA-B8. Opelz et al. (28) typed for D-locus determinants

TABLE II

HLA-A1 and B8 in CAH-A

Author and no. of cases		A1		B8	
		No.	(%)	No.	(% vs. cont.)
Mackay & Morris	37	22	(60)	25	(68 vs. 18)
Freudenberg et al.	56	30	(54)	34	(61 vs. 17)
Galbraith et al.	45	24	(53)	28	(62 vs. 17)
Lindberg et al.	16	9	(56)	10	(62 vs. 23)
Page et al.	21	10	(48)	13	(62 vs. 18)
Scott et al.	17		n.s.	5	(29 vs. 27)

188

in 38 cases of chronic active liver disease and found a very significantly greater frequency of HLA-DW3 (68 %) than among 91 controls (24 %): the association with the B locus (B8) was held to be an indirect result of the DW3 association.

Two studies have been directed towards ascertaining whether the presence of B- or D-locus antigens was associated with a particular clinical subtype of CAH. In Australia, 34 patients with CAH and carrying HLA-B8 were compared with 11 patients negative for HLA-A1 and B8 (26). The latter group contained more males, more older patients, more with long-term remissions after withdrawal of corticosteroid drug treatment, and fewer with auto-immune serological reactions; overall the differences were not significant, apart from the higher mean level of gamma globulin in the B8-positive group. In the United States, CAH patients with DW3 and those without were similar for most clinical characteristics, except that the group positive for DW3 appeared more resistant to treatment (28).

Hepatitis B-associated CAH (CAH-B)
Genetic and familial associations

The carrier state for the hepatitis B surface antigen (HBsAg) exists within families, although there are few reports of multiple intrafamilial cases of CAH-B. With the known high frequency of intrafamilial cross-infection with HBV, it would be difficult to ascertain whether there is a particular genetic predisposition to the carrier state, or to CAH, among carriers of HBsAg.

Racial predisposition

There are marked differences among races in the prevalence of carrier states of HBsAg, and in the frequency of cases of CAH-B compared with all cases of CAH (31). The latter frequency is low (less than 5 %) in Australia (32) and Great Britain (31), somewhat higher (10–25 %) in the United States of America (31), higher still in part of Europe including Austria (31) and Italy (33), and could make a major contribution to all cases of CAH and cirrhosis among certain populations, according to data from Hong Kong (34) and Iraq (35).

Histocompatibility-antigen associations

Analyses of HLA frequencies in CAH-B have given rather variable results, although HLA-B8 is apparently not increased. Bertrams et al. (36) reported on 77 patients with chronic aggressive hepatitis, of whom 48 % were carriers of HBsAg; there was a slight excess of B8, possibly contributed by the HBsAg-negative group. Descamps et al. (37), from a renal dialysis unit, reported on 10 patients with CAH-B of whom three had the phenotype B8, (controls 14 %). Galbraith et al. (21) reported on nine cases of CAH-B and, in marked contrast to CAH-A, none was positive for B8. Lindberg et al. (22), reporting on 13 cases of CAH-B, found HLA frequencies including B8 to be similar to those for controls.

The report of Mazzilli et al. (38) from Rome brings up some interesting points in relation to CAH-B. This series of 42 cases of chronic active hepatitis mostly comprised cases associated with HBsAg (in contrast to Northern European series), and the frequency of HLA-B8 among the controls was relatively low, 7.5 %; 35 patients were persistently antigenaemic, 4 had anti-HBs, and 3 were "cryptogenic". The frequency of HLA-B8 was low, as in the controls, and there was an increased frequency for HLA-B3 of 48 %, compared with 19 % in controls, giving a relative risk for this antigen of 3.83, and the phenotypic association of A3 and BW35 was increased from 6.0 % in controls to 28.5 %.

Cryptogenic CAH (CAH-C)

This term is reserved for those cases of CAH which cannot be assigned to other categories. (The term "cryptogenic CAH" was used by Lindberg et al. (22) in reference to the now designated CAH-A.) The condition is analogous to cryptogenic cirrhosis which is without known cause or antecedents. Possibly some cases of CAH referred to as "cryptogenic" may in fact be ascribed to HBV infection, as judged by an approximately one-third incidence of positive tests for anti-HBcore (39). Scott et al. (24) reported a high frequency of HLA-B8 (11 out of 22 cases) in "cirrhosis" of unspecified nature.

Drug-associated CAH (CAH-D)

Lindberg et al. (22) reported on 13 patients, of whom 8 had presumed oxyphenisatin-induced liver disease. The cases were mostly female (10 out of 13) and, in terms of auto-immune serological reactions, resembled CAH-A. There was an insignificant increase in HLA-A1 and B8 in this group.

HBsAg carriers

Data are available on HLA in carriers of HBsAg without apparent CAH or cirrhosis, in whom there would be no liver disease, non-specific reactive hepatitis, or chronic persisting hepatitis (CPH).

Genetic and familial predisposition

Although differing socio-economic conditions and hygiene could in part account for the wide differences (0.1 %– 15 %) among countries in carrier rates of HBsAg (40), differing racial susceptibility must also contribute. This is strongly suggested by the data of Yap et al. (41) on differing carrier rates in Singapore among racial groups (Indians low, Malays intermediate, and Chinese high) living under similar environmental conditions.

Histocompatibility-antigen associations

Bertrams et al. (36) from West Germany described 51 patients with CPH, of whom 73 % were positive for HBsAg. For this group of cases of CPH, B18 was present in significant excess and there were deficiencies of BW15 (significant) and BW17. Descamps et al. (37), reporting on haemodialysed patients, obtained normal distributions of A1, B8 and B15. Sengar et al. (42) from a dialysis unit, found an excess of B8 in carriers, and a surprising deficiency (0 %) of B8 in 29 "at-risk" subjects with anti-HBs, these findings being seemingly at variance with those of Descamps et al. (37). Gyódi et al. (43) from Hungary examined 83 healthy carriers, predominantly males, and found significant deficiencies of BW17 (as did Bertrams et al. (36)), and B27. Jeannet & Farquet (44) from Switzerland examined 98 healthy carriers and found an increase of HLA-B41.

Boettcher et al. (45), reporting on Australian aboriginals who have high carrier rates of HBsAg, found a deficiency of BW15 and a significant excess of persons homozygous at the B locus; this was considered consistent with the original suggestion of Blumberg that susceptibility to the Au antigen-carrier state was a recessive genetic state controlled by a single autosomal gene (46).

Descamps et al. (37) reported interesting data on 70 uraemic patients capable of eliminating HBsAg after virus-B contamination, the phenotypes B8, and A1, B8 being significantly increased in this group.

Primary biliary cirrhosis (PBC)

Genetic and familial associations

The few reports of multiple cases within families, including a pair of brothers and twin sisters, are cited by Chamuleau et al. (47) who add an interesting sibship in which two sisters had PBC and a third, a monozygotic twin of one of these sisters, had a positive test for antimitochondrial antibody. Galbraith et al. (48) studied 22 families of propositi with PBC, with one family having two cases. This study disclosed a range of associated immunopathic diseases in family members and significant increases above matched controls in the incidence of auto-antibodies to mitochondria, nuclei, and smooth muscle, and was noteworthy in illustrating that within families of propositi with either CAH or PBC, there was overlap of serological characteristics of both diseases.

Racial predisposition

PBC is described almost exclusively from Caucasian areas and the disease does not appear to exist in Asian or African communities. Also, among 146 Asians with various types of chronic liver disease, none had mitochondrial antibodies in the serum (18).

Histocompatibility-antigen associations

Galbraith et al. (21) reported on 73 patients from two different regions of Great Britain and found no significant differences from controls for any HLA antigen. It is of interest that the observed overlap within single patients, and within families, of clinical and serological features of the two major autoimmune liver disease, CAH-A and PBC, is not expressed by HLA phenotypes, in that HLA-B8 is greatly increased in CAH-A but not in PBC. Presumably there is a weak non-HLA-related genetic predisposition to both diseases, and differing "trigger" factors, with that for CAH-A (possibly viral) being dependent on a gene in linkage disequilibrium with HLA-B8.

In a study (29) of 17 patients with PBC, an increased prevalence of BW15 seemed to correlate with an advanced cholestatic form of disease characterized by hepatocellular accumulation of protein-bound copper (8 of 12 patients had BW15), while patients with a benign form of disease did not differ from controls in this respect (1 out of 5 cases had BW15). Lymphocyte responses to different mitogens in vitro showed the same decreased B-cell activity and alterations in T-cell reactions in both subgroups of PBC, in contrast to CAH-A in which the investigators (29) had found normal B-cell reactions and increased T-cell activity.

Alcoholic cirrhosis

Alcoholic cirrhosis was included among "controls" in Melbourne studies on HLA and liver disease. There was an insignificant excess of HLA-B8 in 34 % of 32 cases, compared with 18 % in controls (26).

Haemochromatosis

Genetic aspects of haemochromatosis are reviewed by Bothwell & Charlton (49). They cite the familial occurrence in relatives attributable to genetic predisposition rather than familial exposure to dietary iron. The nature of the genetic abnormality is unknown, but transmission is by a dominant or partly dominant autosomal gene determining a metabolic abnormality resulting in abnormal intestinal absorption of iron; the evidence of consanguinity also raised the possibility of recessive heredity. The excess incidence in males is believed to be due to iron losses in females during menstruation.

Since this disease is regarded as a clear metabolic abnormality, the clearly established association with HLA is most intriguing. Studies from Brittany in France showed a remarkably high association of certain HLA phenotypes with well-documented cases of idiopathic haemochromatosis (50); further data from the same area (51) relate to 84 cases of haemochromatosis, with a contrast group of 204 blood-donor controls. HLA-A3 was present in 75 % *versus* 27 % in controls $(P < 10^{-11})$ and HLA-B14 in 31 % *versus* 3.4 % in controls $(P < 10^{-8})$; the relative risk for haemochromatosis compared with subjects having neither A3 nor B14 was 8.2 for A3, 26.7 for B14, and 90 for A3 and B14 in combination. In studies on five families, there was a haplotype association of A3, B14 with haemochromatosis. The association with A3 has been confirmed in Great Britain (52, 53) and Australia (26).

How may these observations be related to the cause of haemochromatosis? An oligogenic genetic basis for the disease is certainly supported. First, a gene determining iron transport could be present in the same region of chromosome number 6 as the histocompatibility genes, giving a coincidental association of HLA antigens and haemochromatosis; secondly, haemochromatosis could be determined by an as yet unknown immunopathic response, although the usual types of auto-immune serological reactions have not been reported in this disease; and thirdly, if, as suggested (54), HLA molecules facilitate ligand-receptor interactions, there could be facilitation of binding of iron to the intestinal-cell receptor.

Gilbert's disease

This disease is characterized by intermittent unconjugated hyperbilirubinaemia, familial predisposition, and a probably autosomal-dominant heredity. Associations with HLA phenotypes were sought in 19 unrelated patients and 21 first-degree relatives of 7 patients, but no linkages were found (55).

Summary and conclusions

Chronic active hepatitis (CAH) is a progressive destructive liver disease of uncertain pathogenesis, and has generated many controversies in relation to its terminology, causes, histopathological appearances, evolution to cirrhosis, and treatment (1, 8, 9, 10–13). Hence the disease has proved difficult to characterize and classify. However, the existence of subgroups in which different pathogenetic processes may predominate is rendered more likely by differences in HLA frequencies. In the subgroup associated with auto-immune serological reactions, CAH-A, there is a strong association with antigens of the histocompatibility system, A1, B8 and DW3, with the primary association probably being with the D-locus antigen. Another subgroup associated with hepatitis B surface antigen in blood (CAH-B) does not appear to show particular association with any HLA antigen.

The role of the gene(s) associated with B8-DW3 in predisposition is still unknown for CAH and for the various other diseases for which B8-DW3 are markers. This genotype was postulated to confer strong proliferative responses to certain micro-organismal antigens, giving survival advantage, but at the expense of an increased likelihood for auto-reactive cells to be stimulated as forbidden clones (19). It is therefore noteworthy that in a haemodialysis population, HLA-B8 was associated with the capacity to eliminate HBsAg from the blood (37), and, in cases of CAH-A, HLA-B8 and B12 were associated with higher titres of antibody to both viral antigens, rubella and measles, and auto-antigens, smooth muscle, and nuclei (56).

There is another major immunopathic liver disease, primary biliary cirrhosis (PBC), which is claimed from clinical and family studies to share with CAH a similar genetic predisposition; however, there is no indication of any alteration in HLA frequencies in PBC. There is a remarkable association of HLA-A3 and B14 with haemochromatosis and the suggestion is that these antigens segregate with one of the limited number of genes predisposing to the iron-overload characteristic of this disease.

Acknowledgements

The author's work was supported by a grant from the National Health and Medical Research Council of Australia. He is deeply appreciative of advice on the manuscript from Dr. Wolfgang R. Mayr, of the Institut für Blutgruppenserologie der Universität Wien, secretary to the Gastroenterology (Hepatology) Workshop, and to administrative assistance from Drs. J. P. Benhamou and B. Rueff, of the Hôpital Beaujon, Clichy, and Dr. B. Genetet, of the C. T. S., Rennes, during the First International Symposium on HLA and Disease, Paris, June 1976.

References[1]

1. Mackay, I. R. (1975) Chronic active hepatitides. In: *Frontiers of Gastrointestinal Research*, ed. v. Der Reis, L. vol. 1, p. 142, Karger, Basel.
2. Meyer zum Büschenfelde, K-H. & Hopf, U. (1974) Studies on the pathogenesis of experimental chronic active hepatitis in rabbits. I. Induction of the disease and protective effect of allogeneic liver specific proteins. *Brit J. exp. Path.*, **55**, 498.
3. Meyr sum Büschenfelde, K.-H., Kossling, F. K. & Miescher, P. A. (1972) Experimental chronic active hepatitis in rabbits following immunization with human liver proteins. *Clin. exp. Immunol.*, **11**, 99.
4. Mackay, I. R. (1972) Immunosuppressive drugs and chronic hepatitis. *Med. J. Aust.*, **1**, 1207.

[1]Papers indicated by [1] were presented at the 1st Int. Symp. on HLA and Disease, INSERM, Paris, June 1976.

5. Prince, A. M. (1968) An antigen detected in the blood during the incubation period of serum hepatitis. *Proc. nat. Acad. Sci. (Wash.),* **60,** 814.
6. Reynolds, T. B., Peters, R. L. & Yamada, S. (1971) Chronic active hepatitis caused by a laxative oxyphenisatin. *New Eng. J. Med.,* **280,** 813.
7. Rodman, J. S., Deutsch, D. J. & Gutman, S. I. (1976) Methyldopa hepatitis. A report of six cases and a review of the literature. *Amer J. Med.,* **60,** 941.
8. DeGroote, J., Desmet, V. J., Gedigk, P., Korb, G., Popper, H., Poulsen, H., Scheuer, P. J., Schmid, M., Thaler, H., Uehlinger, E. & Wepler, W. (1968) A classification of chronic hepatitis. *Lancet, ii,* 626.
9. International Group (1971) Morphological criteria in viral hepatitis. *Lancet, i,* 333.
10. Geall, M. G., Schoenfeld, L. J. & Summerskill. W. H. J. (1968) Classification and treatment of chronic active liver disease. *Gastroenterology,* **55,** 6.
11. Mackay, I. R. (1976) Chronic active hepatitis, cirrhosis and other diseases of the liver. In: *Immunological Diseases.* 3rd edition, ed. Samster, M. Little, Brown & Co., Boston. (In press.)
12. Hadziyannis, S. J. (1974) Chronic viral hepatitis. *Clin. Gastroenterology,* **3,** 391.
13. Mackay, I. R. (1976) The concept of auto-immune liver disease. *Bull. N.Y. Acad. Med.* **52,** 453.
14. Cavell, B. & Leonhardt, T. (1965) Hereditary hypergammaglobulinemia and lupoid hepatitis. *Acta med. scand.,* **177,** 751.
15. Elling, P., Ranløv, P. & Bildsøe, P. (1966) A genetic approach to the pathogenesis of hepatic cirrhosis. *Acta med. scand.,* **179,** 527.
16. Joske, R. A. & Laurence, B. H. (1970) Familial cirrhosis with auto-immune features and raised immunoglobulin levels. *Gastroenterology,* **59,** 546.
17. Whittingham, S., Mackay, I. R. & Kiss, Z. S. (1970) An interplay of genetic and environmental factors in familial hepatitis and myasthenia gravis. *Gut,* **11,** 811.
18. Whittingham, S., Mackay, I. R., Thanabalasundrum, R. S.. Chuttani, H. K., Manjuran. R., Seah, C. S., Yu, M. & Viranuvatti, V. (1973) Chronic liver disease: Differences in auto-immune serological reactions between Australians and Asians. *Brit. med. J.,* **4.** 517.
19. Mackay, I. R. & Morris, P. J. (1972) Association of auto-immune active chronic hepatitis with HL-A1, 8. *Lancet, ii,* 793.
20. Freudenberg, J.. Erdmann, K. Meyer zum Büschenfelde, K-H., Förster, E. & Berger, J. (1973) HL-A bei Lebererkrankungen. *Klin. Wschr.* **51,** 1075.
21. Galbraith, R. M., Eddleston, A. L. W. F., Smith, M. G. M., Williams, R., MacSween, R. N. M., Watkinson, G., Dick, H., Kennedy, L. A. & Batchelor, J. R. (1974) Histocompatibility antigens in active chronic hepatitis and primary biliary cirrhosis. *Brit. med. J.,* **3,** 604.
22. Lindberg, J., Lindholm, A., Lundin, P. & Iwarson, S. (1975) Trigger factors and HL-A antigens in chronic active hepatitis. *Brit. med. J.,* **4,** 77.
23. Page. A. R., Sharp, H. L., Greenberg, L. J. & Yunis, E. J. (1975) Genetic analysis of patients with chronic active hepatitis. *J. clin. Invest.,* **56,** 530.
24. Scott, B. B., Swinburne, M. L., Rajah, S. M. & Losowsky, M. S. (1974) HL-A8 and the immune response to gluten. *Lancet ii,* 374.
25. Ryder, L. P. & Svejgaard, A. (1976) Associations between HLA and disease. Report from the *HLA and Disease Registry of Copenhagen.*
26. Morris, P. J., Vaughan, H., Tait, B. D. & Mackay, I. R. (1977) Histocompatibility antigen (HLA): associations with immunopathic disease and with responses to microbial antigens. *Aust. N.Z. J. Med.* (submitted).
27. Freudtnberg, J., Baumann, W., Arnold. W., Berger, J. & Meyer zum Büschenfelde, K-H. (1976) HLA in different forms of chronic active hepatitis (CAH): a comparison between adult patients and children, (submitted for publication).[1]
28. Opelz, G., Vogten, A. J. M., Summerskill, W. H. J., Schalm, S. W. & Terasaki, P. I. (1976) HLA determinants in chronic active liver disease: relation of HLA-DW3 to prognosis, (submitted for publication).
29. Salaspuro, M., Makkonen, H., Sipponen, P. & Tiilikainen, A. (1976) HLA-B8, HLA-BW15 and lymphocyte stimulation in chronic active hepatitis and primary biliary cirrhosis, (submitted for publication).[1]
30. Dumble, L. J. & Mackay, I. R. (1976) HLA and chronic active hepatitis (CAH). *Digestion,* (in the press).[1]
31. Prince, A. M. (1971) Role of serum hepatitis virus in chronic liver disease. *Gastroenterology,* **60,** 913.
32. Cooksley, W. G. E., Powell, L. W., Mistilis, S. P.. Mackay, I. R. & Barker, L. F. (1975) Hepatitis B antigen and antibody

in active chronic hepatitis and other liver diseases in Australia. *Amer. J. dig. Dis.,* **20,** 110.

33. Bianchi, P., Porro, C. B., Coltorti, M., Dardanoni, L., Blanco, C. D. V., Fagiolo, U., Farini, R., Menozzi, I., Naccarato, R., Pagliaro, L., Spano, C. & Verme, G. (1972) Occurrence of Australia antigen in chronic hepatitis in Italy. *Gastroenterology,* **63,** 482.

34. Lee, A. K. Y. (1973) Auto-antibodies in cirrhosis and hepatocellular carcinoma. *Aust. N. Z. J. Med.,* **3,** 268.

35. Boxall, E. H., Flewett, T. H., Paton, A. & Rassam, S. W. (1976) Hepatitis-B surface antigen and cirrhosis in Iraq. *Gut,* **17,** 119.

36. Bertrams, J., Reis. H. E., Kuwert, E. & Selmiar, H. (1974) Hepatitis associated antigen (HAA), HL-A antigens and autolymphocytotoxins (Co Co Cy) in chronic aggressive and chronic persistent hepatitis. *Z. Immun. Forsch.,* **146,** 300.

37. Descamps, B., Jungers, P., Naret, C.. Degott, C., Zingraff, J. & Bach, J. F. (1976) HLA-A1, B8-phenotype and HBs antigenemia evolution in 440 hemodialysed patients, (submitted for publication).[1]

38. Mazzilli, M. C., Trabace, S., Di Raimondo, F., Visco, G. & Gandini, E. (1976) HLA and active chronic hepatitis (ACH), (submitted for publication).[1]

39. Benhamou, J-P., Maupas, P. & Pillegand, B. (1976) Core antigen in chronic active hepatitis. *Lancet* **i,** 817.

40. Mackay, I. R. (1976) Liver disease due to infection and allergy. In: *Handbook of Experimental Pharmacology XVI/5: Experimental Production of Liver Disease,* ed. Eichler, O. p. 121, Springer-Verlag, Heidelberg. (In press).

41. Yap, E. H., Ong, Y. W., Simons, M. J., Okochi, K., Mayumi, M. & Nishioka, K. (1972) Australia antigen in Singapore. II. Differential frequency in Chinese, Malays and Indians. *Vox Sang.,* **22,** 371.

42. Sengar, D. P. S., McLeish, W. A., Sutherland, L. T., Couture, R. A. & Rashid, A. (1975) Hepatitis B antigen (HBAg) infection in a hemodialysis unit. I. HL-A8 and immune response to HBAg. *Canad. med. Assoc. J.,* **112,** 968.

43. Gyódi, E., Penke, S., Novák, E. & Hollán, S. R. (1973) HL-A specificities in individuals with persistence of hepatitis-associated antigenaemia. *Haematologia,* **7,** 199.

44. Jeannet, M. & Farquet, J. J. (1974) HL-A antigens in asymptomatic chronic HBAg carriers. *Lancet, ii,* 1383.

45. Boettcher. B. (1975) Some possible causes of associations between HL-A antigens and disease. *Immunogenetics,* **2,** 485.

46. Boettcher, B., Hay, J., Watterson, C. A.. Bashir, H., MacQueen, J. M. & Hardy, G. (1975) Association between an HL-A antigen and Australia antigen in Australian aborigines. *J. Immunogenetics,* **2,** 195.

47. Chamuleau, R. A. F. M., van Berge Henegouwen, G. P., Bronkhorst, F. B. & Brandt, K-H. (1975) Primary biliary cirrhosis in sisters. *Neth. J. Med.,* **18,** 170.

48. Galbraith, R. M., Smith, M., Mackenzie, R. M., Tee, D. E., Doniach, D. & Williams, R. (1974) High prevalence of seroimmunologic abnormalities in relatives of patients with active chronic hepatitis or primary biliary cirrhosis. *New Eng. J. Med.,* **290,** 63.

49. Bothwell, T. H. & Charlton, R. W. (1975) Hemochromatosis. In: *Diseases of the Liver,* 4th edition. ed. Schiff, L. Chapter 28, p. 971. Lippincott, Philadelphia.

50. Simon, M., Bourel, M., Fauchet, R. & Genetet, B. (1976) Association of HLA-A3 and HLA-B14 antigens with idiopathic haemochromatosis. *Gut,* **17,** 332.

51. Fauchet, R., Simon, M., Bourel, M., Genetet, B., Genetet, N. & Alexandre, J. L. (1976 Idiopathic haemochromatosis and HLA anitgens, (submitted for publication).[1]

52. Bomford, A., Eddleston, A. L. W. F., Williams, R., Kennedy, L. & Batchelor. J. R. (1976) HLA-A3 and Idiopathic Haemochromatosis, (submitted for publication).[1]

53. Shewan, W. G., Mouat, S. A. & Allan, T. M. (1976) HLA antigens in haemochromatosis. *Brit med. J.* **1,** 281.

54. Svejgaard, A. & Ryder, L. P. (1976) Interaction of HLA molecules with nonimmunological ligands as an explanation of HLA and disease associations. *Lancet, ii,* 547.

55. Penner, E., Mayr, W. R., Djawan, S., Seyfried, H. & Pacher. M. (1976) Untersuchungen zur Genetik des Gilbert-Syndroms. *Schweiz med. Wschr.,* **106,** 860.

56. Galbraith, R. M., Eddleston, A. L. W. F., Williams, R., Webster, A. D. B., Pattison, J., Doniach, D., Kennedy, L. E. & Batchelor, J. R. (1976) Enhanced antibody responses in active chronic hepatitis: relation to HLA-B8 and HLA-B12 and portosystemic shunting. *Lancet, i,* 930.

HLA and Allergy

A. L. de Weck,[1] M. Blumenthal,[2] E. Yunis[3] & M. Jeannet[4]

I. Introduction

Three important aspects have conditioned the studies of HLA in atopic diseases:

A) Overall susceptibility to allergy (atopic diseases); B) identification of immunoglobulin E (IgE) in the pathogenesis of atopy; and C) knowledge of the genetics of the immune response (Ir).

A. Overall susceptibility to Allergy
(atopic diseases)

A heightened familial incidence of certain inhalation allergies such as asthma or hay fever was first noticed more than a century ago. Since then is has become popular knowledge that there exists a general familial predisposition towards allergic rhinitis, atopic eczema and asthma. Cooke & van der Veer (1) found that 48.4 % of a population of 594 allergic individuals had positive familial histories of allergy, whereas only 14.5 % of 76 non-allergic persons had a similar family history. According to these authors, individuals with a bilateral family history of allergy appeared to manifest symptoms during childhood, whereas those with only one parent suffering from allergy would often only develop symptoms around puberty. Children from asymptomatic parents usually became allergic later in life.

It seems that it is not the allergic disease itself which is hereditary, but rather a general predisposition to develop hypersensitivities to a variety of inhaled allergens. In fact, the studies performed by Cook & van der Veer (1) with relatively crude allergen extracts demonstrated that allergic children often develop different clinical forms of allergic manifestations than their parents, and even become sensitive to different allergens. Many population, family, and twin studies have indicated that familial and probably genetic factors are important in the development of allergic diseases (2–7).

The mode of heredity of atopic diseases remains disputed: studies have produced findings that suggest it is a single dominant gene with partial penetrance (1, 8), a single recessive gene with partial penetrance (9, 10), or multigenic heredity (11). At present, it is generally re-

[1] Institute for Clinical Immunology, University of Bern, Bern, Switzerland.

[2] Department of Medicine, University of Minnesota Medical School, Minneapolis, Minn.

[3] Sidney Farber Cancer Institute, Harvard Medical School, Boston, Mass.

[4] Unité d'Histocompatibilité Hôpital Cantonal, Geneva, Switzerland.

cognized that no one gene hypothesis fits all the available data.

B. Immunoglobulin E (IgE) in allergy and genetic control of serum IgE levels

During the past decade, a number of basic advances in immunology have provided a more solid scientific background for the somewhat empirical clinical definition of atopic diseases. The identification of immunoglobulin E (IgE) as the main antibody involved in atopic hypersensitivity has made it possible to give a better immunological basis to the definition of atopy and to its detection in patients.

After the quantitative measurement of IgE antibodies by various radioimmunological methods became available, it was soon found that atopic people as a group possess much higher IgE levels than normal non-clinically allergic individuals (12). However, some overlapping is always observed in patients with clinical manifestations of allergic rhinitis, asthma or atopic eczema and normal serum IgE levels, or patients without clinical manifestations but moderately elevated IgE levels. Neither has it yet been established whether the serum IgE level is directly controlled by some gene(s) factors, or whether it is only secondarily determined by other factors (such as T-cell recognition, handling of allergens by macrophages, etc.) which would also be genetically controlled and indirectly influence IgE biosynthesis.

Experimental studies dealing with the genetic aspects of reagin (IgE-like antibodies) production have up to now been relatively scarce. In inbred mice sensitized to produce IgE-like antibodies, backcross studies between high and low IgE producers clearly suggest a polygenic rather than a monogenic control (13, 14). Also, studies of the genetic control of reaginic antibody synthesis in inbred rats (15) suggest that genetic control of reagin synthesis is an autosomal trait in which non-responsiveness is dominant.

C. Genetics of the immune response (Ir)

The discovery in experimental animals of genes controlling the immune response to specific antigens (Ir genes) (16, 17) was also a major step in establishing immunogenetics as a new important field of immunology and allergy. A further advance was made when it was discovered (18), in several animal species, that many of the immune-response genes controlling the response to a specific allergen are linked to the major histocompatibility complex (MHC) of the corresponding species. The first Ir gene identified as controlling the immune response to a specific antigen was the "polylysine gene" in guinea pigs (19). The influence of H-linked Ir genes becomes most obvious when inbred strains of animals are submitted to low-grade immunogenic stimulation, e.g., by the use of relatively simple antigens (such as synthetic polypeptides containing a restricted number of antigenic determinants) or by administration of low doses of complex protein antigens (restricting the immune response to a few immunodominant determinants). Most animal studies of the immune responses controlled by Ir genes have used the production of IgG or IgM antibodies or manifestations of T-cell function as parameters. These studies have shown that the majority of H-linked Ir genes hitherto recognized act at the level of specific T-cell recognition (16). Vaz and Levine (13, 14)

197

demonstrated in mice the presence of histocompatibility-linked Ir genes which control specific IgE as well as IgG antibody responses. The presence of murine histocompatibility-linked immune-response genes controlling IgE- and IgG-antibody response to ragweed antigen E, rye-grass group I and Asc-1 allergens has also been demonstrated by Marsh *et al.* (20, 21).

The primary function of Ir genes has been suggested to be coding for specific T-cell receptors. These receptors allow some T cells to function as carrier-specific cells helping B cells in the production of antibodies specific for haptenic determinants on the same antigen (16, 17). T-cell function may also be assessed as T-cell proliferation or production of lymphokines following antigen recognition. In most cases, the Ir genes controlling T-cell function have been characterized as autosomal dominant. Serologic studies in guinea pigs using anti-histocompatibility antigens (22, 23), anti-receptor (24) and anti-idiotype (25) antibodies suggest that the T-cell receptor involved in antigenic recognition is composed of two polypeptide chains, one under the control of Ir *(identical with Ia)* genes, the other under the control of V genes (idiotypes) (26). Other studies in rats and mice suggest the T-cell receptor to be composed of a non-conventional Ig heavy chain, the Ia- and Ir-gene products coded for in the major histocompatibility complex playing merely a regulatory function on T-cell receptors (27). In several cases, however, genes controlling the immune response have been associated with B cells (13, 16). In such cases, there was no frequent association with H antigens. Recently, studies in mice have shown that specific immune responses may be controlled by more than one Ir gene linked to the major histocompatibility complex; complementation of genes may be required for effective response at the T-cell level (28) and/or at the B-cell level (29).

In addition to the Ir genes controlling responsiveness to *specific* antigens, the overall ability of inbred mice to produce an IgE response of any specificity appears to be under a different genetic control (14) involving genes not linked to the MHC (section I.B). In experimental animals, therefore, at least two distinct types of genetic control of IgE responsiveness appear to exist: 1) an antigen-specific control due to Ir genes possibly linked to the major histocompatibility complex; and 2) genes controlling the ability to synthesize IgE of any specificity.

II. Problems in the genetic analysis of allergic diseases

A. Definition of allergy and atopy

Whereas allergic diseases are usually defined as clinical manifestations due to the development of specific immune response and hypersensitivity towards environmental allergens, there are no standard definitions or criteria to be used regarding atopy*. In earlier times, atopy was thought to include many allergic manifestations such as urticaria, migraine, etc. Nowadays it is customary to restrict atopic diseases to allergic rhinitis, asthma and atopic eczema (7).

* Atopy could be defined as a genetically controlled predisposition to the production of specific IgE antibodies upon inhalation of minute amounts of allergen. It has become obvious that the difference observed between atopic and non-atopic individuals only holds for sensitization to inhaled or ingested allergens. The incidence of IgE-mediated hypersensitivity to *injected* allergens, such as insulin, penicillin or insect stings, is not higher in atopic than in non-atopic individuals.

However, since most symptoms of atopic diseases may be mimicked by other causes, genetic studies based on only family histories or questionnaires are rather unreliable. Precise diagnosis of the clinical condition of all patients involved in a study is important before any meaningful genetic analysis is possible. It should also be kept in mind that genetically controlled immune response to an allergen can result in different clinical manifestations. It is important to remain aware that allergic diseases often represent syndromes of many pathogeneses.

B. Role of genetic and non-genetic factors

In atopic diseases it appears that several genetic factors may be involved. Some may be specific for the allergen, and in analogy to findings in other species, the postulated Ir genes are probably related to the HLA system. Other Ir genes could be non-HLA related. Other genetic factors may be of a general nature and not allergen specific (e.g., affecting the ability of the antigen to cross mucosal membranes, controlling immunoglobulin production, or regulating the release and expression of pharmacological mediators). Thus, allergy and atopy are probably an example of diseases in which genetic susceptibility is polygenic. Marsh *et al* (30) have presented evidence to indicate that the association between HLA and skin reactions to purified allergens is greater in allergic individuals with low IgE levels. The suppression or masking of the phenotypic expression of Ir genes (HLA linked) by other genes controlling IgE levels may be an example of epistasis. Therefore, theoretically one could expect that high levels of IgE may be an expression of genes that hamper the specific immune response

to an allergen (hypostasis). These findings may explain the lack of expression of response to ragweed antigen E in members of a family with susceptibility to ragweed allergy (31).

Non-genetic factors will influence the final clinical picture. The time of year the patient is studied (32), antigen exposure, exposure to cross-reacting antigens and the age of the patient are all factors which need to be critically controlled for adequate analysis. The clinical manifestation of a gene may be influenced not only by the genotype but also by the environment. The terms of expressivity and penetrance have been employed to describe the variable manifestations of a gene. Traits most useful for the study of transmission genetics are those in which a genotype expresses itself in approximately the same way despite fluctuations in the environment. In family studies of any disease or trait, one may theoretically consider the degree of penetrance or expressiveness of a dominant gene. In organisms other than man, experimental conditions can be controlled in such a way that a given genotype exposed to different environments shows to what extent environment is responsible for phenotypic variability. On the other hand, a standard environment exposed to different genotypes will reveal the genotype's role in causing the differences observed. In man, neither the environment nor the genotypes are controlled experimentally. Only in identical twins is it possible to determine the influence of a genotype and environment, since in general, homozygotic and dizygotic twins share similar environments before birth and when raised together after birth. Twin studies offer, therefore, the opportunity to test the effect of environment and of genotype upon penetrance and expressivity of a given phenotype.

A penetrance of 0.4 for allergy in

monozygous twins has been calculated by van Arsdel & Motulsky (33), but this is probably an underestimate. This study demonstrated partial penetrance and the evidence for several separate genetic factors is consistent with the recurrent failure to obtain convincing fits with either a factorial, a multifactorial, or a single locus with partial penetrance model (33). Studies of serum IgE levels and of differences in allergic manifestations and immune responses following antigen exposure at different ages in monozygotic twins (34) will be of particular importance for the assessment of the role of genetics *versus* environment.

C. Methodology

The parameters used as well as the methods to determine them are crucial to any genetic analysis. The nature of the allergen studied and its state of purity will influence the results of both *in vivo* and *in vitro* studies. The methods used to determine the immune response to a particular antigen are also to be considered. Whereas the RAST assay and histamine release from leukocytes are undoubtedly correlated to IgE-mediated hypersensitivity and to atopic diseases, several additional causes of error may influence the results of skin tests. The meaning of blast transformation and MIF release tests in relation to atopic disease is not firmly established.

D. Design of genetic analysis in allergic families

A major problem is whether association or linkage is to be found between a genetic marker and an atopic disease. Association between two phenomena (e.g., presence of an HLA antigen and hypersensitivity to a given allergen) may be due to a variety of mechanisms not necessarily involving the presence of a specific genetic marker within a defined linkage group. Linkage, on the other hand, is defined by the presence of a genetic marker to be found in several members of the family studied and directly related to the disease or to the immune response considered.

As previously mentioned, allergic diseases are most likely polygenic. Frequently, only close relatives of an allergic patient are studied and they must be expected to have more genes in common with the proband than unrelated persons. They should, therefore, also have a greater risk of suffering from the same diseases than the proband. Important information will be obtained by studying the immune response to specific allergens in twins. Twin studies may indicate whether genetic variation is present and approximately how much of the total variation is genetic, but they do not reveal how genes operate. If monozygous twins vary in the parameter being studied less than dizygotic twins, there is probably a genetic component to the variation.

Population and family studies are two approaches which may be used to establish whether or not a genotype is involved in the susceptibility or resistance to atopic disease or in the development of an immune response. In general, population studies are easier to perform, but they can only establish associations between genetic markers and the immune response whereas linkage can only be established by family studies. One important bias in family studies is the selection of the families. They are usually selected because they contain two or more affected family members. Accordingly, they are likely to possess more disease-liability genes than families with isolated cases. In addition, families need to be large and preferably studied over at least three generations. One difficult problem in family studies is the establishment of linkage, since some may or may not show linkage. The fact that allergic manifestations may be of different etiologies and pathogenesis should be remembered. Morton (35) has studied families with elliptocytosis. Four showed close linkage between elliptocytosis and the Rh blood group. This was the first suggestion that two different genes can cause elliptocytosis: one locus (El$_1$) closely linked to the Rh locus, and the other (El$_2$) not linked. Therefore, in allergic conditions as well, data from all families should not be systematically pooled since some may show linkage and others may not.

III Studies of the genetics of allergic disease in man

A. Associations between atopic diseases and HLA

In view of the complexity of atopic disease, as far as clinical manifestations, pathogenesis and multiple-allergen specificities are concerned, and in view of the fact that a single-gene mode of heredity of atopy has never been demonstrated, significant associations between HLA antigens and atopic diseases taken as a group appear unlikely. This has not deterred a number of investigators from embarking on population and family studies. The result of such investigations on associations between HLA antigens and various forms of atopic diseases (allergic rhinitis, asthma, atopic eczema), on the basis of clinical diagnosis and without restriction of allergen specificity, are summarized in Table I.

Rachelefsky et al. (36) noted that the linkage of a possible asthma gene could be traced in twelve families. In nine of these haplotypes, the "asthma-susceptibility gene" was linked to haplotypes containing B-cell group 2 H antigens. Geerts et al. (37) studying one family, suggested linkage between HLA loci and a locus for atopic constitution.

The main conclusion to be drawn from most studies is that, in general, associations of a given HLA antigen or haplotype with atopic diseases in unrelated populations are not significant and are not to be expected. However, associations within families of atopic diseases with an HLA haplotype appear much more likely, especially when the criterion used for association is hypersensitivity towards defined allergens.

B. Genetic control of IgE serum levels

Genetic studies of levels of IgE have been difficult because they depend on the definition of normalcy of IgE levels. For instance, age and the type or degree of antigenic exposure will influence the IgE levels. Studies of serum IgE levels in twins (38) showed that monozygous twins possess significantly less mean intrapair variance of IgE levels than the mean intrapair variance of the corresponding groups of dizygous twins. This implies that there is a genetic effect on IgE levels. The mean intrapair variance of monozygous twin children was also significantly less than the intrapair variance of monozygous adult twins, suggesting that differences in serum IgE levels between individuals with the same genotype arise mostly after childhood, presumably under the effect of differences in environmental exposure. The mean intrapair variance of dizygous twins (both adults and children) was also less than the mean intra-

TABLE I

Association between HLA and atopic diseases

Author	References No.	Year	No. of Patients	Comments
Atopic Dermatitis – Population Studies				
Krain	(75)	1973	45	Increased A3, A9 ($p = 0.05$)
Scholz	(76)	1976	103	No significant association
Turner	(77)	1976	40	A1, B8 associated with multiple manifestations of reaginic disease. ($p = 0.02$)
Hoshino	(78)	1976	50	Increased B5 ($p = 0.05$)
Ohkido	(79)	1976	100	Increased B12 (*); BW40 ($p = 0.01$) Decreased BW15 (*)
Goudemand	(80	1976	27	Increased BW35 ($p = 0.01$)
Bronchial Asthma – Population Studies				
Thorsby	(81)	1971	35	Increased A1, B8 ($p = 0.05$); A2, B8 ($p = 0.05$)
Rachelefsky	(36)	1976	71	Increased A2, decreased B8 Increased lymphocyte group 2 (*)
Morris	(82)	1976	47	Increased A1 ($p = 0.02$); B8 ($p = 0.01$) Decreased B12 ($p = 0.02$)
Miscellaneous Disorders – Population Studies				
Thompson	(83)	1976	68	Atopy and nephrotic syndrome: The risk of developing steroid-dependent nephrotic syndrome is four times greater in children with B12; for individuals who are also atopic, the risk is increased 13 times
Tait	(84)	1976	66 + parents	+: parents from infant with death syndrome ("cot death"): A10 was more frequent in mothers ($p = 0.005$) while A9 was less frequent in fathers ($p = 0.001$) and in controls ($p = 0.01$)
Atopic Dermatitis – Family Studies				
Scholz	(76)	1976	19 families 103 patients	Association of atopic dermatitis with HLA haplotypes ($p = 0.000058$)
Goudemand	(80)	1976	27 patients 44 parents	Increased BW35 among 27 patients ($p = 0.01$) and 44 parents ($p = 0.005$)
Bronchial Asthma – Family Studies				
Rachelefsky	(36)	1976	39 families 156 patients	All 5 B-lymphocyte specificities increased in asthma, especially B group 2. ($p = 0.05$)
Geerts	37	1976	1 family 17 patients	Association of atopic constitution with familial haplotypes (*)

(*) No *p* value given.

pair variance expected of random unrelated individuals drawn from the corresponding population. This indicated that the genetic similarity and/or environmental similarity between dizygous twins exert(s) a significant effect on IgE levels. Marsh *et al.* also studied the genetics of serum IgE levels. They used a distribution frequency of serum IgE levels in populations of unrelated allergic and non-allergic subjects to determine a cut-off point between high and low serum IgE levels. On this basis, and following IgE levels in 28 families with a total of 108 children, they concluded that the heredity of total IgE level is recessive and not linked to HLA (30, 39). However, these conclusions can only be accepted with reservation because they were based on arbitrary classification of some of the subjects (with intermediary serum IgE levels between high and low) into high or low IgE phenotypes. They proposed a dominant "R" (IgE regulator) allele which was found to have a gene frequency of 0.48 in the general population.

A point which is not entirely settled is whether the gene(s) controlling serum IgE levels also control(s) serum levels of other immunoglobulins (such as IgG, IgA and IgM). The serum levels of IgG, IgA and IgM in unselected adults are more closely distributed around their mean values than IgE levels (40). Nevertheless, the inheritance of the levels of IgG, IgA and IgM immunoglobulins in twins appears to be quite marked (41, 42). There have been few studies up to now on the correlation of IgG, IgA, IgM and IgE levels in populations of normal and allergic patients (43, 44). In animal studies, the possibility of breeding mice for high or low IgG and IgM responses has been clearly demonstrated by Stiffel *et al.* (45); in addition, inbred mice which develop a high IgE-like response to a number of antigens usually show a high IgG response to the same antigens (14). However, dissociation of IgG and IgM from IgE responses in experimental models has also been observed (46).

The possibility that patients with high IgE levels might be relatively immuno-deficient in IgA (47) reminds one that the demonstration of genetic control for IgE levels does not imply the same gene(s) control(s) biosynthesis of other immunoglobulins.

A study on the incidence of precipitins to *Penicillium casei* in cheese workers placed under conditions of similar allergen exposure (48) also suggested that the formation of IgG antibody must be placed under the control of genes similar, but not identical to those controlling IgE synthesis. A striking familial incidence, associated with HLA-BW 40, of hypersensitivity pneumonitis in families of bird breeders has been reported (49). This allergic disease is dependent upon IgG, not IgE antibodies, and is possibly associated with cellular hypersensitivity to birds' serum proteins.

C. Attempts to identify antigen-specific Ir genes in man with special reference to allergy

In experimental animals, the parameters of immune response used for detection of specific Ir genes have been mostly antibody responses (IgG, IgM or IgE) or cellular immunity reactions, whereas the investigations performed so far in man for detecting Ir genes specific for natural allergens have relied mostly on immediate-type skin reactions (skin tests) due to specific mixtures such as house dust and pollen extracts (known to contain many different antigenic determinants). In a few studies, more purified allergens such as AgE (30, 31, 50, 51), Ra 3 and Ra5 from ragweed pollen, Rye I, II, III and IV of rye-grass pollen and AgB from timothy pollen have been used (30). The results of population and family studies performed to date in order to detect *specific* Ir genes in man are summarized in Table II.

1) Population studies

In most population studies of unrelated allergic patients, no association between a given HLA antigen and the presence of immediate-type skin hypersensitivity (and in some cases specific IgE detected by RAST test and/or lymphocyte transformation detected by ^{3}H-thymidine uptake) towards common

TABLE II

Attempts to identify antigen-specific Ir genes in man with special reference to allergy

Author	Reference No.	Year	Antigen	No. of Patients[a]	Comments
Weeds – Population Studies					
Marsh	(52)	1973	Ag E Ra 5	105	Association of HLA-B7 cross-reacting group with Ra 5 ($p = 0.03$)
Goodfriend	(53)	1976	Ra 5	76	Association of HLA-B7 cross-reacting group with Ra 5 ($p = 0.01$)
Marsh	(30)	1976	Ra 3	76	Association of HLA-A2 – B12 with Ra 3 in patients with low IgE levels ($p = 0.04$ and 0.07)
Roseman	(60)	1976	Staphylococcus toxins Sheep sorrel Lambs qtr. Short ragweed	160	Association of HLA antigen with test allergens (*)
Grass – Population Studies					
Marsh	(30)	1976	Rye grass I	136	Association between HLA-B8 ($p = 0.005$) and A1, B8 haplotype ($p = 0.007$) and Rye I especially in populations with low IgE levels
Jeannet	(67)	1976	Timothy grass	48	No significant association
Schunter	(85)	1957	Timothy grass	110	Increased HLA-A W19 ($p = 0.0012$), decreased HLA-B8 ($p = 0.0025$)
Dust and Mites – Population Studies					
Dasgupta	(86)	1976	mite	37	Association suggested with HLA-A1, B8 ($p = 0.05$)
Perrin-Fayolle	(87)	1976	dust	72	No significant association
Miscellaneous – Population Studies					
Greenberg	(55)		Streptococcal antigen		Associated to HLA-B5
Buckley	(54)		PPD	63	Diminished responsiveness to PPD in patients receiving BCG possessing HLA-B7
Weeds – Family Studies					
Levine	(48)	1972	Ag E	7 families (46)	Association of antigen E sensitivity with familial haplotype
Blumenthal	(50)	1975	Ag E	1 family (57)	Association of ragweed and Ag sensitivity with familial HLA
Marsh	(65)	1975	Ag E and 7 purif. pollen allergens	36 families + (376)	No genetic linkage between familial HLA haplotype and specific Ir to any of the Ag tested
Yoo	(61)	1976	Ag E	1 family (14)	Association of ragweed Ag E with HLA familial haplotype

(*) No p value given.

[a] For familial studies, number of individuals tested given in parentheses.

Author	Reference No.	Year	Antigen	No. of Patients[a]	Comments
Dust and Mites – Family Studies					
Bessot	(63)	1974	dust	7 families	No significant association
Dasgupta	(85)	1976	dust	7 families	Increased frequency of HLA-A1, A7, and A8 (*)
Yoo	(61)	1976	dust	1 family (14)	Association of dust sensitivity with HLA suggested
Grass – Family Studies					
Bessot	(63)	1974	grasses	6 families	Association of grass sensitivity in 4 of 6 families with a familial HLA haplotype
Mercier	(66)	1974	grasses	14 families (63)	Association of grass sensitivity in one of 14 families with a familial HLA haplotype + (in abstract form)
Pillier-Loriette	(64)	1976	cocksfoot	12 families (62)	Association of cocksfoot sensitivity in two of 12 families with a familial HLA haplotype
Buckley	(57)	1975	Natural antigens	3 families	Association of antigen sensitivity with familial haplotypes
Allen	(49)	1976	bird serum protein	4 families (20)	Association of response to bird antigen with familial HLA hyplotype, increased HLA-BW40 ($p = 0.001$)

inhalation allergens has been found. One apperent exception is skin hypersensitivity to antigen Ra 5 from ragweed pollen, which was claimed in two successive studies (52, 53) to be associated with HLA-B7 cross-reacting group (Creg). Antigen Ra 5, whose structure has been elucidated (52), is a low molecular weight (5,000) glycopeptide which probably contains only a restricted number of antigenic determinants and which comprises only a small proportion (about 1 % by weight in comparison to AgE) of the antigens from ragweed pollen.

Marsh *et al.* have recently presented data suggesting that there are two Ir loci: one controlling the response to Rye I which maps closer to the B than to the A locus, and one controlling response to Ra 3 which maps very close to A between A and B. In addition, the gene(s) controlling IgE levels in an allergic individual appear to exert influence on his response to allergens. For instance, IgE-antibody response to Rye I and Ra 3 in allergic persons with low serum IgE levels are associated with two common HLA phenotypes, A1, B8 and A2, B12 respectively (30, 53).

On the other hand, two studies suggest genetic control of the major histocompatibility system and delayed hypersensitivity reactions: i) HLA-B7 with tuberculin unresponsiveness (*in vivo*) (54), and ii) HLA-B5 to high concentrations of a purified streptococcal antigen (55). Association between IgE-mediated hypersensitivity, delayed hypersensitivity reaction and *in vitro* blast transformation of lymphocytes and a particular HLA antigen, although interesting, do not prove the existence of Ir genes in man, but they do suggest their existence in genetic linkage disequilibrium with those HLA-B antigens found in significant association.

2) Family studies

In family studies, Levine *et al.* (50)

were the first to claim a linkage between hypersensitivity to ragweed AgE and HLA haplotypes. In a large family of 57 members, Blumenthal et al. (31) postulated a linkage between hypersensitivity to ragweed AgE and a familial HLA haplotype containing HLA-B12. From the analysis of the pedigree, the authors described one HLA recombinant in which the allergy was associated with the B12 haplotype. Two individuals were assumed to be HLA-IrE recombinants. One of these had a 2–12 haplotype but a negative history of allergy, no reaction on skin testing to antigen E, and 7 non-ragweed-sensitive children. Five of these children were HLA 2–12. The second HLA-IrE recombinant was a member of a family with discordance between haplotype and skin reaction. Using these recombinants, the authors postulated a recombination frequency of 7 %. Four other family members were possible recombinants. This family illustrated some of the problems involved in studies of families with allergies due to the role of several genes, environmental factors and age factors. The conclusions have previously been criticized because of the high incidence of postulated recombinants and because the conventional pedigree analysis based on Morton's lod scores was not used (56). The authors have recently performed further genetic analysis of the distribution of the immune responses in two ragweed-sensitive families. They found evidence for autosomal dominant heredity of positive skin-test reaction to antigen E and/or personal history of seasonal allergy. They also demonstrated by linkage analysis that this locus was linked to HLA-B and the estimated recombination frequency is 0.1 in males and 0.5 in females with a lod score of 2.47.

Buckley et al. (57) described HLA-linked genetic control of the specific response to natural antigens such as alternaria, hormodendrum and mumps virus in three families. In addition, they presented evidence for HLA-linked genetic control of antiviral immunity (58). Further evidence for HLA-linked Ir genes controlling the IgE response to tree pollen antigens in a large family has recently been presented by the authors (59). Roseman et al. (60), Yoo et al. (61, 62) and Bessot et al. (63) have presented evidence in families that there may be HLA-haplotype linkage of Ir to a variety of allergens (including grass pollens, house dust, and others).

On the other hand, Pillier-Loriette et al. (64), when correlating HLA with skin hypersensitivity to cocksfoot and specific anti-cocksfoot IgE levels found segregation of allergy with HLA haplotype in only two out of twelve families. Mercier (65) and Jeannet (66) have also failed to demonstrate linkage of grass-pollen hypersensitivity to familial HLA haplotypes in a limited number of families. Marsh et al. (30) could not confirm linkage between HLA haplotype and hypersensitivity to a number of purified allergens in 36 families, some of them alledgedly large. Unfortunately, these data have not yet been published in extenso (65). These authors did find HLA-identical sibling pairs who showed marked differences in their pattern of specific sensitivity, as well as HLA-distinct pairs who showed very similar patterns. In fact, sibling pairs with high IgE levels but different HLA antigens showed a greater concordance in their pattern of skin sensitivity than HLA-identical sibling pairs where one has a high and the other a low IgE level.

Black et al. (68) also failed in a study of ten families to demonstrate genetic linkage between familial HLA haplotypes and immune responsiveness to any of four extensively studied allergens, even when antigen-induced lymphocyte proliferation was used in addition to measurement of IgE-mediated skin hypersensitivity and serum IgG antibody as parameters of specific immune responsiveness.

The difficulties involved in family studies have already been discussed. It is possible that linkage exists in some but not all of the families. Some of the discrepancies in the reported studies may be related to the size of the family, the selection of families and a possible hypostatic effect of the level of IgE. It has become clear from the many studies that the issue of linkage of HLA haplotypes to hypersensitivity towards purified allergens will be resolved only through studies of large families over at least three generations. Each family needs to be analyzed individually. Investigators will have to use pure allergens, control the exposure to antigens, and analyze the level of serum IgE.

Although additional formal proof is required, present evidence points to the existence of two possible genetic controls; one linked to HLA which controls the specific immune response and one controlling the level of IgE not linked to HLA.

IV. Perspectives

Greater effort should be made to evaluate the associations of HLA antigens with the immune response to chemically defined antigens. However, no significant HLA association was found in a preliminary study of 40 unrelated individuals allergic to penicillin and showing sensitization to the benzylpenicilloyl group (69). The use of chemically well-defined allergens would be of advantage and the observation that contact sensitization to chemical contactants in guinea pigs is genetically controlled (70) in an MHC-linked fashion (71) is therefore of particular interest. Studies on association of HLA and contact dermatitis in selected groups of patients professionally exposed to contact sensitizers could be quite rewarding.

One of the most important variables in the study of the immune response is exposure to the antigen. Retrospective studies using natural allergens, as hitherto performed, are subject to severe limitations, since the degree of allergen exposure cannot be quantitatively assessed and since most natural allergens are chemically poorly characterized.

The best approach to the detection of specific Ir genes in humans would probably involve investigations of primary sensitization to chemically defined antigens *in vitro*, since programmes of large-scale experimental sensitization to chemically defined compounds in families or populations will probably be considered unethical. There is, therefore, a need to develop *in vitro* methodology to establish and assess immune response *in man*.

It has already been demonstrated in experimental animals that primary sensitization of T cells *in vitro* to chemically defined antigens is technically feasible (72, 73). Preliminary experiments on the induction of cytotoxic cells by penicillin *in vitro*, using cultures of peripheral blood lymphocytes from people showing no evidence of previous sensitization of penicillin, might also afford a tool for such studies (74). In any case, prospective studies *in vitro* under conditions of graded allergenic exposure and using chemically well-defined allergens would probably yield a greater contribution to the demonstration of Ir genes and to the study of their physicochemical nature in man than any retrospective studies on sensitization to natural allergens performed in populations or families of allergic patients.

References

1. Cooke, R. A. & van der Veer, A. (1916) Human sensitization. *J. Immunol.* 1, 201.
2. Schwartz, M. (1952) Heredity in bronchial asthma: a clinical and genetic study of 191 asthma probands and 50 probands with baker's asthma. *Acta Allerg.* Suppl. 2, 215.
3. Black, P. L. & Marsh, D. G. (1976) The genetics of allergy. In: *Bronchial Asthma: Mechanisms and Therapeutics,* eds. Segal, M. S. & Weiss, E. B. Little Brown Publ. Co., Boston, Mass., (in press).
4. Sherman, W. B. (1968) *Hypersensitivity, Mechanisms and Management,* W. B. Saunders Co, Phil.
5. Spaich, D. & Ostertag M. (1936) Untersuchunge nüber allergische Erkrankungen bei Zwillingen. *Z. Menschl. Vererb. Konstitutionslehre* 19, 731.
6. Bowen, R. (1953) Allergy in identical twins. *J. Allergy* 24, 236.
7. Schnyder, U. W. (1960) Neurodermitis, Asthma, Rhinitis: Eine genetisch-allergologisch Studie. *Int. Arch. Allergy,* Suppl. 17.
8. Ratner, B. & Silberman, D. E. (1952) Allergy – its distribution and the hereditary concept. *Ann. Allergy* 9, 1.
9. Weiner, A. S., Zieve, J. & Fries, J. H. (1936) The inheritance of allergic disease. *Ann. Eugen.* 7, 141.
10. Adkinson, J. (1920) The behaviour of bronchial asthma as an inherited character. *Genetics* 5, 363.
11. Tips, R. L. (1954) A study of the inheritance of atopic hypersensitivity in man. *Amer. J. Hum. Genet.* 6, 328.
12. Berg, T. & Johansson, S. G. O. (1969) IgE concentrations in children with atopic disease. *Int. Arch. Allergy Appl. Immunol.* 36, 219.
13. Vaz, N. M. & Levine, B. B. (1970) Immune responses of inbred mice to repeated low doses of antigens: relationship to histocompatibility (H-2) type. *Science* 168, 852.
14. Levine, B. B. & Vaz, N. M. (1970) Effect of combinations of inbred strain, antigen and antigen dose on immune responsiveness and reagin production in the mouse. A potential mouse model for immune aspects of human atopic allergy. *Int. Arch. Allergy* 39, 156.
15. Murphey, S. M., White, C., Waters, T. & Fireman, P. (1975) Genetic control of reaginic antibody synthesis in inbred rats. *J. Allergy clin. Immunol.* (abstract) 55, 109.
16. Benacerraf, B. & McDevitt, H. O. (1972) Histocompatibility-linked immune response genes. *Science* 175, 273.
17. McDevitt, H. O. & Landy, M. (1972) *Genetic Control of Immune Responsiveness,* Academic Press, New York.
18. McDevitt, H. O. & Chinitz, A. (1969) Genetic control of the antibody response: relationship between immune response and histocompatibility (H-2) type. *Science* 163, 1207.
19. Levine, B. B., Ojeda, A. & Benacerraf, B. (1963) Studies on artificial antigens. III. The genetic control of the immune response to hapten poly-L-lysine conjugates in guinea pigs. *J. exp. Med.* 118, 953.
20. Chang, E. B. & Marsh, D. G. (1974) Immune responsiveness of inbred mice to pollen allergens. *J. Allergy clin. Immunol.* (abstract) 53, 65.
21. Patrucco, R. & Marsh, D. G. (1974) Immune response to ascaris antigen in inbred mice. *J. Allergy clin. Immunol.* (abstract) 53, 65.
22. Schwartz, B. D., Paul, W. E. & Shevach, E. M. (1976) Guinea pig I antigens: functional significance and chemical characterization. *Transplant Rev.* 30, (in press).
23. Geczy, A. F., de Weck, A. L., Schwartz, B. D. & Shevach, E. M. (1975) The major histocompatibility complex of the guinea pig. I. Serologic and genetic studies. *J. Immunol.* 115, 1704.
24. Geczy, A. F., Geczy, C. L. & de Weck, A. L. (1975) Histocompatibility antigens and genetic control of the immune response in guinea pigs. II. Specific inhibition of antigen-induced lymphocyte proliferation by anti-receptor alloantisera. *Europ. J. Immunol.* 5, 711.
25. Geczy, A. F., Geczy, C. L. & de Weck, A. L. (1976) Histocompatibility antigens and genetic control of the immune response in guinea pigs. III. Specific inhibition of antigen-induced lymphocyte proliferation by strain-specific anti-idiotypic antibodies. *J. exp. Med.* 144, 226.
26. de Weck, A. L. & Geczy, A. F. (1976) Attempts to elucidate the molecular structure of Ir gene products and T-cell receptor in guinea pigs with anti-histo-

compatibility, anti-receptor and anti-idio-type antisera. *Immunopothology VII,* (in press).

27. Rajewsky, K. & Eichmann, K. (1976) Antigen receptors of T helper cells. In: *Contemporary Topics in Immunobiology,* (in press).

28. Katz, D. H., Dorf, M. E. & Benacerraf, B. (1976) Control of T-lymphocyte and B-lymphocyte activation by two complementing Ir-GL immune response genes. *J. exp. Med.* **143,** 906.

29. Munro, A. J. & Taussig, M. J. (1975) Two genes in the major histocompatibility complex control immune response. *Nature (Lond.)* **256,** 103.

30. Marsh, D. G. (1976) Allergy: a model for studying the genetics of human response. In: *Nobel Symposium No. 33 Molecular and Biological Aspects of the Acute Allergic Reactions,* eds. Johansson, S. G. O., Strandberg, J., & Urnäs, B. Plenum Press.

31. Blumenthal, M. N., Amos, D. B., Noreen, H., Mendell, N. R. & Yunis, E. J. (1974) Genetic mapping of Ir locus in man: linkage to second locus of HL-A. *Science* **184,** 1301.

32. Yunginger, J. W. & Gleich, G. (1973) Seasonal changes in serum and nasal IgE concentrations. *J. Allergy. clin. Immunol.* **51,** 174.

33. van Arsdel, P. P. & Motulsky, A. G. (1959) Frequency and hereditability of asthma and allergic rhinitis in college students. *Acta. genet.* **9,** 101.

34. Falliers, C. J., Cardoso, R. R. de A., Bane, H. N., Coffey, R. & Middleton, E. Jr. (1971) Discordant allergic manifestations in monozygotic twins: genetic identity versus clinical, physiologic, and biochemical differences. *J. Allergy* **47,** 207.

35. Morton, N. E. (1956) The detection and estimation of linkage between the genes for elliptocytosis and the Rh blood type. *Amer. J. Human Genet.* **8,** 80.

36. Rachelefsky, G. S., Terasaki, P. I., Katz, R. M. & Siegel, S. C. (1976) B-lymphocyte and histocompatibility antigens in extrinsic asthma. In: HLA and Allergy, ed. de Weck, A. *Monogr. Allergy* **11.**

37. Geerts, S. J., Pöttgens, H., Limburg, M. & van Rood, J. J. (1975) Predisposition for atopy or allergy linked to HLA. *Lancet* **i,** 461.

38. Bazaral, M., Orgel, A. H. & Hamburger, R. N. (1974) Genetics of IgE and allergy: serum IgE levels in twins. *J. Allergy clin. Immunol.* **54,** 288.

39. Marsh, D. G., Bias, W. B. & Ishizaka, K. (1974) Genetic control of basal serum immunoglobulin E level and its effect on specific reaginic sensitivity. *Proc. nat. Acad. Sci. (Wash.)* **71,** 3588.

40. Buckley, R. H., Dess, S. C. & O'Fallon, W. M. (1968) Serum immunoglobulins. I. Levels in normal children and in uncomplicated childhood allergy. *Pediatrics* **41,** 600.

41. Allensmith, M., McCellan, B. & Butterworth, M. (1969) The influence of heredity and environment on human immunoglobulin levels. *J. Immunol.* **102,** 1504.

42. Kalff, M. W. & Hijmans, W. (1969) Serum immunoglobulins in twins. *Clin. exp. Immunol.* **5,** 469.

43. Orgel, H. A., Lenoir, M. A. & Bazaral, M. (1974) Serum IgG, IgA, IgM and IgE levels and allergy in Filipino children in the United States. *J. Allergy clin. Immunol.* **53,** 213.

44. Lichtman, M. A., Vaughan, J. H. & Hames, C. G. (1967) The distribution of serum immunoglobulins, anti-y-G globulin ("rheumatoid factor") and anti-nuclear antibodies in White and Negro subjects in Evans Country, Georgia. *Arthritis Rheum.* **10,** 204.

45. Stiffel, C., Mouton, D., Bouthilier, Y., Heumann, A. M., Decreusefond, C., Mevel, J. C. & Biozzi, G. (1974) Polygenic regulation of general antibody synthesis in the mouse. *Prog. Immunol. II,* **2,** 203.

46. Revoltella, R. & Ovary, Z. (1969) Reaginic antibody production in different mouse strains. *Immunology* **17,** 45.

47. Soothill, J. F. (1974) Immunodeficiency and allergy. *Prog. Immunol. II,* **5,** 183.

48. Minnig, H. & de Weck, A. L. (1972) Die "Käsewascherkrankheit". Immunologische Studien. *Schweiz. Med. Wschr.* **102,** 1205.

49. Allen, D. H., Basten, A., Woolock, A. J. & Guinan, J. (1976) HLA and bird breeder's hypersensitivity pneumonitis. In: HLA and Allergy, ed. de Weck, A. *Monogr. Allergy* **11.**

50. Levine, B. B., Stember, R. H. & Fotino, M. (1972) Ragweed hay fever: genetic control and linkage to HL-A haplotypes. *Science* **178,** 1201.

51. Yoo, R. J., Flink, R. J. & Thompson, J. S. (1976) The relationship between HL-A antigens and lymphocyte response in ragweed allergy. *J. Allergy clin. Immunol.* **57,** 25.

52. Marsh, D. G., Bias, W. B., Hsu, S. H. & Goodfriend, L. (1973) Association of the

HL-A7 cross-reacting group with a specific reaginic antibody response in allergic man. *Science* **179**, 691.

53. Goodfriend, L., Santilli, J. Jr., Schacter, B., Bias, W. B. & Marsh, D. G. (1976) HLA B7 cross-reacting group and human IgE-mediated sensitivity to ragweed allergen Ra 5. In: HLA and Allergy, ed. de Weck, A. *Monogr. Allergy* **11**.

54. Buckley, C. E., White, D. & Siegler, H. (1976) HL-A B7 associated tuberculin unresponsiveness in BCG treated patients. In: HLA and Allergy, ed. de Weck, A. *Monogr. Allergy* **11**.

55. Greenberg, L., Gray, E. & (1975) Association of HL-A5 and immune responsiveness in vitro to streptococcal antigens. *J. exp. Med.* **141**, 935.

56. Bias, W. B. & Marsh, D. G. (1975) HLA linked antigen E immune response genes: an unproved hypothesis. *Science* **188**, 375.

57. Buckley, G., Dorsey, F., Corley, R. Ralph, W., Woodberry, M. & Amos, D. (1973) HLA-linked human immune response genes. *Proc. nat. Acad. Sci. (Wash.)* **70**, 2175.

58. Buckley, R. H. & McGeady, S. J. (1975) Repression of cell-mediated immunity in atopic eczema. *J. Allergy clin. Immunol.* **56**, 393.

59. Buckley, E. C., Haysmann, M. L., Johnson, A. R., Cohen, H. J., McMillan, C. W. & Amos, D. B. (1976) Immune response genes, immunity deficiency and autoimmunity in an HLA recombinant family. *Ann. Int. Med.* (in press).

60. Roseman, J., Buckley, C. & Amos, D. B. (1976) Human immune response polymorphisms detectable with 4 common allergens. *J. Allergy clin. Immunol.* **57**, 228.

61. Yoo, T. J., Kuo, C. Y., Thompson, J. S., Flink, R., Faster, F. & Schindler, M. S. A family study of HLA antigen and immune response (Ir) gene linkage in ragweed and dust allergy. *J. Allergy clin. Immunol.* (abstract) **57**, 229.

62. Yoo, T. J., Flink, R. J. & Thompson, J. S. (1976) The relationship between HLA antigens and lymphocyte response in ragweed allergy. *J. Allergy clin. Immunol.* **57**, 25.

63. Bessot, J. C., Mayer, S., Tongio, M. M. & Pauli, G. (1974) IgE, contrôle génétique et système HL-A. *Lyon Méd. Med.* **10**, 1363.

64. Pillier-Loriette, C., Marcelli-Barge, A., Dausset, J., Treich, L., Gervais, P., Raffard, M., Hemocq, E., Berman, D. & de Moutis, G. (1976) Search for a correlation between familial allergy to dactyl (pollen hypersensitivity) and HLA antigens. In: HLA and Allergy, ed. de Weck, A. *Monogr. Allergy* **11**.

65. Mercier, P., Anfosso-Capra, F., Autran, P., Boutin, C., Aubert, J. & Charpin, J. (1974) Génétique, système HLA et atopie. *Lyon Méd. Med.* **10**, 1371.

66. Jeannet, M., Girard, J. P., Varonier, H. S., Mirinanoff, P. & Joyce, P. (1976) HLA antigens in grass pollinosis. In: HLA and Allergy, ed. de Weck, A. *Monogr. Allergy* **11**.

67. Marsh, D. G., Jaretti, B. S., Black, P. L., Amerson, J. B., Chase, G. A. & Bias, W. B. (1975) Genetic complexity of immune response (Ir) in man. *J. Allergy clin. Immunol.* (abstract) **55**, 81.

68. Black, P. L., Marsh, D. G., Jarret, E., Delespesse, G. J. & Bias, W. B. (1974) Family studies of lymphocyte responses to highly purified pollen antigens. *Proc. IXth Leukocyte Culture Conference, 1974.*

69. de Weck, A. L. & Spengler, H. (1976) Evaluation of genetic control of the immune response to penicillin in man. In: HLA and Allergy, ed. de Weck, A. *Monogr. Allergy* **11**.

70. Polak, L., Barnes, J. M. & Turk, J. L. (1968) The genetic control of contact sensitization to inorganic metal compounds in guinea pigs. *Immunology* **14**, 707.

71. Geczy, A. F. & de Weck, A. L. (1975) Genetic control of sensitization to structurally unrelated antigens and its relationship to histocompatibility antigens in guinea pigs. *Immunology* **28**, 331.

72. Shearer, G. M. (1975) Recognition of chemically modified autologous cells: importance of the murine major histocompatibility complex. In: *Immune Recognition,* ed. Rosenthal, A. S., p. 21, Academic Press, New York.

73. Ben-Sassoon, S. Z., Paul, W. E., Shevach, E. M. & Green, I. (1975) In vitro selection and extended culture of antigen-specific T lymphocytes I. Description of selection culture procedure and initial characterization of selected cells. *J. exp. Med.* **142**, 90.

74. de Weck, A. L. & Spengler, H. (1976) Experimental approaches to a study of the relationship between HLA and penicillin allergy. In: HLA and Allergy, ed. de Weck, A. *Monogr. Allergy* **11**.

75. Krain, L. S. (1974) Histocompatibility antigens: a laboratory and epidemiologic tool. *J. Invest. Derm.* **62**, 67.

76. Scholz, S., Ziegler, E., Braun-Falco, O.,

Wüstner, H., Knutz, B. & Albert, E. D. (1976) HLA family studies in patients with atopic dermatitis. In: HLA and Allergy, ed. de Weck, A. *Monogr. Allergy* 11.

77. Turner, M. W., Brostoff, J., Wells, R. S. & Soothill, J. F. (1976) HLA in eczema and hayfever. In: HLA and Allergy, ed. de Weck, A. *Monogr. Allergy* 11.

78. Hishino, K., Inouye, Unokuchi, T., Ito, M., Tamaoki, N. & Tsuji, K. (1976) HLA and diseases in Japan. In: HLA and Allergy, ed. de Weck, A. *Monogr. Allergy* 11.

79. Ohkido, M., Ozana, A., Matsuo, I., Niizunia, K., Nakano, M., Tsuji, K., Nose, Y., Ito, M., Kato, S. & Yamamoto, K. (1976) HLA antigens and susceptibility to atopic dermatitis. In: HLA and Allergy, ed. de Weck, A. *Monogr. Allergy* 11.

80. Goudemand, J., Deffrenne, C. & Desmons, F. (1976) HLA antigens and atopic dermatitis. In: HLA and Allergy, ed. de Weck, A. *Monogr. Allergy* 11.

81. Thorsby, E. & Lie, S. O. (1971) Relationship between the HLA system and susceptibility to disease. *Transplant. Proc.* 3, 1305.

82. Morris, M., Vaughan, J., Lane, D. & Morris, P. J. (1976) HLA and asthma. In: HLA and Allergy, ed. de Weck, A. *Monogr. Allergy* 11.

83. Thompson, P. D., Barratt, T. M., Stokes, C. R., Soothill, J. F. & Turner, M. W. (1976) HLA typing and atopic features in steroid sensitive nephrotic syndrome of childhood. In: HLA and Allergy, ed. de Weck, A. *Monogr. Allergy* 11.

84. Tait, B. D., Williams, A. L., Mathews, J. D. & Cowling, D. C. (1976) HLA and the sudden infant death syndrome. In: HLA and Allergy, ed. de Weck, A. *Monogr. Allergy* 11.

85. Schunter, F., Schieferstein, G., Tchorz, P., Fischer, H. & Schneider, W. (1975) Histokompatibilitätsantigene bei pollinosis. *Z. Immun. Forsch.* 150, 105.

86. Dasgupta, A. & Misim, N. (1976) Population and family studies to demonstrate Ir genes: HLA haplotype in atopic allergy. In: HLA and Allergy, ed. de Weck, A. *Monogr. Allergy* 11.

87. Perrin-Fayolle, M., Betuel, H., Biot, N. & Groselaude, M. (1976) HLA antigens in patients allergic to pollen and to house dust. In: HLA and Allergy, ed. de Weck, A. *Monogr. Allergy* 11.

HLA and Malignant Diseases

M. J. Simons[1] & J. L. Amiel[2]

Introduction

Malignant diseases have had an important role in the development of HLA studies of diseases in two main ways. First, the discovery of associations between the H-2 histocompatibility system in mice and the occurrence of cancer following exposure to oncogenic viruses (1, 2) was a major stimulus to investigation of HLA type and diseases in man. The H-2 associations strengthened the argument for a substantial influence of genetic predisposition in the development of natural cancer and in susceptibility to environmental carcinogens. Secondly, the earliest studies seeking an association between HLA antigens and human disease involved patients with malignancies. Amiel's finding in 1967 (3) of an increased frequency of the 4c antigen in Hodgkin's disease patients encouraged the hope that HLA studies would provide an insight into the role of genetic factors in malignant diseases. In the years since Amiel's report, evidence has accumulated in support of an association between Hodgkin's disease and antigens of the 4c system (HLA-B5, BW35, B18 and BW15), and probably also with the antigens HLA-A1 and B8 (4–11). However, the situation has been complicated by the inability of some groups

to detect altered frequencies of these or of other antigens. Furthermore, reports claiming to confirm an association usually implicated a different one or two of the six antigens, and the strength of the association with any of the six was relatively weak. It was hoped that a co-operative study conducted as part of the 5th International Histocompatibility testing workshop would resolve the issue, but the results, while again implicating some of the same six antigens, were generally regarded as disappointing (12).

Acute lymphocyte leukaemia (ALL) was the first leukaemia to be investigated by HLA typing. In the earliest report, Kourilsky and colleagues were unsuccessful in their search for an association with any of 10 HLA antigens (13). Walford et al. (14) were the first to report a significant association involving an increase in *HLA-A2, B12* haplotype, and a decrease in A1, although Thorsby et al. (15) had earlier found a numerical but not statistically significant increase in the *HLA-A2, B12* haplotype. Rogentine and associates (16, 17) also found an increased frequency of HLA-A2 in ALL patients while other studies found differences in frequencies of other antigens [e.g. HLA-A9- (18)] or no apparent differences at all.

HLA studies of a variety of solid tumours (9) revealed alterations of antigen frequencies in six of ten carcinomata, but the differences did not attain

[1] WHO Immunology Research & Training Centre, Faculty of Medicine, University of Singapore, McAlister Road, Singapore 3.

[2] Institut Gustave-Roussy, 94800 Villejuif, France.

statistical significance. Among patients with solid malignant neoplasms, Tarpley and colleagues detected a significant increase in HLA-B8 in salivary gland adenocarcinoma, and in B5 in connective-tissue sarcomas (19). As in the study of Takasugi et al. (9), several other deviations from control antigen frequencies were detected, but were not statistically significant after correction for the number of antigens studied.

In 1974 the first evidence of an HLA association with nasopharyngeal carcinoma (NPC) in the Chinese was published (20, 21). The association was unusual in that it involved blank, unde--tected antigen(s) at locus B, in addition to A2 at locus A. Subsequently, the blank gene was identified and designated Singapore 2 [Sin 2, (22)]. The existence of this locus B gene was independently confirmed by Payne et al., who referred to it as Hsieh (23). The associated with a relative risk (RR) of the order of 3.5 (i.e. individuals with the HLA type have a 3.5 fold increased risk for developing NPC). When compared with the strong associations between HLA and diseases such as ankylosing spondylitis, even that of HLA-A2, Sin 2 and NPC is relative weak. In general, then, HLA studies of malignant diseases have failed to show the strong associations that many had expected on the basis of findings in the mouse model systems, and some doubt has arisen as to the merit of HLA typing in cancer.

In this review, an optimistic viewpoint will be taken of the progress achieved in the 10 years since Amiel's original study. Far from being disappointed with the apparently poor yield of positive results, the findings of HLA associations in no less than three types of malignancy (Hodgkin's disease, ALL and NPC) support the original hope that HLA typing would provide some insight into the heritable nature of cancer. Whether a pessimistic or an optimistic viewpoint is taken is largely a matter of level of expectation. Up to the 1st International Symposium, the strongest and best established association so far reported was that between the Chinese-related haplotype A2, Sin 2 and NPC (24). Data from the HLA and Disease Registry of Copenhagen (25) indicated highly significant associations of four HLA antigens in Hodgkin's disease. The antigens and the relative risks associated with them, are: B18 (1.85), B5 (1.59), A1 (1.42) and B8 (1.33). Three antigens are associated with lower relative risks for ALL [A2 (1.34), B12 (1.24) and B8 (1.28)]. One way of regarding these values is that they are less than twice the normal risk. The alternative view is that they are one-third to one-half the maximum relative risk so far identified in a human cancer. Undoubtedly, these HLA results represent a substantial improvement on previous blood group findings in malignant diseases in which blood group A has been found to confer only a slightly increased risk for carcinoma of the stomach (RR approx. 1.24), and in which no certain correlations have been demonstrated in lymphomas or leukaemias.

The basis for an optimistic view of the HLA findings so far obtained is that the associations with at least the three diseases and possibly others have been achieved despite the heterogeneity and relatively small size of patient and comparison groups, despite serological problems which have complicated HLA typing-pattern interpretation, and despite the application of conservative statistical procedures for calculation of the significance of altered HLA gene frequencies. The workshop on HLA and Malignant Diseases at the First International Symposium revealed that several studies are in progress which have been designed to overcome these difficulties. Application of the information arising from the workshop can be expected to clarify suspected associations and, hopefully, to reveal the existence of hitherto unsuspected associations.

Rather than review the chronological sequence of HLA studies in malignancy over the past 10 years, it is more useful to consider the current position in relation to data presented at the workshop. For this purpose, malignant diseases will be considered under four headings:

1. Lymphomas
2. Leukaemias
3. Carcinomata
4. Other malignancies

In discussing results in each of these groups, attention will be directed to some principles of HLA studies which should be considered in the planning of future studies.

1. Lymphomas

1.1 Hodgkin's disease

There have been numerous reports of HLA associations with Hodgkin's disease. A common pattern has been the increased frequency of HLA antigens of the 4c system (B5, BW35, B18, and BW15), supporting the original finding of Amiel (3) and the confirmatory report of Forbes & Morris (4). Increased frequencies of HLA-A1 and -B8 have also been implicated in several studies (see 25 for a review). However, not all studies have revealed statistically significant alterations in gene frequencies. A likely explanation for the apparent inconsistencies in results is that the patients in the different studies, although having the same diagnosis, varied in respect of factors involved in the cause and natural history of the malignancy. As Bodmer (10) has written, "If the disease has a heterogenous aetiology it is quite likely that only some forms of the disease and not others will show a given (HLA) association". If a particular HLA type is associated with only some patients with a certain malignancy, the association may not be strong enough to be recognised by HLA typing the total patient group. Where possible it is desirable to subgroup patients in the hope of achieving sufficient restriction of the heterogeneity of HLA type in one of the subgroups for differences in gene frequencies to be detected.

In Hodgkin's disease, four histopathological subtypes are recognised. The lymphocyte predominant and nodular sclerosing forms portend a poor outcome, whereas the lymphocyte depleted and mixed cellularity types have a more favourable progosis. Based on findings of associations involving B5 and B18, and A1 and B8, Graff and associates (7) proposed that the clinical and pathological pattern of Hodgkin's disease was influenced by the HLA phenotype of the host.

Histopathological type is only one of the known factors that influence survival in Hodgkin's disease. Falk & Osoba (5) recognised that, in addition to histological variety, sex and age, Hodgkin's disease patients were heterogeneous with respect to duration of disease at the time of typing. In retrospect it is obvious that patients with any malignancy vary in their length of survival, and HLA typing using fresh lymphocytes can only be undertaken on patients who are still living at the time of the study. If any HLA association with a malignancy was with processes affecting survival from the disease, as distinct from those concerned with susceptibility to the malignancy, then variation in the results of retrospective studies may have arisen solely because of heterogeneity in the duration of survival of the patients being typed. In the study of Falk & Osoba (5) the frequencies of A1 and B5 were high, irrespective of disease duration, whereas B8 was increased in frequency only in those having the disease for more than 5 years.

The Canadian study of Hodgkin's disease, and the findings of Rogentine and co-workers (16, 17) of an increased frequency of HLA-A2 in surviving acute lymphocytic leukaemia patients, focused attention on a basic question: the nature of HLA associations with malignant diseases. It was realised that prospective studies of patients typed at the time of diagnosis were necessary to establish whether:

1. there is an association between HLA antigens and a disease,
2. any association is with disease susceptibility and/or survival,
3. there is a relation between HLA type of patients and response to initial therapy.

In the case of Hodgkin's disease, there are two extensive studies of a prospective design in progress. Osoba & Falk (26) have found that the proportion of patients with the specificities AW19 and B5 (present either singly or together) who achieved complete remission following the initial course of therapy was lower than in the "AW19, B5-negative" group. Furthermore, a lower proportion of the "AW19, B5-positive" patients stayed in remission

without any maintenance therapy than did the "negative" patients. The study will need to be continued for 2 to 3 years more before the previous finding of a better survival of B8-positive patients can be reassessed.

In Denmark, 368 patients have been entered into a prospective study. Kissmeyer-Nielsen provided information at the workshop indicating an association between A1 and B8, and possibly B7, with survival from Hodgkin's disease. However, only some 20 % of patients have succumbed to the disease so it is not yet possible to analyse the results on the basis of mean survival times.

1.2 Burkitt's lymphoma

There have been three reports of HLA studies in Burkitt's lymphoma (27–29). The results, whether taken separately or combined (30), were negative. However, the failure to detect alterations in HLA antigen frequencies should be accepted with reservations. First the number of patients studied, even when combined, was relatively small. Secondly, the proportion of undetected antigens at the A and B loci was relatively large. As discussed in the papers, this may represent a common occurrence of homozygosity or the existence of gene(s) which are unique to or more frequent in Africans than Caucasians. The more extensive use of sera of African origin may help in resolving the matter. Whatever the case proves to be, any HLA association would probably have to be stronger than that with NPC for it to have been detected. Thus, while recognising the difficulties involved in studying BL patients, an investigation designed to overcome the problems preventing any HLA association from being recognised has yet to be performed.

1.3 Other lymphomas

The position is essentially unchanged from that reviewed by Morris in 1974 (31), when the strongest indication of an association was that between HLA-B12 and follicular lymphoma (32). Dick *et al.* (33) also detected an increased frequency of B12 in a retrospective study of lymphoma patients.

2. Leukaemias

2.1 Acute lymphocytic leukaemia (ALL)

The findings of Walford and of Thorsby and their associates (14, 15) that the *HLA-A2, B12* haplotype was increased in ALL rekindled interest in HLA and leukaemias. Rogentine *et al.* (16) were able to confirm the locus A finding of an increased frequency of HLA-A2. Subsequently, they reconfirmed the A2 association with ALL and, in addition, presented evidence that the association affected patient survival rather than susceptibility to ALL (17). The American study is continuing and at the workshop a preliminary analysis of the results of a prospective study of 372 children with ALL was presented (34). The gene frequencies of *HLA-A2* and *AW24* were increased, while the frequencies of *A1, AW25, AW26* and *AW31* were decreased. This perturbation of frequencies only applied to genes of locus *A,* and not of locus *B* or *C.* When correction was made for the number of individual antigens studied, none of the differences between ALL patients and controls remained statistically significant. An alternative approach is to regard the current prospective investigation as a test of hypotheses arising from previous studies that A2 and B12 occur with increased frequency in ALL. The frequencies of these two specificities in ALL patients and controls were 58 and 48 %, and 27 and 21 % respectively. For A2, the difference was not as marked as that of 65 % and 44 % in the previous study, but the p value (one-sided) for the difference is nonetheless significant at 0.01. For B12, p = 0.07.

Further support for the association between HLA-A2 and ALL was provided by Pollack & DuBois (35) who detected A2 in 62 % of patients (26/42) and 47 % of the controls (165/355). The French group of Gluckman and colleagues (36) obtained similar results. When this group published the first report on HLA and ALL in 1967 (13), no differences in HLA antigen frequencies were detected. In the latest study the frequency of A2 in the group of 126 patients (57 %)was of the same order as before, whereas that in the control group of 591 subjects was now 44 %. In addition to providing more evidence for the A2-ALL association, the French study is noteworth in several respects. First, it illustrates the importance of the composition of the comparison group in the detection of HLA associations with disease. In the current study, more attention had been given to matching patients and controls with respect to variables such as place of origin. Secondly, by revealing that ALL patients may have an increased frequency of homozygosity at locus *A,* it indicated another way of analysing data for evidence of alterations in HLA antigen patterns.

Based on a prospective study, Klouda *et al.* (37) found a trend towards a low frequency of A9, and showed that pa-

216

tients with A9 had a higher median survival time. They suggested that "the HLA-A9 antigen may be associated with both a diminished susceptibility to ALL in childhood and a better prognosis in those children who develop the disease, compared with those who lack the antigen". A reduced frequency of A9 in ALL has been observed in at least four studies (15, 16, 38, 39), so the possibility has to be considered that both A2 and A9 antigens may be associated with different aspects of the development and course of ALL.

As in Hodgkin's disease, there is scope for diminishing the heterogeneity of patients grouped with the single diagnosis of ALL. Subdivision into T-cell, B-cell and 'null'-cell leukaemias would be a first step, with the prospect of further divisions according to subpopulations of T and possibly other lymphocytes involved in leukaemic processes.

2.2 Other leukaemias

HLA studies in leukaemias other than ALL have been less frequent. At the workshop, Oliver *et al.* (40) reported on studies of 150 patients with acute myelogenous leukaemia (AML). The patients who were HLA typed represented 61 % of the 246 treated during the 5-year study period. There was a slight increase in A2 in the patients (53 % *vs.* 45 %), and patients with the phenotypes A1 and B8 and/or A2 and B12 survived longer than patients without either of these pairs of antigens. These differences did not withstand statistical correction. Benbunan *et al.* (41) found an increase in HLA-B5 frequency in promyelocytic leukaemia. Both the English and French reports merit further investigation by prospective studies.

HLA antigen frequencies in patients with chronic lymphocytic (CLL) or chronic leukaemias (CML) have not been notably different from comparison groups (see 11) but the chronic leukaemias have been less intensively studied than ALL or even AML. Recently Pollack & DuBois (35) detected increased frequencies of A9, A28 and AW29 in 34 CLL patients. The A9 association is in agreement with the previous finding of Jeannet & Magnin (42).

2.3 Anomalous serological reactions

A phenomenon that was initially a complication of HLA typing in leukaemia now promises to provide information on leukaemia-associated antigens. Some HLA typing sera, which show the expected pattern of reactivity with cells from normal individuals, react more frequently with lymphocytes from leukaemia patients. An example is Walford's finding of an increased reactivity of Thorsby's anti-FJH (anti-B27) serum with lymphocytes from patients with CLL (11). Several laboratories have reported similar kinds of increased frequencies of HLA antigens in leukaemias (e.g. 16, 42, 43). Pollack & DuBois (35) found that the majority of typing sera used by them gave "extra" reactions with leukaemia cells, so the presence of non-HLA activity in "monospecific" HLA-typing sera may not be an unusual event.

Analysis of sera showing anomalous reactions by absorption studies has established that some of the reactivity represents antibodies to B-cell-specific alloantigens. Pollack & DuBois (35) found that some sera react with leukaemia cells from patients with myelocytic and with lymphocytic forms of leukaemia. They suggested that the non-HLA antigens being detected may be related to B-cell Fc receptor alloantigens. With other sera, absorption with leukaemic cells, but not with normal lymphocytes, removed reactivity. Sera which react predominantly, if not exclusively with leukaemic cells, and in which the reactivity does not segregate among the normal members of leukaemia case families, are likely to be useful as typing reagents for putative leukaemia-associated antigens. There is an indication from the results presented by Cohen *et al.* (44) that some sera distinguish between antigens associated with lymphocytic and with myeloid leukaemias. Other human sera lacking anti-HLA activity have been found to react with normal peripheral-blood granulocytes. Using a microgranulocytotoxic assay and alcohol-treated granulocytes, Drew *et al.* (45) have detected normal human granulocyte alloantigens on chronic myelogeneous, acute myeloblastic leukaemia cells, and on a cell line of chronic myeloblastic origin. Chronic lymphocytic leukaemia cells were unreactive, and most acute lymphoblastic leukaemia cells also seemed to lack granulocyte antigens. Thus, while the presence of normal granulocyte antigens may prove to be useful as leukaemic cell markers, their occurrence should be considered before claims are made for the existence of leukaemia-associated antigens.

It is likely that more normal tissue isoantigenic polymorphisms will be discovered by analysis of human sera. At this stage it is clear that reactions of HLA typing sera may be due to the presence of non-HLA antibodies. While the reactions may be spurious with respect to HLA loci A and B gene typing, in the broader context of cell-surface antigenic determinants they provide interesting possibilities for analysis of non-HLA polymorphisms and of leukaemia-associated antigens.

3. Carcinomata

Terasaki and his colleagues (9, 46, 47) have conducted the most extensive investigations of HLA and cancers. In the first study of 1996 Caucasian patients, differences in HLA antigen frequencies were detected between controls and patients in nine out of a total of 14 malignancies (9). "Application of the most conservative statistical correction of p values, however, caused all differences to fall short of statistical significance". Nonetheless, certain points are of interest, such as the finding that in cervical carcinoma, as in Hodgkin's disease, three HLA antigens showed altered frequencies.

In a second study of HLA frequencies in 2005 cancer patients (46), significant deviations ($p < 0.05$) of HLA antigen frequencies were observed in 14 out of the 17 cancers but, as before, none of the alterations remained significant when corrected for the number of specificities tested. The authors thought that cancer of the prostate was the most likely cancer to have an association with HLA among those tested. In both series, A1 and B8 were low, and A28 and BW22 were both high. AW29 was positively associated with cancers of the kidney, liver and lung and there were HLA associations with leukaemias, including an increased A2 in ALL.

A different approach was adopted in an analysis of HLA data of patients with 19 types of cancer and 12 non-malignant diseases (47). Rather than using HLA phenotype frequencies alone, Terasaki & Mickey estimated haplotype frequencies from phenotype frequencies. Differences significant at p less than 0.05 level were derived for cancer of the stomach (*A3, B7; W28, B12*), bladder (*A2, BW21*), prostate (*A1, B8*), ovary (*A9, BW35*), colon (*A1, B8*), tongue *(A1, B8)* and kidney (*A2, B12*). Only for cancer of the larynx, rectum, endometrial and mouth were no frequency differences from those of the controls observed, although the A1, B8 haplotype was often linked to susceptibility to mouth cancer.

In the studies by Terasaki, cancers were mainly divided into broad anatomical location categories. It seems probable that the lack of diagnostic precision resulted in the grouping of patients who were heterogeneous with respect to tumor type, thereby diminishing the likelihood that any HLA association(s) would be detected. That altered HLA antigen frequencies were observed despite the drawbacks of patient pooling favours the prospect that at least some of the associations were real.

Tarpley and associates (19) sought to achieve a more discriminating subdivision of patients with solid malignant neoplasms based on histopathologic as well as on anatomic site. They found an increase in HLA-B8 in salivary gland adenocarcinoma patients and in all solid malignant neoplasm patients taken together. There was also a three-fold increase in B5 in patients with connective-tissue sarcomas. The authors recognised that the finding of an increased frequency of B8 was not observed by Takasugi, Terasaki et al. Also, the trends noted by the latter group in cervix, lung and breast carcinoma, and in melanoma, were not observed in the Tarpley study.

In thinking about the possibility of HLA associations with malignant diseases, it is important to remember that the occurrence rate of most, if not all, malignancies varies in different parts of the world and among different ethnic groups. This feature is best established in those centres where the incidence of particular cancers is known. Differences in incidence of a particular cancer between populations, and changes in incidence within a population, underlie the view that the majority of malignancies are caused by environmental agents. The relation between smoking and carcinoma of the lung is a well-established example. In the context of HLA studies, the main issue is whether the incidence patterns of any cancers indicate an important role for genetic factors.

3.1 Nasopharyngeal carcinoma (NPC)

The high incidence among the Chinese and Chinese-related peoples compared with Caucasian and most other populations in the world has given rise to the proposal that there is a prominent genetic element in susceptibility to this malignancy (48, 49, 50). The first study of only 28 NPC-positive Singapore Chinese patients and 27 NPC-negative controls (clinically suspected of having NPC, but with no histological evidence of malignancy) revealed an increased frequency of *undetectable* antigens at locus B. In a subsequent study of a larger number of NPC patients and controls, the existence of a larger locus B blank in the NPC patients was confirmed (21). An increased frequency of the locus A allele A2 was also observed. It was hypothesized that the increased risk associated with the locus B blank reflected the presence of further HLA antigen(s), undetected by the antisera used which were largely of Caucasian origin, and predicted that at least one of the antigens would be associated with a high risk for NPC and found mainly in Chinese-related populations. Subsequently, sera were identified which defined a new locus B antigen termed Singapore 2 (Sin 2), and preliminary evidence was obtained for an asociation of Sin 2 with NPC (22). This was achieved by screening sera from multiparous women with lymphocytes from NPC patients and controls, seeking a higher frequency of reaction of a serum with the patients that could not be ascribed to the presence of antibody to known specificities. The strategy of looking for alterations in lymphocyte-antigen frequencies which are disease associated by using uncharacterised sera, rather than simply typing patients for known antigent with sera characterised for anti-HLA activity, is likely to be especially useful in studying diseases where the size of the blank differs in patients and controls as in Burkitt's Lymphoma in Africans, and carcinoma of the stomach in the Japanese.

The most recent study of 110 Singapore Chinese NPC patients and 91 NPC-negative controls (24) provided confirmation of the association between an increased risk for NPC and the HLA genes HLA-A2 and Sin 2. The risk was found to be restricted to the co-occurrence of A2-Sin 2, suggesting that the genotype predisposing to the the development of NPC was the A2. Sin 2 haplotype. Evidence has been obtained that a similar association existed in Malaysian and Hong Kong Chinese (51). The findings indicated that the increased risk for NPC associated with the A2-Sin 2 phenotype was a feature common to Asian Chinese in at least three geographic locations.

HLA patterns have also been studied in American Chinese. Jing *et al.* (52) investigated 37 patients and 48 control subjects and found a significantly high-er frequency of A2 and a deficit of locus B antigens in the patients. A2 and less than 2 locus B antigens co-occurred frequently in both Chinese cases and controls, and were associated with a high risk for NPC (RR = 3.53; p = 0.0062). These results were very similar to those obtained in the Singapore studies. The frequencies of A2 blank among the Singapore Chinese patients and controls (76/144 − 53 %; 68/236 − 29 %) were also comparable to the U.S. Chinese patients and comparison subjects (20/37 − 54 %; 12/48 − 25 %). In the American study, A2 alone conferred a higher risk for NPC (RR = 3.40; p = 0.021) than that associated with less than 2 locus B antigens (RR = 1.68; p = 0.23). The authors concluded that the data obtained from the study of U.S. Chinese strongly agreed with results from the studies conducted in Southeast Asia. Preliminary observations indicate that Sin 2 is present in U.S. Chinese patients but it remains to be determined whether the locus B blank will be substantially filled by the Sin 2 gene as in Asian Chinese patients. It does seem very probable, though, that the HLA phenotype of A2-Sin 2 will be found to be associated with an increased risk for NPC in American as well as in Asian Chinese.

In a review on HLA patterns and NPC, Simons & Day (53) developed the hypothesis that the high risk for NPC found among the Southern Chinese had a genetic basis mediated by alleles of the HLA system. The haplotype A2 . Sin 2 is not itself the main "Chineseness" factor associated with NPC, since over half the Chinese NPC cases do not have the haplotype. The existence of an NPC disease susceptibility (DS) gene in linkage disequilibrium with A2 . Sin 2 was therefore postulated which carried a high risk for NPC and which would be found predominantly among Southern Chinese. An important corollary of the hypothesis was that the A2 . Sin 2 haplotype would only be associated with an increased risk for malignancy in those ethnic groups among whom A2-Sin 2 occurred in linkage disequilibrium. This situation has only been established for the Chinese. However, the hypothesis of an NPC-DS locus allele common to most, if not all, NPC patients does imply a relation between the frequency of that allele and the incidence of NPC in the ethnic group. The question is whether the putative NPC-DS allele is sufficiently closely linked with detectable HLA genes for its existence to be inferred from results of HLA typing.

Malays and Tunisians are two medium NPC-incidence peoples of great interest in immunogenetic studies of NPC since Malays have a history of genetic admixture with mongoloid peoples, while Tunisians are a mixed population of maghrebian type with no known appreciable intermingling with mongoloid genes. Sin 2 was not detected in any of 109 Tunisian NPC patients by Betuel *et al.* (54). There was a higher frequency of B locus blanks among NPC cases (46 % *vs.* 37 %) but the difference only attained marginal statistical significance. However, close examination of locus B phenotypes revealed considerable differences between patients and controls. While the study was inconclusive, the results were consistent with the existence of an altered HLA profile among the Tunisian NPC cases.

In normal Malays, Sin 2 occurs in low frequency (approximately 3 %). None of 40 Malay NPC patients had Sin 2 (53). Since the HLA association in Chinese patients involved a haplotype that was in linkage disequilibrium among normal Chinese, the Malay HLA data was examined for evidence of a similar phenomenon. There does appear to be linkage between A9-B18 in normal Malays ($\Delta \div 0.019$). Among the 40 Malay NPC patients, the delta value for A9 − B18 was 0.061. If these preliminary findings of an HLA association involving a haplotype that was in linkage disequilibrium in normal Malays can be confirmed, the hypothesis of an HLA genetic basis to NPC predisposition would be even further strengthened.

The Singapore studies have indicated that the A2-Sin 2 association is mainly with increased susceptibility to NPC, but it may also be associated with poor survival. Sin 2 was present in 29 (46 %) of 63 newly diagnosed Chinese NPC patients, and in 7 (37 %) of 19 patients surviving for more than five years, compared with 23 (25 %) of 91 controls. The number of patients in the surviving group was relatively small, but there was a trend of a decreased survival of Sin 2-positive patients.

3.2 Other Carcinomata

3.2.1 Lung carcinoma

Dellon and colleagues (55) found AW19 and B5 associated with bronchogenic carcinoma in that patients with either or both of these antigens had prolonged survival. A similar association between AW19 and/or B5 was found when 69 of the patients were reassessed two years after diagnosis and therapy (56). The observations are being further investigated in a prospective study involving a larger number of patients with the same histology, clinical stage and prognostic factors.

3.2.2 Oesophageal carcinoma

A new finding reported at the workshop was the relatively strong association of HLA-B40 and oesophageal carcinoma (57). Among Iranian peoples living south of the Caspian Sea, carcinoma of the oesophagus is a common malignancy. It shows geographic and ethnic variation, the highest incidence occurring among Turkish-Mongol peoples in the northeastern areas. BW40 was detected in 13 (18.3 %) out of 71 patients, and in 7 (4.2 %) out of 168 control subjects, a difference corresponding to a χ^2 (Mantel-Haenzel) of 9.5, a p value (corrected) of 0.03, and an RR of 5.1. The relative risk revealed by this preliminary study is the highest so far reported for a human malignancy. If the comparison is restricted to the highest risk Mazandarani and Turks, the frequency difference of BW40 is even greater, being 8 (26 %) out of 31 patients in contrast to 3 (3 %) out of 107 controls. The Iranian study is ongoing, so clarification of the preliminary observations should not be long in forthcoming.

3.2.3 Gastric carcinoma

The high incidence of gastric carcinoma among the Japanese is well established. In a study of 256 Japanese patients with carcinoma of the stomach, Tsuji and colleagues (58) found altered frequencies of HLA antigens at both loci. At locus A, AW30/31 was decreased in frequency, while at locus B, B18 was increased and B5, BW16 and BW35 all decreased in frequency. An alternative way of analysing the data is to calculate the size of the 'blank' at both loci. For locus A, the gene frequency corresponding to the blank was 22.1 % vs. 8.6 % for the 137 normal subjects. At locus B the respective figures were 45.2 % and 10.9 %. Decreased frequencies of the cross-reacting antigens B5 and BW35 account for 21.6 % of the 34.1 % difference at locus B. The pattern is reminiscent of that found in NPC, where the first indication of an HLA association was the relatively greater frequency of undetected locus B antigens. Sin 2, which was not typed for in this study, has a gene frequency of approximately 7 % in normal Japanese (23). The frequency in gastric carcinoma patients of Sin 2, and possibly of other gene(s) yet to be detected, is awaited with interest.

3.2.4 Cervical carcinoma

In the studies of Takasugi et al. (9), cervical carcinoma patients showed altered frequencies of 3 antigens (increased A1 and B12, decreased A9). Koenig & Muller (59) have now reported an increased frequency of B12 in 121 patients with carcinoma of the cervix. The increase was present both in patients with localised and with invasive carcinoma. In a smaller study of 42 patients, Dostal & Mayr (60) found an increase of BW15 which remained statistically significant after correction. Previously, Bertrams et al (61) did not detect any differences in HLA antigen frequencies in any of 64 patients.

Squamous-cell carcinoma of the cervix is related to sexual practices in that it occurs more frequently among women who begin heterosexual activity at an early age and who have multiple sex partners. In keeping with the concept that cervical carcinoma may be caused by a venereally transmitted carcinogen is the considerable seroepidemiological and molecular virological evidence for a relationship between genital infection with herpes simplex virus 2 (HSV − 2) and cancer of the cervix. A prospective HLA study of cervical cancer patients is now required to resolve the question of whether there are HLA associations. The number of patients to be studied should be large enough to enable patient hererogeneity to be diminished by subgrouping according to suspected risk factors such as exposure to HSV − 2, age at

222

first intercourse, number of sex partners, as well as according to tumor histology, response to therapy and duration of survival.

3.2.5 Breast carcinoma

Bertrams et al (61) combined their data with that of four previous studies and revealed a possible association of HLA-A10 and BW 18, or of the haplotype A10-BW18, with breast cancer. A study by de Jong-Bakker et al. (62) directed attention at the combination A9-B27. At the workshop, preliminary results of two ongoing studies were reported. In a prospective survey, Osoba is finding an increased frequency of B8 among longer-term survivors (63). Deneufbourg & Bouillenne (64) are in the process of prospectively examining 141 patients who have been subgrouped as parous/non-parous, and according to pre- and post-menopausal onset. There are identifications of altered antigen frequencies so the final results are awaited with interest.

3.2.6 Laryngeal carcinoma

The Belgian pair of Bouillenne & Deneufborg (65) also have an ongoing study of HLA type in laryngeal carcinoma patients. Seventy-five patients have been studied retrospectively, and the survivors followed for 3 years; an additional 92 cases were typed at the time of diagnosis and studied prospectively. Broad subgrouping based on anatomic location (glottic and supra-glottic utmours) and histologic type (differentiated and non-differentiated) has been made. As in the breast cancer studies there are some alterations of antigen frequencies. The studies are noteworthy because they represent an attempt to maximise the likelihood of identifying one or more subgroups of patients in whom an HLA association may exist.

3.2.7 Choriocarcinoma

Choriocarcinoma is a unique type of malignancy in that the tumour arises from foetal trophoblast and grows in a genetically different maternal host. As an allogeneic graft, the tumour might be expected to provoke an allograft reaction. Since HLA genes are involved in allograft reactions, choriocarcinoma was an obvious malignancy for HLA studies. Klouda et al. (66) obtained an indication that HLA incompatibility was related to prognosis in that survival was more prolonged among patients who were most incompatible with their husbands. Lewis & Terasaki (67), in proposing that the incidence of possible HLA-compatible matings was higher than would be expected in random matings, also drew attention to the possible importance of HLA antigens. However, Mittal et al. (68) found no increase in the occurrence of HLA-compatible couples among patients than among healthy people. The position is thus unresolved and further studies are required.

4. Other malignancies

4.1 Multiple myeloma

There have been four reports (see 69) on a total of 149 patients with multiple myeloma. In all four studies there have been increases in one or more of the 4c group of cross-reacting antigens, findings recognised by Mason & Cullen (69) to be reminiscent of the position in Hodgkin's disease.

4.2 Malignant melanoma

In view of the known role of immuno-logic processes in malignant melanoma, there seemed to be a good prospect of finding HLA associations. To date it is far from clear whether HLA genes are associated with the malignancy. Tarpley et al. (19) found an increase in B8 but several groups have failed to show significant associations between patients and controls (9, 70, 71). Clark et al. (72) did report a reduced frequency of HLA-BW35 but, when typing families of patients was performed, the inherit-ance of BW35 was found to be ano-malous. The explanation appeared to be that sera from patients with pro-gressing melanoma, but not in those who are free of disease, were able to mask BW35, rendering the antigen un-detectable by certain antisera (73). This phenomenon may be relevant to the area of serum-blocking factors, but it is a complication to HLA genetic typ-ing and should be taken into account in future studies.

4.3 Retinoblastoma

Retinoblastoma is a childhood malig-nancy of genetic interest since there is an hereditary form due to an autosomal dominant-gene mutation with relative-ly high penetrance, and a sporadic form of unknown aetiology. Among 122 German children, the frequency of BW35 was increased, whilst that of B12 was decreased (74). Furthermore, there was an excess of BW35 homozy-gotes, suggesting that the presence of BW35-associated gene(s) was connect-ed with retinoblastoma. However, the fact that the altered frequencies of BW35 and B12 were also seen in the non-hereditary form of the disease pre-cluded a simple interpretation of the findings. For a discussion of the com-plexity of the genetic considerations, reference should be made to the paper of Bertrams and associates (74). At the workshop Gallie et al. (75) reported finding no difference in the frequencies of BW35, B12 or any other antigen. They also showed that, in families where several members were affected with retinoblastoma, the tumour did not segregate with the HLA type. Nor was there any linkage with the occurrence of spontaneous regression since, in several families in which one parent showed spontaneous regression, child-ren inheriting each of these haplotypes had tumours that did not regress.

Considerations in HLA studies

Arising from the studies to date, nume-rous factors have been identified which should receive consideration in the planning of future HLA studies. The importance of careful selection and subgrouping of patients according to identified or suspected risk factors in order to reduce the heterogeneity of those to be studied has been referred to. The necessity of matching patients and controls for features such as ethnic and sub-ethnic type has been noted.

The limitations of retrospective studies, and the merits of prospective surveys, in identifying any HLA association and in determining whether an association is with disease susceptibility or survival, have been mentioned. Two other areas of importance in HLA genetics and malignant diseases are HLA typing strategies and methods, and statistical approaches to the analysis of HLA typ-ing data.

1. HLA genetic typing

Most studies of HLA type in malignant diseases have been limited to locus A and locus B genes. As in NPC, the majority of patients lack the A and B locus genes associated with an increased risk for the malignancy. It has therefore been proposed (76) that other genes exist, which were called DS genes following McDevitt & Bodmer (77), which are more intimately involved in disease. Since some HLA associations, such as that of A2 and ALL, are with survival rather than susceptibility, it is prudent to use the broader term 'disease associated', and to refer to the genes as DA genes pending clarification of the nature of the association(s) in each case.

Alleles of the *C* locus, situated between the *A* and *B* loci, have been investigated in only a few studies. Wentzel *et al.* (78) reported differences in the reactions of acute myeloid leukaemic cells compared with lymphocytes from normal controls with certain *C*-locus antisera but were careful to note that some of the reactions could be attributed to changes in leukaemic cell membrane antigens. It can be expected that typing for *C*-locus alleles in linkage disequilibrium with A and/or B locus genes, which are known to be associated with a risk for a disease, will also reveal associations. C1/C3 has been shown by Payne *et al.* (79) to be linked to Hsieh (Sin 2), so it is likely that C1/C3 will be associated with NPC in the Chinese, but only as part of the *A2, Sin 2* haplotype. *C* locus gene associations with cancers are unlikely to be of notable strength since there is strong linkage between the *C* and *B* loci, yet all *B* locus gene associations with cancer are relatively weak.

As in non-malignant diseases, typing cancer patients for genes of the *D* locus and of the B-cell (Ia) alloantigenic system(s) holds the best promise of enabling the existence of DA genes to be identified. There is preliminary evidence for a *D* locus gene, termed *Singapore 2a*, which appears to be more strongly associated with NPC rather than the corresponding B locus gene, *Sin 2* (80). However, initial results of *D* locus typing in Hodgkin's disease (81) and in malignant melanoma (71) have been unrevealing. B cell typing of patients with malignant diseases has only just begun. While there are some interesting observations, particularly with the leukaemias, no studies have been completed, so further comment is premature.

2. Statistical analysis

The traditional approach to establishing an association between HLA and disease is to show alterations in the frequencies of particular HLA antigens in studies of unrelated patients. This procedure is most suited to detecting associations of single antigens with diseases, when the strength of the association is sufficient to withstand correction of the significance levels for the number of specificities tested. In those situations where a previously claimed association is being tested (e.g. ↑A2 in Caucasians with ALL; ↑Sin 2 in Chinese NPC patients) and where the direction of the alteration is given, it is probably appropriate to use an uncorrected, one-sided p value. While this may result in the identification of some new HLA associations with malignant diseases, the fact remains that any associations are likely to be relatively weak. Furthermore, the traditional method is insensitive to minor departures from the null hypothesis involving several antigens. Such a situation might exist where a disease association involves linkage disequilibrium with more than one HLA locus allele, or where the association was with one or more allele of a cross-reacting group (e.g. 4c Hodgkin's disease).

Mathews (82, 83) has formulated a more discriminative test of the null hypothesis in which the existence of heterogeneity over all allelic and linked antigens is assessed by combining individual probabilities. Briefly, a modified χ^2 is calculated for the 2×2 table for each antigen, and χ^2 is summed over all antigens. The expected value of the summary χ^2 is known, and the variance is computed by randomly drawing notional samples of cases from the combined pool of cases and controls. The randomization procedure automatically allows for the non-independence of allelic and linked antigens. The signnificance of the observed heterogeneity is assessed by comparing the observed value of the summary χ^2 with its expected mean and variance. The method can be readily extended to provide heterogeneity testing of all A and B locus phenotypes or possible haplotypes as estimated by the Terasaki-Mickey method (47). It is important that patients and controls are well matched for ethnic type and other variables since the method is so powerful that significant heterogeneity in antigen frequencies can be detected between quite small groups which are poorly matched for ethnic type.

Both the traditional approach and that of Mathews depend on linkage disequilibrium between observable HLA genes and a disease-associated gene, and cannot give an estimate of the full risk associated with the HLA complex. Reference has been made to the approach developed by Terasaki & Mickey for computing HLA haplotype frequencies from phenotype data (47). The approach is provocative in that it seems to offer a more sensitive means for detecting the existence of DA genes linked to HLA based on data derived from studies of unrelated subjects than has been achieved from analysis of HLA specificities *per se*. However, the approach depends on the validity of the assumption of random mating, so it must be used with caution when cases and controls are sampled from ethnically mixed populations.

Day & Simons have recently described an alternative approach which involves investigating the HLA similarity of related cases with the disease by HLA haplotyping of multiple case family members (84).

Whether the study to be undertaken is of individual patients or of multiple case families is mainly influenced by cancer records and the availability of new and surviving cancer patients. In both cases, the recent advances in statistical analysis of HLA data have increased the likelihood that real associations will be recognized.

Applications of HLA association data

The knowledge of HLA associations with malignant diseases can be applied in many ways. For the clinician, an HLA genetic marker may be helpful in identifying different types of a malignancy, hence contributing to an improvement in disease classification. If the associations of HLA type with survival can be substantiated (e.g. A2 with ALL, AW19-B5 with lung cancer, B8 with breast cancer), the results of HLA typing will be useful to clinicians in providing information on prognosis. If an HLA pattern is associated with poor survival, it may be appropriate for different regimens of therapy to be considered as part of the management of those patients with the HLA type.

In the near future, HLA markers of cancer susceptibility may be useful in population screening programmes seeking to identify persons at high risk. Bringing high cancer risk individuals under closer surveillance will facilitate earlier diagnosis, and consequently earlier and more effective treatment. However, at present, the relative risk for NPC associated with *A2, Sin 2* in the Chinese is barely strong enough as a basis for screening normal individuals. If D locus and B lymphocyte alloantigen typing reveals HLA patterns associated with relative risks of 5 or more, it may become realistic to search for individuals with high cancer risk, provided advances in mass screening technology can also be achieved.

For the cancer scientist, discovery of HLA types associated with increased risk for certain malignancies raises exciting possibilities. One prospect is that the information can be employed in testing hypotheses concerning the role of environmental agents in cancer causation. Some viruses are prime suspects as aetiological agents in certain cancers. Approaches to examining the role of viruses, such as Epstein-Barr virus (EBV) in NPC, by combined HLA typing and immunological testing, have been described (85). The suspected causal relation between herpes simplex virus 2 (HSV 2) and cervical cancer, and between EBV and Burkitt's lymph-

oma could be similarly investigated. Concerning the relation between hepatitis B virus (HBV) and hepatocellular carcinoma, it has been proposed that identification of patients according to HBV immune status subgroups is an important first step in HLA and other blood genetic studies seeking evidence of genes controlling HBV immunoresponsiveness and genes in association with hepatocellular carcinoma (86). Particularly in the leukaemias, viruses are thought to be important as causal factors but the existence of human leukaemia viruses remains to be established. Also, the action of different agents may result in a similar disease process. Since A2 is only associated with a proportion of ALL patients, subgrouping may aid in the identification of aetiological factors.

If the preliminary evidence for an association between HLA-BW40 and oesophageal carcinoma (57) is confirmed, HLA typing could be used in the search for dietary carcinogens in this diet-associated cancer. Similar hopes can be held for stomach cancer in the Japanese.

It is widely held that DA genes are involved in immune responses (Ir). Circumstantial evidence for this view can be obtained by concurrent immunological testing and HLA typing. Twomey *et al.* (87) investigated lymphocyte function and HL-A antigen frequency in patients with gynaecologic squamous cancer, and found a high frequency of lymphocyte hyporesponsiveness among patients in whom B8 was more than two-fold more frequent than controls. Similarly, Chan and colleagues (88) have demonstrated diminished responsiveness to *in vitro* stimulation with mitogens of lymphocytes obtained from NPC patients who had been previously shown to be characterized by a high frequency of A2 – Sin 2 (24). Determination of whether immunodeficiency is associated with the high hisk HLA type prior to the development of malignancy, or is part of the malignancy process, can be achieved by prospective studies of unrelated individuals or, more simply, by family studies. If immunodeficiency is present in unaffected family members of cancer patients, and co-segregates with the HLA type, it is strong evidence that the DA genes which are linked to HLA genes are involved in immunity.

Instead of concentrating exclusively on cancer patients, it might be informative to study elderly subjects who have been exposed to environmental factors which are known to be associated with cancer causation, yet who have not developed cancer. In these individuals immunoresistance may be subserved by Ir genes which are linked to HLA genes. Final proof as to whether DA genes are involved in immunity must await the development of direct methods for immune response gene identification.

Summary

HLA associations have been established with NPC in the Chinese, and with Hodgkin's disease and ALL in Caucasians. Promising results have also been reported for carcinoma of the oesophagus, lung, stomach, prostate, breast and cervix, as well as for NPC in Malays and Tunisians, and for AML. Prospective studies can be expected to resolve whether associations exist in these as well as in other malignancies, and whether any association is with susceptibility to the disease, survival from the disease, or both. For the clinician, application of knowledge concerning HLA associations with cancers might prove to be helpful in achieving earlier diagnosis and improved prognosis. For the cancer scientist, the potential usefulness of genetic markers in the search for environmental oncogens, and in elucidating the mechanisms of cancer development, is an exciting prospect.

Acknowledgements

We are greateful to Drs. N. Rogentine and R. T. Oliver for assisting us during the Malignancy Workshop of the HLA and Disease Symposium.

References

1. Lilly, F., Boyse, E. A. & Old, L. J. (1964) Genetic basis of susceptibility to viral leukemogenesis. *Lancet* **ii**, 1207.
2. Lilly, F. (1971) The influence of H-2 type on Gross virus leukemogenesis. *Transplant. Proc.* **3**, 1239.
3. Amiel, J. L. (1967) Study of the leucocyte phenotypes in Hodgkin's disease. *Histocompatibility Testing 1967*, p. 79. Munksgaard, Copenhagen.
4. Forbes, J. F. & Morris, P. J. (1970) Leukocyte antigens in Hodgkin's disease. *Lancet* **ii**, 849.
5. Falk, J. & Osoba, D. (1971) HL-A antigens and survival in Hodgkin's disease. *Lancet* **ii**, 1118.
6. Kissmeyer-Nielsen, F., Kjerbye, K. E. & Lamm, L. U. (1975) HL-A in Hodgkin's disease III. A prospective study. *Transplant. Rev.* **22**, 168.
7. Graff, K. S., Simon, R. M., Yankee, R. A., DeVita, V. T. & Rogentine, G. N. (1974) HL-A antigens in Hodgkin's disease: Histopathologic and Clinical Correlations. *J. Nat. Cancer Inst.* **52**, 1087.
8. Bjorkholm, M., Holm, G., Johansson, B.,

Mellstedt, M. & Moller, E. (1975) A Prospective study of HLA antigen phenotypes and lymphocyte abnormalities in Hodgkin's disease. *Tissue Antigens* **6**, 247.

9. Takasugi, M., Terasaki, P. I., Henderson, B., Mickey, M. R., Menck, H. & Thompson, R. W. (1973) HL-A antigens in solid tumours. *Cancer Res.* **33**, 648.

10. Bodmer, W. F. (1973) Genetic factors in Hodgkin's disease: Association with a disease susceptibility locus (DSA) in the HL-A region. *Nat. Cancer Inst. Monogr. No.* **36**, p. 127.

11. Walford, R. L., Waters, H. & Smith, G. D. (1971) *Human histomocpatibility system and neoplasia.*

12. Marris, P. J., Lawler, S. & Oliver, R. T. (1972) HL-A and Hodgkin's disease. *Histocompatibility Testing 1972,* p. 669, Munksgaard, Copenhagen.

13. Kourilsky, F. M., Dausset, J., Feingold, N., Dupuy, J. M & Bernard, J. (1967) Etude de la repartition des antigenes leucocytaires chez des malades atteints de lecemie aigue en remission. In: *Advance in Transplantation,* eds. Dausset, J., Hamburger, J. & Mathé, G., p. 515. Munksgaard, Copenhagen.

14. Walford, R., Finkelstein, S., Neerhout, R., Konrad, P. & Shanbrom, E. (1970) Acute childhood leukemia in relation to the HL-A human transplantation genes. *Nature (Lond.)* **225**, 461.

15. Thorsby, E., Bratlie, A. & Lie, S. O. (1969) HL-A genotypes of children with acute leukemia. *Scand J. Haematol.* **6**, 409.

16. Rogentine, G. H., Yankee, R. A., Gart, J. J., Ham, J. & Arapani, R. J. (1972) HLA antigens and disease – acute lymphocytic leukemia. *J. Nat. Cancer Inst.* **51**, 2420.

17. Rogentine, G .N., Trapani, R. J., Yankee, R. J. & Menderron, E. S. (1973) HLA antigens and acute lymphocytic leukemia: The nature of the HLA-A2 association. *Tissue Antigens* **3**, 470.

18. Lawler, S. D., Klouda, P. T., Smith, P. G., Till, M. M. & Hardisty, R. M. (1974) Survival and the HL-A system in Acute Lymphoblastic Leukemia. *Brit. Med. J.* **1**, 547.

19. Tarpley, J. L., Chretien, P. B., Rogentine, G. N., Twomey, P. L. & Dellon, A. L. (1975) Histocompatibility antigens and solid malignant neoplasms. *Arch. Surg.* **110**, 269.

20. Simons, M. J., Day, N. E., Wee, G. B., Shanmugaratnam, K., Ho, J. H. C.,

Wong, S. H., Ti, T. K., Yong, N. K., Dharmalingam, S. & de-Thé, G. (1974) Nasopharyngeal carcinoma: V. Immunogenetic studies of South East Asian ethnic groups with high and low risk for the tumour. *Cancer Res.* **34**, 1192.

21. Simons, M. J., Wee, G. B., Day, N. E., Moris, P. J., Shanmugaratnam, K. & de-Thé, G. (1974) Immunogenetic aspects of nasopharyngeal carcinoma: I. Differences in HL-A antigen profiles between patients and comparison groups. *Int. J. Cancer* **13**, 122.

22. Simons, M. J., Wee, G. B., Chan, S. H., Shanmugaratnam, K., Day, N. E. & de-Thé, G. (1975) Probable identification of an HLA second locus antigen associated with a high risk of nasopharyngeal carcinoma. *Lancet* **i**, 142.

23. Payne, R., Radvany, R. & Grumet, C. (1975) A new second locus HL-A antigen in linkage disequilibrium with HL-A2 in Cantonese Chinese. *Tissue Antigens* **5**, 69.

24. Simons, M. J., Wee, G. B., Goh, E. H., Chan, S. H., Shanmugaratnam, K., Day, N. E. & de-Thé, G. (1976) Immunogenetic aspects of nasopharyngeal carcinoma: IV. Increased risk in Chinese for nasopharyngeal carcinoma associated with a Chinese-related HLA profile (A2, Singapore 2). *J. Nat. Cancer Inst.* **57**, 977.

25. Svejgaard, A., Platz, P., Ryder, L. P., Nielsen, L. S. & Thomsen, M. (1975) HL-A and disease associations – a survey. *Transplant. Rev.* **22**, 3.

26. Osoba, D. & Falk, J. A. (1976) *HLA antigens and survival in Hodgkin's disease.*

27. Dausset, J., Singh, S., Gourand, J. L., Degos, L., Solal, C. H. & Klein, G. (1975) HL-A and Burkitt's disease. *Tissue Antigens* **5**, 48.

28. Dick, H M., Steel, C. M., Levin, A. G. & Henderson, N. (1975) Burkitt's lymphoma and HL-A antigens. *Tissue Antigens* **5**, 52.

29. Bodmer, J. G., Bodmer, W. F., Ziegler, J. & Magrath, I. T. (1975) HL-A and Burkitt's tumour – a study in Uganda. *Tissue Antigens* **5**, 59.

30. Bodmer, J. G., Bodmer, W. F., Dickbourne, P., Degos, L., Dausset, J. & Dick, H. M. (1975) Combined analysis of three studies of patients with Burkitt's lymphoma. *Tissue Antigens* **5**, 63.

31. Morris, P. J. (1974) Histocompatibility systems, immune response and disease

in man. In: *Contemporary Topics in Immunobiology* **3**, p. 141. Plenum Press, New York.

32. Forbes, J. F. & Morris, P. J. (1971) Transplantation antigens and malignant lymphomas in man. Follicular lymphoma, reticulum cell sarcoma and lymphosarcoma. *Tissue Antigens* **1**, 265.

33. Dick, F. R., Fortuny, I., Athanasios, T., Greally, J., Wood, N. & Yunis, E. J. (1972) HLA and lymphoid tumours. *Cancer Res.* **32**, 2608.

34. Johnson, A. H., Ward, F. E., Amos, D. B., Leikin, S. & Rogentine, G. N. (1976) HLA and acute lymphocytic leukemia: A prospective study of 372 patients. Abstracts, p. 227.

35. Pollack, M. S. & DuBois, D. (1976) The effects of non-HLA antibodies in common typing sera on HLA antigen frequency data. Abstracts, p. 232.

36. Gluckman, E., Lemarchand, F., Nunez-Roldan, A., Hors, J. & Dausset, J. (1976) Possible excess of HLA-A homozygous among aplastic anemia and acute lymphoblastic leukemia. Abstracts, p. 226.

37. Klouda, P. T., Lawler, S. D., Till, M. M. & Hardisty, R. M. (1974) Acute lymphoblastic leukemia and HL-A: A prespective study. *Tissue Antigens* **4**, 262.

38. Batchelor, J. R., Edwards, J. H. & Stuart, J. (1971) Histocompatibility and acute lymphoblastic leukemia. *Lancet* **i**, 699.

39. Sanderson, A. R., Mahour, G. H., Jaffe, N. & Das, L. (1973) Incidence of HL-A antigens in acute lymphocytic leukemia. *Transplantation* **16**, 672.

40. Oliver, R. T. D., Pillai, A., Klouda, P. T. & Lawler, S. D. (1976) HL-A linked resistance factors and survival in acute myelogenous leukemia. Abstracts, p. 231.

41. Benbunan, M., Saglier, M., Owens, A., Husson, N., Bussel, A., Reboul, M., Dastot, H. & Czazar, E. (1976) Acute myelocytic leukemia (AML), chronic myeloid leukemia and HLA antigens. Abstracts, p. 217.

42. Jeannet, M. & Magnin, C. (1971) HLA antigens in malignant diseases. *Transplant. Proc.* **3**, 1301.

43. Dausset, J. & Hors, J. (1975) Some contributions of the HL-A complex to the genetics of human diseases. *Transplant. Rev.* **22**, 24.

44. Cohen, E., Gregory, S. G., Weinreb, N. & Minowada, J. (1976) Antibodies to "leukemia" associated antigen in sera of plasmapheresis donors. Abstracts, p. 220.

45. Drew, S. I., Billing, R,, Bergh, O. J. & Terasaki, P. L. (1976) Human granulocyte antigens detected on leukemia cells and a chronic myelogeneous cell line. Abstracts, p. 224.

46. Terasaki, P. I., Perdue, S. T. & Mickey, M. R. (1976) HLA frequencies in cancer. A second study. (Genetics of Human Cancer).

47. Terasaki, P. I. & Mickey, M. R. (1975) HL-A haplotypes of 32 diseases. *Transplant. Rev.* **22**, 105.

48. Shanmugaratnam, K. (1971) Studies on the etiology of nasopharyngeal carcinoma. *Int. Rev. exp. Path.* **10**, 361–413.

49. Ho, J. H. C. (1972) Current knowledge of the epidemiology of nasopharyngeal carcinoma – A review. In: *Oncogenesis and Herpesviruses,* eds. Biggs, P. M., de-Thé, G. & Payne, L. N., p. 357. Lyon, France (IARC Scientific Publications No. 2).

50. Simons, M. J., Kwa, S. B., Day, N. E., Wee, G. B., Hawkins, B.R., de-Thé, G. & Shanmugaratnam, K. (1973) Immunogenetic studies of South East Asian ethnic groups with high and low risk for nasopharyngeal carcinoma. In: *Analytic and experimental epidemiology of cancer,* eds. Nakahara, W., Hirayama, T., Nishioka, K. & Sugano, H., p. 171. University of Tokyo Press, Tokyo.

51. Simons, M. J., Wee, G. B., Singh, D., Dharmalingam, S., Yong, N. K., Chau, J. C. W., Ho, J. H. C., Day, N. E. & de-Thé, G. (1976) Immunogenetic aspects of nasopharyngeal carcinoma (NPC): V. Confirmation of a Chinese-related HLA profile (A2 – Singapore 2) associated with an increased risk in Chinese for NPC. In: *Proc. Symp. on Epidemiology and Cancer Registries in the Pacific Basin,* Hawai, Nov. 10–14, 1975, ed. Henderson, B. E., (in Press).

52. Jing, J., Louie, E., Henderson, B. E. & Terasaki, P. (1976) HL-A patterns in Nasopharyngeal Carcinoma cases from California. In: *Proc. Symp. Epidemiology and Cancer Registries in the Pacific Basin.* ed. Henderson, B. E., (in Press).

53. Simons, M. J. & Day, N. E. (1976) HLA patterns and NPC. In: *Proc. Sym. Epidemiology and Cancer Registries in the Pacific Basin,* ed. Henderson, B. E., (in Press).

54. Betuel, H., Camoun, M., Colombani, J., Day, N. E., Ellouz, R. & de-Thé, G. (1976) The relationship between nasopharyngeal carcinoma and the HLA sy-

stem among Tunisians. *Int. J. Cancer* **16**, 249–254.

55. Dellon, A. L., Rogentine, G. N. & Chretien, P. B. (1975) Prolonged survival in bronchogenic carcinoma associated with HL-A antigens W-19 and HL-A5: A preliminary report. *J. Nat. Cancer Inst.* **54**, 1283.

56. Rogentine, G. N., Dellon, A. L. & Chretien, P. B (1976) Prolanged disease-free survival in bronchogenic carcinoma associated with HLA-AW19 and HLA-B5. A 2-year prospective study. Abstracts, p. 234.

57. Mohaghegpour, N., Dolatshahi, K., Hashemi, S., Modabber, F. & Tagasuki, M. (1976) HLA-BW40 in Iranian patients with oesophageal cancer. Workshop communication.

58. Tsuji, K., Nose, Y., Hoshino, K., Inouye, H., Ho, M., Ito, Y., Yasuda, N. & Tamaoki, N. (1976) Comparative study between gastric cancer patient and normal healthy control against HLA antisera. Abstracts, p. 237.

59. Koenig, U. D. & Muller, N. (1976) Cervical carcinoma and HLA-antigens. Abstracts, p. 228.

60. Dostal, V. & Mayr, W. R. (1976) HLA SD antigens in cervix cancer and in recurrent herpes genitalis patients. Abstracts, p. 223.

61. Bertrams, J., Thraenhart, O., Feldmann, U. & Kuwert, E. (1975) HL-A antigens in carcinoma of the breast, ovarium, cervix and endometrium: Possible association of haplotype HL-A10 – W18 with carcinoma of the breast. *Z. Krebsforsch.* **83**, 219.

62. de Jong-Bakker, M., Cleton, F. J., D'Amaro, J., Keuning, J. J. & van Rood, J. J. (1974) HL-A antigens and breast cancer. *Europ. J. Cancer* **10**, 555.

63. Osoba, D. (1976) Workshop communication. (Verbal presentation - no title).

64. Deneufborg, J. M. & Bouillenne, C. (1976) Larynx cancer. Abstracts, p. 222.

65. Bouillenne, C., Deneufborg, J. M. (1976) Breast cancer. Abstracts, p. 219.

66. Klouda, P. T., Lawler, S. D. & Bagshawe, K. D. (1972) HL-A matings in trophoblastic neoplasia. *Tissue Antigens* **2**, 280.

67. Lewis, J. L. & Terasaki, P. I. (1971) HL-A leukocyte antigen studies in women with gestational trophoblastic neoplasms. *Amer. J. Obstet. Gynec.* **111**, 547.

68. Mittal, K. K., Kachru, R. B. & Brewer, J. I. (1975) The HL-A and ABO anti-gens in Trophoblastic disease. *Tissue Antigens* **6**, 157.

69. Mason, D. Y. & Cullen, P. (1975) HL-A antigen frequencies in myeloma. *Tissue Antigens* **5**, 238.

70. Bergholtz, B., Klepp, O., Kaakinen, A. & Thorsby, E. (1976) HLA antigens in malignant melanoma. Abstracts, p. 218.

71. Lamm, L. U., Kissmeyer-Nielsen, K., Kjerbye, J. E., Mogensen, B. & Petersen, N. C. (1974) HL-A and ABO antigens and malignant melanoma. *Cancer* **33**, 1458.

72. Clark, D. A., Necheles, T., Nathanson, L. & Silverman, E. (1973) Apparent HL-A5 deficiency in malignant melanoma. *Transplantation* **15**, 326.

73. Clark, D. A., Necheles, T. F., Nathanson, L., Whitten, D., Silverman, E. & Flowers, A. (1976) Apparent HL-A5 deficiency in human malignant melanoma. II. HL-A5 masking activity in sera of patients with progressing disease.

74. Bertrams, J., Schildberg, P., Hopping, W., Bohme, U. & Albert, E. (1973) HL-A antigens in retinoblastoma. *Tissue Antigens* **3**, 78.

75. Gallie, B. L., Dupont, B., Whitsett, C., Kitchen, F. D., Ellsworth, R. M. & Good, R. A. (1976) Histocompatibility typing in spontaneous regression of retinoblastoma. Abstracts, p. 225.

76. Simons, M. J., Chan, S. H. & Day, N. E. (1974) Genes, Immunity and Nasopharyngeal Cancer. In: *Cancer Today,* eds. Kirk, R. L. & McCullagh, P. J., pp. 115–126. John Curtin School of Medical Research, Australian National University, Canberra, Australia.

77. McDeivtt, H. O. & Bodmer, W. F. (1974) HL-A, Immune-Response Genes, and Disease. *Lancet* **i**, 1269.

78. Wentzel, J., Carvalho, A. S., Freeman, C. B., Taylor, G. M. & Harris, R. (1975) HL-A and acute myeloid leukemia. *Histocompatibility Testing 1975*, p. 813. Munksgaard, Copenhagen.

79. Payne, R., Radvany, R., Grumet, F. C., Feldman, M. & Cann, H. (1975) Two third series antigens transmitted together – a possible fourth SD locus? *Histocompatibility Testing 1975*, p. 343. Munksgaard, Copenhagen.

80. Simons, M. J., Chan, S. H., H, J. H. C., Chau, J. C. W., Day, N. E. & de-Thé, G. (1975) A Singapore 2-associated LD antigen in Chinese patients with nasopharyngeal carcinoma. *Histocompatibility*

Testing 1975. Munksgaard, Copenhagen, (in Press).

81 Hansen, J. A., Young, C. W., Whitsett, C., Case, D. C., Jersild, C., Good, R. A. & Dupont, B. (1976) HLA and MLC typing in patients with Hodgkin's disease. Workshop communication.

82. Mathews, J. D. (1976) New method for heterogeneity testing over several antigens by combining probabilities. Abstracts, p. 276.

83. Mathews, J. D. (1976) Heterogeneity testing by analysis of possible haplotype frequencies. Abstract, p. 277.

84. Day, N. E. & Simons, M. J. (1976) Disease susceptibility genes – their identification by multiple case family studies. *Tissue Antigens* **8**, 109.

85. Simons, M. J., Wee, G. B., Chan, S. H., Shanmugaratnam, K., Day, N. E. & de-Thé, G. (1975) Immunogenetic aspects of nasopharyngeal carcinoma (NPC) III. HL-A type as a genetic market of NPC predisposition to test the hypothesis that Epstein-Barr virus is an etiological factor in NPC. In: *Oncogenesis and Herpesviruses II,* eds. de-Thé, G., Epstein, M. A. & zur Hausen, H., pp. 249–258. Lyon, France (IARC Scientific Publications No. 11).

86. Simons, M. J., Yu, M. & Shanmugaratnam, K. (1975) Immunodeficiency to Hepatitis B virus infection and genetic susceptibility to development of hepatocellular carcinoma. *Ann. N. Y. Acad. Sci.* **259**, 181.

87. Twomey, P. L., Rogentine, G. N. & Chretien, P. B. (1974) Lymphocyte function and HL-A antigen frequency in gynecologi squamous cancer. *Int. Surg.* **59**, 468.

88. Chan, S. H., Chew, T. S., Goh, E. H., Simons, M. J. & Shanmugaratnam, K. (1976) Impaired general cell-mediated immune functions *in vivo* and *in vitro* in patients with nasopharyngeal carcinoma. *Int. J. Cancer* **18**, pp. 139–144.

Immunopathology, Immunodeficiencies, and Complement Deficiencies

B. Dupont, R. A. Good, G. Hauptmann, I. Schreuder & M. Seligmann

The diseases to be included in this chapter on immunopathological diseases are: systemic lupus erythematosus, Sjögren's disease, sarcoidosis, glomerulonephritis, autoimmune hemolytic anemia, primary immunodeficiency diseases, and complement-deficiency diseases.

The assumption that disease associations with the HLA complex may reflect the presence of abnormal immune-response genes within the major histocompatibility complex (MHC), and the assumption that these genes are characteristic for certain diseases, has led to the study of several autoimmune diseases for HLA antigen associations. The early studies by Grumet *et al.* (1) indicated that patients with systemic lupus erythematosus had increased frequencies of the HLA-B8 and BW15 antigens. This initially promising observation was, however, not established in other studies prior to this symposium on HLA and Disease. A slight increase in HLA-B8 has been demonstrated in Caucasian patients with Sjögren's disease (2, 3, 4). In sarcoidosis, the findings have not convincingly demonstrated an association with the HLA complex. In patients with glomerulonephritis, autoimmune hemolytic anemia, and in different groups of patients with primary immune-deficiency diseases, it

Memorial Sloan-Kettering Cancer Center, 1275 York Avenue, New York 10021.

has not been possible to establish a clear association between disease entities and the HLA system. It is suprising that these diseases, which all develop as a result of abnormal immunological reactions or where the underlying genetic defects cause serious immunological deficiency syndromes, do not show clear associations with the major histocompatibility complex. Many of these diseases, however, probably have multifactorial etiological components and may even, in addition, depend on polygenic factors.

Most of the positive findings in relation to associations between autoimmune diseases and the HLA complex have been obtained from the study of patients with genetically determined selective deficiencies in the synthesis of the different serum-complement components. The complement system plays a major role in the development of inflammatory reactions. It has been shown that complement activation plays an important part in retaining granulocytes at the inflammatory sites. The study of C5-deficient mice and C6-deficient rabbits has demonstrated that fixation of C3 is important for the production of acute allergic inflammation. It is indeed characteristic that genetically determined deficiency syndromes involving the early serum-complement components (C1, C2, and C4) are frequently associated with systemic lupus erythematosus syndromes and glomerulonephritis. It was, therefore, of major interest when it was shown that genetically determined deficiency of complement C2 was associated with the HLA complex (5–10). Subsequently it was found that selective C4 deficiency which also occurs together with systemic lupus syndromes and glomerulonephritis was linked to the HLA complex (11, 12). These findings have added a new dimension to the understanding of the mechanisms by which HLA-disease associations can be caused. A simple interpretation involving only abnormalities in immune-response genes affecting T-lymphocyte or B-lymphocyte differentiation as the explanation for these associations is not likely. The observation of associations between genetically determined complement-deficiency syndromes, autoimmune-disease entities and the HLA complex indicates that several different mechanisms may cause these associations.

Systemic lupus erythematosus

Systemic lupus erythematosus (SLE) is a disease featured by a pleomorphic clinical picture including involvement of the skin, joints, kidney, heart, nervous system, respiratory tract, etc. Diffuse proliferative glomerulonephritis, and involvement of the central nervous system are of major prognostic significance. The borders of the disease are difficult to define. Attempts to establish minimal criteria for diagnosis have not been very successful. For instance, in the classical criteria of the American Rheumatism Association, possibly the most important biological feature, that is, the presence of antibodies to native DNA, has not been included. There is an important prevalence in females. The predisposing role of a poorly defined genetic background is obvious, as well as the triggering role of environmental factors such as several drugs. It is also known that the prevalence of SLE is increased in Black Americans compared with the Caucasian population (13).

Studies in the canine SLE syndrome indicate that C-type viruses may be the etiological agent in a genetically susceptible host (14). Attempts to isolate specific viruses from patients with SLE have, however, led to conflicting results (15). Viruses, in particular oncorna viruses, have been suspected as the etiological agents in the NZB-mouse syndrome manifesting an SLE-like syndrome with antinuclear antibodies and immune-complex glomerulonephritis. The genetic host component in the disease development is established, but it has not been demonstrated that the predominant genetic host factor is associated with the H-2 complex (16).

A number of studies have been performed in order to establish whether the major genetic components in the development of SLE is associated with the genetic determinants within the HLA complex (1, 17–27). Initially it was indicated that HLA-B8 and BW15 were increased among Caucasian patients with SLE (1). A slight increase in BW15 was observed by other groups of investigators (17). Subsequently studies seem to indicate that probably B8 is slightly increased in SLE (20, 23–26). HLA-D-locus typing in Caucasian patients with SLE using homozygous typing cells for the HLA-D specificities associated with B8 (DW3) and BW15 (DW4) has not demonstrated an increase in these determinants among Caucasian SLE patients (27). It now seems established that B8 is slightly increased in Caucasian patients with SLE.

Studies of HLA-antigen distribution among SLE patients of other ethnic groups have not demonstrated a clear association to any specific HLA antigens. Forty Black American SLE patients were studied and a slight increase in HLA-B5 was demonstrated (18). This was, however, not confirmed in another study of 60 Black American patients (21).

Studies of HLA-antigen frequencies in patients with SLE have been complicated by the presence of antilymphocyte antibodies in serum from the patients. Increased incidence of positive reactions with anti-A1 and anti-B8 antisera has been observed in patients showing IgG or complement coating on their red cells (28). Similar observations have been observed in the study of lymphocytes obtained from SLE patients (29). Most of these antibodies are of the IgM type. Some of the antibodies are directed against B lymphocytes and others against T lymphocytes (30–33).

In spite of the fact that twin studies in SLE strongly suggest genetic components in the pathogenesis of the disease (34), is has not been possible to demonstrate that the major genetic component in this multifactorial disease is strongly associated with the HLA complex.

Sjögren's disease

Sjögren's syndrome which occurs mostly in females is a disorder in which the combination of rheumatoid joint disease and dryness of the eyes and mouth are associated. The kerato-conjunctivitis sicca and xerostomia may, however, occur in the absence of arthritis. Other connective-tissue disorders including systemic lupus erythematosus, scleroderma or polymyositis, may occur or develop in such patients. Rheumatoid factors are regularly demonstrable in serum and the blood may contain any of several other autoantibodies. Reticulum-cell sarcoma develops in a greater frequency than normal.

The initial three reports on HLA-antigen frequencies in Sjögren's syndrome have demonstrated an increase in the HLA antigen B8 among the patients. The relative risk for disease development for individuals with B8 is calculated to 3.25 based on these three studies (2, 3, 4). This association has been confirmed in three additional studies (35, 36, 37). Recent studies with HLA-D homozygous typing cells for the HLA-B8-associated HLA-D-specificity DW3 have demonstrated that the association with this D-locus determinant is stronger than the association with the B8 determinant (36, 37).

Sarcoidosis

Sarcoidosis is a chronic granulomatous disease of unknown etiology, involving especially eyes, lymph nodes, spleen, lungs, liver, skin and brain. Ocular lesions usually reflect an anterior uveitis, but posterior uveitis and/or retinitis may occur. Sarcoid nodules, however, may involve any tissues, and the disease is usually a multisystem disorder. The basic pathology is noncaseating granulomata comprising epitheloid cells, Langhan's giant cells, plasma cells, and a peripheral ring of small lymphocytes. Clinical manifestations are highly variable and are featured by spontaneous remissions and exacerbations; erythema nodosum may occur in certain populations. There is regular depression of delayed allergic responses and diminished numbers and functions of T lymphocytes in the circulating blood. Proliferation of lymphoid cells is prominent in the lymph nodes and spleen. Kveim test, representing an indurative reaction to saline suspensions of heat-inactivated sarcoid tissue injected intradermally, is positive. Calcium metabolism may be abnormal. The disease in the U.S. is more prevalent in Blacks than Whites, but Black Africans are spared since the disease occurs predimonantly in Western populations and in highly developed industrial countries. Familial incidence has occurred and a recessive heredity of susceptibility has been suggested. When Kveim antigen is placed in tissue culture with peripheral-blood lymphocytes, macrophage-migration-inhibiting factor is produced by patients with the disease. It seems likely that the disease represents an infection with an as yet undefined organism.

Initial studies of HLA antigens in Caucasian patients with sarcoidosis have not demonstrated significant association with any HLA antigen (38–40). HLA genotyping and MLC testing in familial sarcoidosis have not revealed an association with HLA-D determinants (40). In a study of 80 patients with sarcoidosis is was, however, demonstrated that none of the patients who had positive delayed-hypersensitivity reactions to tuberculin were HLA-B7. The PPD-negative patients, however, had an increased incidence of B7 (41). This could imply that immune-response genes associated with the HLA complex are significant for the severity of the disease development but that the HLA system or associated genes do not influence the susceptibility to the disease-causing agent. In a recent study of 28 Black American patients with sarcoidosis, it has been demonstrated that an increase in B7 exists among the patients from this ethnic group compared with a matched normal control population (42).

Glomerulonephritis

Studies by Mickey et al. (43) have indicated an increase in HLA-A2 in patients with chronic glomerulonephritis. Another study also demonstrated a slight but insignificant increase in A2 (44), but this could not be demonstrated in the Dutch material (45).

Glomerulonephritis with IgA deposits in renal mesangium

At the HLA-Disease Symposium in Paris 1976, it became clear during the Immunopathology Workshop that a subgroup of patients with glomerulon-

ephritis associated with BW35 may exist:

Schönlein-Henoch syndrome

Schönlein-Henoch anaphylactoid purpura is a disease occurring almost exclusively in children in whom nondeforming arthritis occurs together with swelling of the gut, bloody diarrhea, abdominal pain, painful swellings of face and head, glomerulonephritis and a characteristic purpuric nonthrombopenic-rash involving the buttocks and lower extremities. The pathogenesis appears to involve deposition of IgA and complement components in the renal mesangium and in vessels in the skin lesions. The syndrome seems sometimes to have been provoked by infections, food, and insect stings or bites.

Balkan nephritis

Balkan Nephritis is a progressive renal disease featured by interstitial inflammation, fibrosis and tubular damage which occurs in river-valley regions of Rumania, Bulgaria and Yugoslavia. The disease progresses in advanced stages to a nephronophthisis. The condition clearly relates to the geographic region and is not only determined by genetic factors, since persons moving out of the region do not develop the disease while those moving into the area do. The onset is insidious, without initiating episode of edema or hematuria. Available evidence dissociates the condition from provoking streptococcal infection, intoxication with known nephrotoxic drugs, e.g. phenacetin, or other recognized nephrotoxins.

Berger's disease

This disease is characterized by idiopathic mesangial deposition of IgA. This is a form of glomerulonephritis with diffuse mesangial deposits containing IgA and C3. The patients present with recurrent gross hematuria or with microscopic hematuria and a light proteinuria. Their serum IgA level is usually elevated. The course of the disease is chronic but often mild. However, some patients develop hypertension and renal insufficiency. Recurrence after transplantation is very common.

Necrotizing venulitis associated with other autoimmune manifestations

This disease is characterized by cutaneous necrotizing venulitis and can be associated with rheumatoid arthritis, systemic lupus erythematosus, Sjögren's disease, lymphoma and glomerulonephritis (46).

It has been reported in a study from Paris that 14 out of 30 patients with Berger's disease had BW35 (47). MacDonald et al. (48) from Australia found BW35 in 6 out of 13 patients with the same disease, and in another study from Czechoslovakia 8 out of 29 patients with Schönlein-Henoch nephritis had BW35 (49). It was also observed that BW35 is increased among patients with Balkan nephritis and subacute thyroiditis (50). Finally, Glass et al. have demonstrated that necrotizing cutaneous venulitis complicated with other autoimmune manifestations, including glomerulonephritis, is associated with the antigens A11 and BW35 (46). It is possible that these cases of glomerulonephritis of nonstreptococcal etiology can all be grouped together as *BW35-associated nephritis*. A common component in the pathogenesis is IgA deposits in the mesangial tissue and in the skin. A specific susceptibility of BW35-positive individuals to a presently unknown virus is a possibility.

Autoimmune hemolytic anemia

Studies by Clauvel et al. have indicated a significant increase in HLA-A3 in patients with idiopathic and autoimmune hemolytic anemia (51). Additional information on this disease entity does not exist.

Idiopathic paraproteinemia

So-called benign monoclonal immunoglobulins, that is, those without any evidence of malignant lymphoplasmacytic proliferation are not uncommonly encountered. They are found in close to 3 % of elderly healthy individuals (more than 80 years old). In younger patients, such homogenous immunoglobulins may be associated with primary or secondary (for instance iatrogenic) immunodeficiencies or with various peculiar diseases such as papular mucinosis, a dermatologic disease. The level of monoclonal immunoglobulin usually remains stable through the years. The transient character of these monoclonal components can be observed. Very rare instances of familial occurrence of benign monoclonal immunoglobulins have been reported. A single study has demonstrated a slight increase in B7 among patients with benign monoclonal immunoglobulins (52).

Primary immunodeficiency diseases

The primary immunodeficiency diseases comprise a heterogeneous group of conditions generally genetically determined in which one or another of the specific immunological defense mechanisms is lacking or severely compromised. Except for the complement-component deficiencies described elsewhere, the specific gene responsible for each of the entities remains unknown. Thus, for the most part, definitions of these diseases must be based on description of symptom complexes and complexes of immunologic perturbations often genetically transmitted.

Severe combined immunodeficiencies in which both B cells and T cells fail to develop normally may have one of at least five separate genetic bases, and it is in this group of diseases that a beginning has been made in defining gene products which may underlie the diseases. Apparently autosomal-recessive heredity or absence of adenosine deaminase, nucleosidephosphorylase, or inosinephosphorylase has been associated with a broadly based immunodeficiency disease involving both T and B lymphocytes and accompanied by poor thymic development. Autosomal recessive inheritance of an abnormal inhibitor for adenosine deaminase has been linked to apparent adenosine-deaminase deficiency. Autosomal and x-linked heredity of severe combined deficiency of both T- and B-cell function in which adenosine deaminase is not disturbed also occur.

Bruton's disease

Bruton's disease is an x-linked infantile agammaglobulinemia in which B cells are absent from blood and lymphoid tissue. These patients, who also lack germinal centers, fail to produce antibodies and Ig normally. By contrast, thymus and T lymphocytes, and cell-mediated immunity seem quite normal. These patients experience increased frequency of infections, especially with encapsulated bacterial pathogens.

DiGeorge-athymic syndrome

DiGeorge-athymic syndrome is a primary immunodeficiency in which the thymus and parathyroid derivatives of the third and fourth paryngeal pouches fail to develop normally. These patients lack T lymphocytes, have excessive numbers of B lymphocytes, and often present as hypoparathyroid hypocalcemic tetany in the neonatal period. These patients frequently have vascular abnormalities that reflect failure of normal development of the outflow tracts of the heart and major blood vessels attributable to the maldevelopment of the aortic arches. Correction of the immunodeficiency has regularly been accomplished by transplantation of fetal thymus.

Wiskott-Aldrich syndrome

Wiskott-Aldrich syndrome is an x-linked recessive disorder featured by the clinical triad of increased susceptibility to a wide range of pathogens, eczema, and propensity to bleeding due to deficient numbers and morphological abnormality of platelets. The basic immunologic defect involves both cell-mediated and humoral immunity and particular deficiency of responses to polysaccharide antigens, but the fundamental cellular or molecular basis is unknown.

Common variable immunodeficiency

Common variable immunodeficiency with hypogammaglobulinemia represents a variety of diseases which may be sporadic or transmitted either as autosomal recessives or apparently dominant Mendelian traits. Immunodeficiencies are largely humoral, but B lymphocytes are present in blood and tissues and numbers of both cell types may be normal. Deficiencies of synthesis and secretion of Ig and antibodies sometimes associated with suppressor influences of T lymphocytes or adherent cells have been described. This is perhaps the most frequent of the primary immunodeficiency diseases. Frequent associations with infections, autoimmune diseases, malabsorption and malignancies have been reported.

Ataxia telangiectasia

Immunodeficiency with ataxia telangiectasia is transmitted as an apparent autosomal-recessive trait. In this disease, maldevelopment of thymus, T-cell immunodeficiency, and frequent absence of IgA and/or IgE are associated with progressive cerebellar ataxia and form telangiectases, especially in sclera, ear, popliteal and antecubital spaces. Survival is usually limited to a few years, and respiratory infection is the most frequent cause of death. Malignancies occur in high frequency.

Thymoma

Immunodeficiency associated with thymoma is a syndrome in which stromal-epithelial thymus tumor is associated with progressive immunologic failure, usually involving both cell-mediated and humoral immunodeficiencies. This disease occurs later in life and has not been shown to be hereditary. The pathogenetic mechanism is unknown.

Selective deficiency of immunoglobulin

Selective deficiency of immunoglobulin, e.g. IgA, IgG or IgE, has been shown in some instances to be transmitted as Mendelian autosomal-recessive traits, and generally these have not been associated with defects in structural genes associated with Ig synthesis. B lymphocytes which produce the Ig in which the patients are deficient are usually present in normal numbers in peripheral blood.

Transient immunodeficiencies of infancy

Transient immunodeficiencies of infancy that derive from slow development of immunological systems have also been described and have been linked to pathogenesis of certain forms of familial allergy.

Original studies by Hors et al. (53) indicated that HLA-A1 was significantly increased among patients with primary immunodeficiency diseases. The material consisted of at least seven different disease entities. A recent study of 52 patients with primary immunodfieficiency diseases of ten different entities did not confirm this observation (54). HLA typing of patients with ataxia telangiectasia (55) and selective IgA deficiency, (56, 57) have not demonstrated significant associations to the HLA complex. Studies by Sanderson et al. (58) and by Terasaki et al. (59) have indicated that patients with severe combined immunodeficiency (SCID) present extraneous HLA antigens on their lymphocytes. It is, however, possible that these reactions are caused by additional antibodies in the HLA antisera which are directed against subpopulations of lymphocytes (B lymphocytes and other non-T lymphocyytes). An abnormal distribution of subpopulations of lymphocytes in the peripheral blood of patients with different primary immune-deficiency diseases could very well present a problem for the correct interpretation of the positive reactions obtained during the HLA-typing procedures.

Complement-component deficiencies

The complement system has been defined as a group of at least 18 distinct serum proteins including 11 proteins of the classical complement system(C1q, C1r, C1s, C4, C2, C3, C5, C6, C7, C8, C9) at least four proteins of the alternate or properdin pathway, and at least three control proteins (inhibitors). The occurrence of isolated genetic deficiencies of complement has been increasingly recognized over the last few years, and has provided important information on the role of complement in the inflammatory process, host resistance to infection and immune response in vivo. Hereditary deficiencies (autosomal recessive), have been described for all classical components except C1q and C9. In addition, genetic deficiencies of proteins of the control mechanisms have also been documented: decreased C1-inhibitor resulting in hereditary angio-edema (the most common deficiency encountered), and decreased C3b inactivator causing chronic C3 hypercatabolism (only one case described). On the other hand, no deficiencies have yet been found of the alternative-pathway factors.

The recognition of a genetic linkage between genes controlling the serum levels or the polymorphism of important components of the classical and alternate pathways of complement activation and the genes of the major histocompatibility complex (MHC) has given rise to new interest in genetic aspects of the complement system and in the diseases associated with hereditary complement deficiencies. At the present time, it is established that C2 deficiency, C4 deficiency, and the polymorphism of factor B of the alternate pathway are controlled by genetic determinants closely linked to the HLA complex.

C2 deficiency is the most common deficiency of a classical complement component described in man. Heterozygous deficiency for C2 was estimated to occur at a frequency of approximately 1 % (60). The first cases of homozygous C2 deficiency were found among healthy individuals, but more recently the defect has been found in patients with a variety of diseases with immunological manifestations. Two cases have been reported showing most or all of the clinical and laboratory characteristics

240

of systemic lupus erythematosus (61, 62). One of these two cases has had recurrent infections during childhood in addition to the lupus syndrome (61). Other patients have shown discoid lupus erythematosus (63). Several patients presented with a disease resembling systemic lupus erythematosus but without the characteristic serological findings (63, 64, 71). This "lupus erythematosus-like syndrome" is clinically characterized by the occurrence of skin rashes on the face, chest, and arms with solar sensitivity and the occurrence of arthralgias. The skin biopsy is characteristic for systemic lupus erythematosus (SLE) on light microscopy, but immunofluorescence staining shows no deposits of immunoglobulins or C3 as in classical SLE. LE cells, anti-nuclear antibodies and antibodies to natural DNA are lacking. Renal involvement is frequently minimal or absent. One patient with C2 deficiency died of dermatomyositis (65). Three others had manifestations of anaphylactoid purpura (66–68). The association with chronic glomerulonephritis has also been reported in three patients (69, 70). Other patients have shown chronic vasculitis (72), rheumatic disease (69, 9) and Hodgkin's disease (73).

Two cases of homozygous C4 deficiency have now been discovered. The first cases described were reported by Hauptmann et al. (74). The patient was an 18-year-old German girl who presented with a lupus erythematosus-like syndrome, mild urinary abnormalities, without anti-nuclear antibodies and absence of immunoglobulin, and C3 deposits in the skin lesions. A second case was studied by Ochs et al (11): the C4 homozygous patient was a 5-year-old boy with a lupus erythematosus-like syndrome, nephritis and anti-nuclear antibodies.

Recent studies have demonstrated that genes controlling the synthesis of complement component C2 (5), C4 (12), as well as the polymorphism of factor B of the alternate pathway of complement activation (75), are linked to the HLA complex. These observations demonstrate a considerable homology between the genetic components within, or closely linked to, the HLA complex and the genetic determinants within the H-2 complex in the mouse. It has been known for several years that the level of a serum globulin, Ss, and its allotypic variant, Slp, was controlled by genetic determinants within the H-2 complex (76). Demant and coworkers demonstrated that the level of hemolytic complement in mice was under genetic control by determinants within the H-2 region (77–79). Subsequently, it was reported that the genetic control of complement C1, C2 and C4 was controlled by genes within the H-2 complex of the mouse (80). Even the C3 levels may be controlled by the H-2 complex, at least during ontogeny (81, 82). It now seems likely that the Ss protein of the mouse is a serum-complement component (83), and that the Ss protein may be identical to the murine complement C4 (84–86). Meo et al. (86) have demonstrated immunological crossreactivity between murine Ss protein and the human C4.

The association between genetic determinants controlling certain serum-complement components and the major histocompatibility complex have subsequently also been demonstrated to exist in the guinea pig and rhesus monkey (87–89).

The linkage between HLA determinants and C2 deficiency has now been established in a large number of families (5–10, 60, 69, 70, 90, 91). The C2 deficiency is intimately linked to the HLA alleles A10, B18, DW2 and to the Bf-S allele. The association with

DW2 seems much more intimate than the association with A10, B18. Indeed, the association of C2 deficiency with the antigen B18 seems to be secondary to a primary association with DW2. No clear evidence for strong linkage disequilibrium between DW2 and B18 was found by Dupont et al. (92) in an extensive study of a normal population in New York. It is possible that the haplotype B18, BW2, C2 deficiency is selectively increased in C2-deficient patients. The selection of patients and the small number of observations does not, however, make such a conclusion possible at present. It is likely that the C2-deficiency gene is located outside the HLA complex close to the HLA-D determinant based on the observation of DW2-C2-deficiency recombinants (7, 69).

The association between the HLA complex and the genetic determinants for C4 deficiency has now been established in two unrelated families described by Ochs et al. 11) and Rittner et al. (12). In both cases, C4 deficiency was clearly linked to the HLA. The patient and other members of the family described by Ochs et al. have been studied in HLA-D-typing experiments with the HLA-D homozygous-typing cells obtained from the family described by Hauptmann et al. (12, 74). These studies demonstrated that the two C4 homozygous-deficient patients did not share HLA-D determinants (11). The study indicates that the C4-deficiency gene is probably located outside the HLA complex in a distance of approximately 10 centimorgans. It is not presently possible to determine on which side of the HLA complex the C4- deficiency gene is located.

The following serum-complement components do not seem to be associated with the HLA complex: C1r deficiency (93), C7 deficiency (94, 95), C1-inhibitor deficiency (96, 97). Studies by Mittal et al. (98) indicate that C6 deficiency is not associated with the HLA complex. Hobart & Lachmann (99) found no linkage between C6 polymorphism and other genetic markers, including HLA. Recent studies by Carpenter et al. (100) indicate, however, that C6 deficiency seems to be associated but not linked with the MHC, and that the C6 polymorphism is linked to the MHC. Finally, it has been shown that C8 deficiency in one large family in Tunisia is not associated with the HLA complex (101), whereas in another family study attributed Merritt et al. (102), C8 deficiency was said to be linked to the MHC. These differences may be explained by virtue of the fact that the C8 molecule is composed of three polypeptide chains and the control of the synthesis of one chain may be closely linked to the MHC.

The studies of genetically determined deficiencies in isolated serum-complement components have added considerably to the understanding of the etiological and pathogenic mechanisms in the development of diseases such as systemic lupus erythematous, glomerulonephritis and Hodgkin's disease. Individuals who are homozygous or heterozygous deficient for C2 manifest a considerable increase in these diseases (60, 63, 103). When randomly selected SLE patients are studied for the HLA determinants which are selectively increased in C2 deficiency, e.g. B 18 and DW2 it is demonstrated that the C2-deficient patients only constitute a minor fraction of the patients with these diseases (27).

Conclusions

Systemic lupus erythematosus is not strongly associated with any HLA determinants. A slight increase in the frequency of B8 in Caucasian patients with SLE is observed. Individuals with serum-complement C2 deficiency and C4 deficiency frequently demonstrate SLE syndromes, glomerulonephritis and Hodgkin's disease. An increased incidence of atopic diseases and gluten sensitivity is also observed (103). The genes for C2 deficiency and C4 deficiency are closely linked to the HLA complex. C2 deficiency can be specifically mapped outside the HLA complex close to the HLA-D locus. This complement-deficiency syndrome is nearly always associated with DW2 and/or B18. A similar mapping of the C4 deficiency gene cannot be made at present.

Sjögren's disease is clearly associated in Caucasian patients with B8. A much stronger association, however, is observed for the DW3 specificity which in the normal population is in strong positive genetic linkage disequilibrium with B8. This demonstrates that the genetic determinant responsible for susceptibility to the disease development is probably closely associated with DW3 rather than the B8 determinant.

Sarcoidosis is not significantly associated with any HLA determinants. The observation of an increase in B7 in Black American patients with sarcoidosis, and the increase in B7 in Caucasian sarcoid patients who are PPD nonresponsive by skin testing, demonstrates the probable involvement of histocompatibility-linked immune-response genes in the development of disease severity.

Patients with glomerulonephritis do not demonstrate significant deviation in HLA antigens. It is likely, however, that this heterogeneous disease entity can be subdivided. The BW35-associated non-streptococcal glomerulonephritis characterized by IgA deposits in the mesangial tissue may constitute a disease entity. Chronic glomerulonephritis in some patients with serum-complement deficiencies associated with certain HLA determinants may represent another subgroup.

No significant and consistent association between primary immunodeficiency syndromes and HLA determinants have been demonstrated in population studies or in family studies. It is possible, however, that the varying phenotypic expression of these different disease entities may be determined in part by genetic determinants within the HLA complex. The heredity of certain HLA haplotypes may supply the patient with Ir genes which will influence the severity of the immunodeficiency. Future studies of HLA-haplotype segregation in families with multiple cases of primary immunodeficiency diseases may clarify such critical questions.

References

1. Grumet, F. C., Coukell, A., Bodmer, J. G., W. F. & McDevitt, H. O. (1971) Histocompatibility (HL-A) antigens associated with systemic lupus erythematosus. *New Eng. J. Med.* **285,** 193.
2. Sturrock, R. D., Banesi, B. A., Dick, H. M. & Dick, W. C. (1974) HL-A antigens and the sicca syndrome. *Ann. rheum. Dis.* **33,** 165.
3. Ivanyi, D., Drizhal, I., Erbenova, E., Horejs, J., Salavec, M., Macurova, H., Dostal, C., Balik, J. & Juran, J. (1976) HL-A in Sjögren's Syndrome. *Tissue Antigens* **7,** 45.
4. Gershwin, M. E., Terasaki, P. I., Graw, R. & Chused. T. M. (1975) Increased frequency of HL-A8 in Sjögren's Syndrome. *Tissue Antigens* **6,** 342.
5. Fu, S. M., Kunkel, H. G., Brushman, H. P., Allen, F. J. & Fotino, M. (1974) Evi-

dence for linkage between HL-A histocompatibility genes and those involved in the synthesis of the second component of complement. *J. exp. Med.* **140**, 1108.

6. Day. N. K., L'Esperance, P., Good, R. A., Michael, A. F., Hansen, J. A., Dupont, B. & Jersild, C. (1975) Hereditary C2 deficiency: genetic studies and association with the HL-A system. *J. exp. Med.* **141**, 1464.

7. Friend, P., Kim, Y., Handwerger, B., Reinsmohen, N., Michael, A. & Yunis, E. (1975) C2 deficiency in man. Relationship, including probable genetic mapping, to the mixed lymphocyte reaction stimulator (S or D) determinant short 7a. In: *Histocompatibility Testing 1975*, p. 928, Munksgaard, Copenhagen.

8. Fu, S. M., Stern R., Kunkel, H. G., Dupont, B., Hansen. J. A., Day, N. K., Good, R A., Jersild, C. & Fotino, M. (1975) Mixed lymphocyte culture determinants and C2 deficiency: LD-7a associated with C2 deficiency in four families. *J. exp. Med.* **142**, 495.

9. Gibson, D. J., Glass, D., Carpenter, C. B. & Schur, P. H. (1976) Hereditary C2 deficiency: diagnosis and HLA gene complex associations. *J. Immunol.* **116**, 1065.

10. Wolski, K. P., Schmid, F. R. & Mittal, K. K. (1975) Genetic linkage between the HL-A system and a deficit of the second component (C2) of complement. *Science* **188**, 1020.

11. Ochs, H. D., Rosenfeld, S. I., Thomas, E. D., Giblett, E. R., Alper, C. A., Dupont, B., Hansen, J. A., Grosse-Wilde, H. & Wedgwood, J. (1976) Linkage between the gene(s) controlling the synthesis of C4 and the major histocompatibility complex. In: *HLA and Disease*, eds. Dausset, J. & Svejgaard, A., Inserm, Paris, p. 208.

12. Rittner, C, Hauptmann, G., Grosse-Wilde, H., Grosshans, E., Tongio, M. M. & Mayer, S. (1975) Linkage between HL-A (major histocompatibility complex) and genes controlling the synthesis of the fourth component of complement. In: *Histocompatibility Testing 1975*, p. 945, Munksgaard, Copenhagen.

13. Lee, S. L. & Siegel, M. (1976) Systemic lupus erythematosus: epidemiological clues to pathogenesis. In: *Infection and immunology in the rheumatic diseases*, p. 307, Blackwell Scientific Publications, Oxford, London.

14. Lewis, R. M. & Schwartz, R. S. (1976) Caine systemic lupus erythematosus: a communicable disease? In: *Infection and immunology in the rheumatic diseases*, p. 259, Blackwell Scientific Publications, Oxford, London.

15. Phillips, P. E. (1976) Recent attempts at implicating viruses in systemic lupus erythematosus (SLE). In: *Infection and immunology in the rheumatic diseases*, p. 265, Blackwell Scientific Publications, Oxford, London.

16. Lerner, R. A., Dixon, F. J., Croker, B. P., Del Villano, B. C., Jensen, F. C., Kennel, S. J. & McConahey, P. J. (1974) The possible role of oncorna-viruses in the etiology and pathogenesis of murine lupus. *Adv. Biosciences,* **12**, 356.

17. Waters, H. Konrad, P. & Walford, R. L. (1971) The distribution of HL-A histocombatibility factors and genes in patients with systemic lupus erythematosuu. *Tissue Antigens* **1**, 8.

18. Niel. K. M., Brown, J. C., Dubois, E. L., Quismorio, F. P., Friou, G. J. & Terasaki, P. I. (1974) Histocompatibility (HL-A) antigens and lymphocytotoxic antibodies in systemic lupus erythematosus (SLE). *Arthritis Rheum.* **17**, 397.

19. Kissmeyer-Nielsen, F., Kjerbye, K. E., Andersen, E. & Halberg, P. (1975) HL-A antigens in systemic lupus erythematosus. *Transplant. Rev.* **22**, 164.

20. Goldberg, M. A., Arnett, F. C., Bias, W. B. & Shulman, L. E. (1976) Histocompatibility antigens in systemic lupus erythematosus. *Arthritis Rheum.* **19**, 129.

21. Stastny, P. (1972) The distribution of HL-A antigens in black patients with systemic lupus erythematosus (SLE). *Arthritis Rheum.* **15**. 455.

22. Bitter, T. (1972) HL-A antigens associated with lupus erythematosus. *New Eng. J. Med.* **286**, 435.

23. Szegedi, G. & Stenszky, V. HLA and systemic lupus erythematous (1976) In: *HLA and Disease,* eds. Dausset, J. & Svejgaard, A., Inserm, Paris, p. 292.

24. Nakagawa, J., Ikehara, Y., Ito, K. & Fukase, M. (1976) HLA antigens in various autoimmune and related diseases. Ibid, p. 205.

25. Van den Berg-Loonen. E. M., Swaak, A. J. G., Nijenhuis, L. E., Feltkamp, T. E. & Engelfriet, C. P. (1976) Histocompatibility antigens and other genetic markers in patients with systemic lupus erythematosus. Ibid, p. 214.

26. Dostal, C., Ivanyi, D., Macurova, H., Hana, I. & Strejcek, J. (1976) HLA-B8 antigen in systemic lupus erythematosus (SLE). Ibid, p. 199.

27. Hansen, J. A., Rothfield, N. F., Jersild. C., Wernet, P. & Dupont, B. (1976) MLC determinants (HLA-D) in patients with systemic lupus erythematosus (SLE). Ibid, p. 201.

28. Da Costa, J. A. G., White, A. G.. Parker, A. C. & Brigor, G. B. (1974) Increased incidence of HL-A1 and 8 in patients showing IgG or complement coating on their red cells. *J. clin. Pathol.* **27**, 353.

29. Mittal, K. K., Rossen R. D., Sharp, J. T., Lidsky, M. D. & Butler, W. T. (1970) Lymphocyte cytotoxic antibodies in systemic lupus erythematosus. *Nature (Lond.)* **225**, 1255.

30. Wernet, P. & Kunkel, H. G. (1973) Demonstration of specific T-lymphocyte membrane antigens associated with antibodies inhibiting the mixed leukocyte culture in man. *Transplant. Proc.* **5**, 1875.

31. Suciu-Foca, N., Buda, J., Almojera, P. & Reemtsa, K. (1974) HL-A antigens and MLC responsiveness in systemic lupus erythematosus. *Lancet* **ii**, 726.

32. Winfield, J. B., Winchester, R. J., Wernet, P., Fu, S. H. & Kunkel, H. G. (1975) Nature of cold-reactive antibodies to lymphocyte surface determinants in systemic lupus erythematosus. *Arthritis Rheum.* **18**, 1.

33. Del Giacco, G. S., Locci, F., Loy, M.. Leone, A. L., Batzella, M. G., Mantovani, G. & Ibba, G. (1976) HLA and collagen diseases: Frequency studies and correlation with anti-T-lymphocyte antibodies. In: *HLA and Disease,* eds. Dausset, J. & Svejgaard, A. Inserm, Paris, p. 198.

33. Stefanova, G. (1976) Relationship between HLA and other immunological tests in nephropathy due to SLE. Ibid, p. 211.

34. Block, S. R., Winfield, J. B., Lockshin, M. D., D'Angelo, W. A.. Weksler, M. E., Fotino, M. & Christian, C. L. (1975) Twin studies in systemic lupus erythematosus (SLE). *Arthritis Rheum.* **18**, 285.

35. Clough, J. D., Aponte, C. J. & Braun, W. E. (1976) HLA-B8 and clinical features of Sjögren's Syndrome. In: *HLA and Disease,* eds. Dausset, J. & Svejgaard, A. Inserm, Paris, p. 196.

36. Ivanyi, D., Hincova, E., Sula, K., Drizhal, I., Erbenova, E., Macurova, H., Dostal, C., Horejs, J. & Balik, J. (1976) Increased frequency of HLA-B8 and HLA-DW3 in Sjögren's Søndrome (SS). Ibid, p. 202.

37. Opelz, G., Terasaki, P., Vogten, A., Schalm, S., Summerskill, W., Kassan, S., Chused, T. & Fye, K. (1976) Association of HLA-DW3 with chronic active liver disease and Sjögren's disease. Ibid, p. 167.

38. Hedfors, E. & Möller, E. (1973) HL-A antigens in sarcoidosis. *Tissue Antigens* **3**, 95.

39. Kueppers, F., Mueller-Eckhardt, C., Heinrich, D., Schwab, B. & Brackertz, D. (1974) HL-A antigens of patients with sarcoidosis. *Tissue Antigens* **4**, 56.

40. Möller, E., Hedfors, E. & Wiman, L. G. (1974) HL-A genotypes and MLR in familial sarcoidosis. *Tissue Antigens* **4**, 299.

41. Persson, I., Ryder, L. P., Staub Nielsen, L. & Svejgaard, A. (1975) The HL-A7 histocompatibility antigen in sarcoidosis in relation to tuberculin sensitivity. *Tissue Antigens* **6**, 50.

42. McIntyre, J., McKee, K. & Loadholt. C. (1977) Increased HLA-B7 antigen frequency in the South Carolina black population in association with sarcoidosis. *Transplant. Proc.* (in press).

43. Mickey, M. R., Kreisler, M. & Terasaki, P. I. (1970) Leukocyte antigens and disease. II. Alterations in frequencies of haplotypes associated with chronic glomerulonephritis. In: *Histocompatibility Testing 1970,* p. 239, Munksgaard, Copenhagen.

44. Jensen, H., Ryder, L. P., Staub Nielsen, L., Clausen, E., Jørgensen, F. & Jørgensen, H. E. (1975) HLA antigens and glomerulonephritis. *Tissue Antigens* **6**, 368.

45. van Rood, J. J., van Hooff, J. P. & Keuning, J. J. (1975) Disease predisposition, immune responsiveness and the fine structure of the HL-A supergene. *Transplant. Rev.* **22**, 75.

46. Glass, D., Soter, N. A., Gibson, D., Carpenter, C. B. & Schur, P. H. (1976) An association between HLA and Cutaneous Necrotizing Venulitis. *Arth. and Rheum.* (in press).

47. Noel, L. H., Descamps, B., Jungers, P., Bach, J. F., Busson, M., Guillet, V, & Hors, J. (1976) HLA Serotyping in 5 well defined Kidney Diseases. In: Ibid.

48. Macdonald. I. M., Dumble, L. J. & Kincaid-Smith, P. (1976) HLA and glomerulonephritis. Ibid, p. 203.

49. Nyulassy, S., Buc, M.. Sasinka, M., Pavlovic, M., Hrischova, V., Kaiserova, M., Stefanovic, J. (1976) HLA system in glomerulonephritis. Ibid, p. 207.

50. Kostelan, A. Personal communication.

51. Clauvel, J. P., Marcelli-Barge. A., Cog-

gia, I. G., Poirier, J. C., Benajam, A. & Dausset, J. (1974) HL-A antigens and idiopathic autoimmune hemolytic anemias. *Transplant. Proc.* **6**, 447.

52. Van Camp, B., Dergent-Cole & Petermans, M. (1976) HLA-B7 and idiopathic paraproteinemia. In: *HLA and Disease,* eds. Dausset, J. & Svejgaard, A. Inserm, Paris, p. 213.
53. Hors, J., Griscelli, C.. Schmid, M. & Dausset, J. (1975) HL-A antigens and immune deficiency states. *Brit. Med. J* **4**, 45.
54. Buckley, R. H., MacQueen, J. M. & Ward, F. E. (1976) HLA antigens in primary immunodeficiency disease. In: *HLA and Disease,* eds. Dausset, J. & Svejgaard, A. Inserm, Paris, p. 195.
55. Berkel, A. I. & Ersoy, F. (1976) HLA antigens i nataxia-telangiectasia. Ibid, p. 194.
56. Bajtai. G., Hernadi, E. & Ambrus, M. (1976) HLA-A1 and B8 in selective IgA deficiency. Ibid, p. 193.
57. Hägele, R., Evers, K. G., Leven, B. & Krüger. J. (1976) HLA frequencies in primary immunodeficiency diseases (IDD). Ibid, p. 200.
58. Sanderson, A. R., Gelfand, E. W. & Rosen, F. S. (1972) A change in HL-A phenotype associated with a specific blocking factor in the serum of an infant with severe combined immunodeficiency disease. *Transplantation* **13**, 142.
59. Terasaki, P. I., Miyapima, T., Sengar. D. P. S. & Stiehm, E. R. (1972) Extraneous lymphocytic HL-A antigens in severe combined immunodeficiency disease. *Transplantation* **13**, 250.
60. Fu, S. M., Stern, R.. Kunkel, H. G., Dupont. B., Hansen, J. A., Day, N. K. Good, R. A., Jersild, C. & Fotino, M. (1975) LD-7a association with C2 deficiency in five of six families. In: *Histocompatibility Testing 1975,* p. 933, Munksgaard, Copenhagen.
61. Day, N. K., Geiger, H., McLean, R., Michael, A. & Good. R. A. (1973) C2 deficiency. Development of lupus erythematosus. *J. clin. Invest.* **52**, 1601.
62. Osterland, C. K., Espinoza, L.. Parker, L. P. & Schur, P. H. (1975) Inherited C2 deficiency and systemic lupus erythematosus: studies on a family. *Ann. Int. Med.* **82**, 323.
63. Agnello, V. (1976) Association of C2 deficiency and HLA genes with systemic and discoid lupus erythematosus. In: *HLA and Disease,* eds. Dausset, J. & Svejgaard, A. Inserm, Paris, p. 296.
64. Agnello, V., De Bracco, M. M. E. & Kunkel, H. G. (1972) Hereditary C2 deficiency with some manifestations of lupus erythematosus. *J. immunol.* **108**, 837.
65. Leddy, J. P., Griggs, R. C., Klemperer, M. & Frank, M. M. (1975) Heredity complement deficiency with dermatomyositis. *Amer. J. Med.* **58**, 83.
66. Einstein, L. P., Alper, C. A., Bloch, K. J., Herrin, J. T., Rosen, F. S., David, J. R. & Colten, H. R. (1975) Biosynthetic defect in monocytes from human beings with genetic deficiency of the second component of complement. *N. Eng. J. Med.* **292**, 1169.
67. Gelfand, E. W., Clarkson, J. E. & Minta, J. O. (1975) Selective deficiency of the second component of complement in a patient with anaphylactoid purpura. *Clin. Immunol. Immunopathol.* **4**, 269.
68. Sussman, M., Jones, J. H., Almeida, J. D. & Lachmann, P. J. (1973) Deficiency of the second component of complement associated with anaphylactoid purpura and presence of myoplasma in the serum. *Clin. exp. Immunol.* **14**, 531.
69. Friend, P. S., Handwerger, B. S., Kim, Y.. Michael, A. F. & Yunis, E. (1975) C2 deficiency in man. Genetic relationship to a mixed lymphocyte reaction determinant (7a*). *Immunogenetics* **2**, 569.
70. Hauptmann, G., Tongio, M. M.. Lang, J. M., Grosse-Wilde, H. & Mayer, S. (1976) Linkage between C2 deficiency and the HLA-A10, B18/Bfs haplotype in a French family. In: *HLA and Disease,* eds. Dausset, J. & Svejgaard, A. Inserm, Paris, p. 306.
71. Pickering, R. J., Michael, A. F., Herdman, R. C., Good. R. A. & Gewurz, H. J. (1971) The complement system in chronic glomerulonephritis: three newly associated aberrations. *J. Paed.* **87**, 30.
72. Friend, P., Repine, K. E., Kim, Y., Clawson, C. C. & Michael, A. F. (1975) Deficiency of the second component of complement (C2) with chronic vasculitis. *Ann. Int. Med.* **83**, 813.
73. Day, W. K., Rubinstein, P., Case, D., Hansen, J. A., Good, R. A., Walker, M. E., Tulchin, N., Dupont, B. & Jersild, C. (1976) Linkage of gene for C2 deficiency and the major histocompatibility complex (MHC) in man: family study of a further case. *Vox Sang.* **31**, 96.
74. Hauptmann, G., Grosshans, E. & Heid, E. (1974) Lupus erythemateux aigus et défi-

246

cits héréditaires en complément. A propos d'un cas par déficit complet en C4. *Ann. Derm. Syph.* **101**, 479.

75. Allen, F. H. Jr. (1974) Linkage of HL-A and GBG. *Vox Sang.* **27**, 382.

76. Schreffler, D. C. & David, C. S. (1975) The H-2 major histocompatibility complex and the I immune response region: genetic variation, function, and organization. *Adv. immunol.* **20**, 125.

77. Hinzova, E., Demant, P. & Ivanyi, P. (1972) Genetic control of haemolytic complement in mice: association with H2. *Folia biol.* **18**, 237.

78. Demant, P., Capkova, J., Hinzova, E. & Voracova, B. (1973) The role of the histocompatibility-2-linked Ss-S1p region in the control of mouse complement. *Proc. nat. Acad. Sci. (Wash.)* **70**, 863.

78. Hauptmann, G., Sasportes, M., Tongio, M. M., Mayer, S. & Dausset, J. (1976) The localization of the Bf locus within the MHS region on chromosome no. 6. *Tissue Antigens* **7**, 52.

79. Lamm, L. U., Jørgensen, F. & Kissmeyer-Nielsen, F. (1976) Bf maps between the HLA-A and D loci. *Tissue Antigens* **7**, 122.

79. Capkova, J. & Demant, P. (1974) Genetic studies of the H-2 associated complement gene. *Folia biol.* **20**, 101.

80. Goldman, M. B. & Goldman, J. N. (1975) Relationship of levels of early components of complement to the H2 complex in mice. *Fed. Proc.* **34**, 979.

81. Ferreira, A. & Nussenzweig, V. (1975) Genetic linkage between serum levels of the third component of complement and the H-2 complex. *J. exp. Med.* **141**, 513.

82. Ferreira, A. & Nussenzweig, V. (1976) Control of C3 levels in mice during ontogeny by a gene in the central region of the H-2 complex. *Nature (Lond.)* **260**, 613.

83. Hansen, T. H., Shin, H. S. & Shreffler, D. C. (1975) Evidence for the involvement of the Ss protein of the mouse in the hemolytic complement system. *J. exp. Med.* **141**, 1216.

84. Curman, B. Östberg, L., Sandberg, L., Malmheden-Erikson. I., Stalenheim, G., Rask, L. & Peterson. P. A. (1975) H-2 linked Ss protein in C4 component of complement. *Nature (Lond.)* **258**, 243.

85. Lachmann, P. J., Grennan, D., Martin. A. & Demant, P. (1975) Identification of Ss protein as murine C4. *Nature (Lond.)* **258**, 242.

86. Meo, T., Krasteff, T. & Shreffler, D. C.

(1975) Immunochemical characterization of murine H-2 controlled Ss (serum substance) protein through identification of its human homologue as the fourth component of complement. *Proc. nat. Acad. Sci. (Wash.)* **72**, 4536.

87. Sevach, E., Green, I. & Frank, M. M. (1976) Linkage of C4 deficiency to the major histocompatibility locus in the guinea pig. *VIth Int. Complement Workshop J. immunology* **116**, 1750.

88. Ziegler, J. B., Alper, C. A. & Balner, H. (1975) Properdin factor B and histocompability in the rhesus monkey. *Nature (Lond)* **254**, 609.

89. Ziegler, J. B., Watson, L. & Alper, C. A. (1975) Genetic polymorphism of properdin factor B in the Rhesus: evidence for single subunit structure in primates. *J. Immunol.* **114**, 1649.

90. Fu, S. M., & Kunkel, H. G. (1975) Association of C2 deficiency and the HL-A haplotype 10, W18. *Transplantation* **20**, 179.

91. Wolski, K. P., Schmid. F. R. & Mittal, K. K. (1976) Genetic linkage between the HLA system and a deficit of the second component (C2) of complement in four generations of a family. *Tissue Antigens* **7**, 35.

92. Dupont, B., Hansen, J. A., Whitsett, C.. Slater, L. & Lee, T. D. (1977) Population genetics for five HLA-D determinants in Caucasians (New York City). *Transplant. Proc.* (in press).

93. Day. N. K., Rubinstein, P.. De Bracco, M., Moncada, B., Hansen, J. A., Dupont, B., Thomsen, M., Svejgaard, A. & Jersild, C. (1975) Hereditary C1r deficiency: lack of linkage to the HL-A region in two families. In: *Histocompatibility Testing 1975*, p. 960, Munksgaard, Copenhagen.

94. Prochazka, E., Lehner-Netsch, G., Simard, J., Bergeron, P. & Delage, J. M. (1976) HLA antigens and heredity deficiency of the seventh component of complement in a family. In: *HLA and Disease*, eds. Dausset, J. & Svejgaard, A. Inserm, Paris, p. 210.

95. Rittner, Ch., Opferkuch, W., Wellek, B., Grosse-Wilde, H. & Wernet, P. Lack of linkage between gene(s) controlling the synthesis of the seventh component of complement and the HLA region on chromosome no. 6 in man. *Hum. Genetics* (to be published).

96. Ohela, K., Tiilikainen, A., Kaakinen. A. & Rasanen, J. (1975) Lack of association between HL-A haplotypes and HANE.

XIVth Congress of the Int. Soc. Blood Transfusion, Helsinki 1975, Abstract.

97. Tanimoto, K., Horiuchi, Y., Juji, T., Yamamoto, K., Kodama, J., Murata, S., Funahashi, S. & Nagaki, K. (1976) HLA types in the two families with hereditary angioneurotic edema. In: *HLA and Disease,* eds. Dausset, J. & Svejgaard, A. Inserm, Paris, p. 212.

98. Mittal, K. K., Wolski, K. P., Lim, D., Gewurz, A., Gewurz, H. & Schmid, F. R. (1976) Genetic independence between the HL-A system and deficits in the first and sixth components of complement. *Tissue Antigens* **7,** 97.

99. Hobart, M. J. & Lachmann, P. J. (1976) Allotyping of complement components in whole serum by isoelectric focusing in gel followed by specific hemolytic assay. *J. Immunol.* **116,** 1736.

100. Raun, D., Glass, D., Carpenter, C. B. & Schur, P. H. (1976) C6 deficiency – HLA association. *Fed. Proc.* **35,** 655.

101. Day, N. K., DeGos, L., Beth, E., Sassportes, M., Gharbi, R. & Giraldo, G. (1976) C8 deficiency in a family with xeroderma pigmentosum. Lack of linkage to the HL-A region. In: *HLA and Disease,* eds. Dausset, J. & Svejgaard, A. Inserm, Paris, p. 197.

102. Merrit, A. D., Petersen, B. H., Biegel, A. A., Meyers, D. A., Brooks, G. F. & M. E. Hodes (1976) Chromosome 6: Linkage of the Eight Component of Complement (C8) to the Histocompatibility Region (HLA). In: *Human Gene Mapping.* **3.** Baltimore Conference. S. Krager, Basel, (in press).

103. Mowbray, J. F. (1976) Association of heterozygous C2 deficiency with both diseases and HLA. In: *HLA and Disease,* eds. Dausset, J. & Svejgaard, A. Inserm, Paris, p. 204.

Other Diseases

P. J. Morris, J. Hors, P. Royer & L. P. Ryder

In this section very diverse groups of diseases have been covered, basically representing all those diseases which do not fit into one of the more well-defined disease groups. Thus, studies of HLA range from those in the Vogt-Koyanagi-Harada syndrome to gonococcal urethritis. Nevertheless, some interesting associations have appeared, and the failure to find association in the majority of diseases discussed in this section is not without relevance in the overall picture of HLA and disease.

Ophthalmology (excluding uveitis and Behcet's disease)

The most interesting association in this whole section is that of HLA with the Vogt-Koyanagi-Harada syndrome in the Japanese. This syndrome is characterised by depigmentation of the skin and hair, inflammatory ocular lesions (usually consisting of iridocyclitis or exudative retinal detachment), and meningitis. Neurological involvement is common and often precedes the ocular inflammation. This disease is not uncommon in the Japanese (7 % of uveitis patients), but is rare in Caucasians (less than 1 % of uveitis patients). Furthermore, the prognosis is relatively good in Japanese but is poor in Caucasians. Both viral

University of Oxford, Nuffield Dept. of Surgery, Radcliffe Infirmary, Oxford.

and allergic aetiologies have been discussed, but no definite evidence for either exists. Tagawa et al. (1) from Japan have studied 42 patients and found that an antigen BW22J (SA1), which is found only in the Japanese and is a split of the antigen BW22, was present in 45 % of these patients compared with 13 % of the control population. But even more striking was the association of a D-locus antigen, LD-Wa (again probably occurring only in the Japanese, and apparently linked to SA1), with this disease. There were 67 % of the patients who were LD-Wa positive compared with 16 % of the control population. Thus, here is another example of a disease which is more closely related to the D locus than the B locus. As the cause of this disease syndrome is likely to prove to be either viral or allergic, this association would best be explained by linkage to an immune-response gene, although as mentioned above no real evidence for this suggestion exists at present. The relative risks of the association with BW22J and LD-Wa are 5.4 and 10.5 respectively (Table I).

Interesting observations have been made in primary open-angle glaucoma and ocular hypertension by Shin et al. (2) and Becker & Shin (3). First, they showed that B7 and B12 occurred more frequently in patients with primary open-angle glaucoma (Table II), and

TABLE I

The frequency of BW22J and LD-Wa in the Vogt-Koyanagi-Harada syndrome in Japanese (Togawa et al. 1976)

	Control population n positive/n Studied (%)	Patient population n positive/n Studied (%)	Rel. risk
BW22J	10/76 (13)	19/42 (45)	5.4
LD-Wa	13/81 (16)	28/42 (67)	10.5

TABLE II

The frequency of HLA-A3, B7 and B12 in Caucasians with and without primary open-angle glaucoma (Shin et al. 1976).

	Normal (n = 50)	Primary open-angle glaucoma (n = 50)
HLA-A3	18 %	46 %
HLA-B7	16 %	52 %
HLA-B12	16 %	50 %

secondly, that the presence of B7 or B12 in patients with ocular hypertension predisposed to the development of glaucomatous damage to the optic nerve in these patients. These findings would be of great clinical significance if proved to be correct, but confirmation is not yet available. If primary open-angle glaucoma does indeed have an immunologic component in its aetiology as suggested by Becker et al. (4) and Waltman & Yarian (5), this association again might be explained most satisfactorily on the basis of a linkage with immune-response genes. It should be noted that Hoshino et al. (6) found no association of HLA with glaucoma in 52 Japanese patients.

Genetic disorders

A number of genetic disorders have been extensively studied. Three studies

of HLA in cystic fibrosis are available. Kaiser et al. (7) showed an increased frequency of B18 in 12 patients and in 32 heterozygotic gene carriers, while Polymenidis et al. (8) showed an increased frequency of B5 in 24 patients. As B18 and B5 are cross-reacting antigens, these findings could be considered suggestive of a possible association, but the failure of Lamm et al. (9) to show any association with HLA in detailed family studies probably means that HLA plays no part in the expression of this common genetic condition.

von Willebrand's disease, a familial haemorrhagic disorder transmitted by a dominant autosomal-mutant gene, has been studied by Goudemand et al. (10) and Muller et al. (11) in a total of 62 patients, and in addition, very extensive family studies have been performed by the former workers. No association with HLA appears to be present.

A fascinating family of 20 subjects, covering three generations, in whom six have hereditary haemorrhagic telangiectasia (Osler-Weber-Rendu disease) has been studied by Kissel et al. (12). The haplotype HLA-A2/BW17 was found in all six patients but in only two healthy members of the third generation, in whom visceral angiomatosis cannot be excluded. This observation is very suggestive of a possible HLA linkage, and further families with this rare condition need to be studied.

Single studies of relatively small numbers of patients with other genetic disorders such as acute porphyria, familial Mediterranean fever, Hurler's disease, and G-6-PD deficiency have been performed but no striking associations have appeared.

Congenital disorders

A number of congenital anomalies have been studied in relation to HLA. These include disorders such as Down's syndrome, brachymetacarpy, pyloric stenosis and congenital heart anomalies. The only association with HLA that has been reported is that of HLA-A2 with heart anomalies (Buc et al. (13)), but this has not been confirmed.

One promising observation by Couillin et al. (14) has been made in triploid conceptuses which result in spontaneous abortion. A triploid karyotype may result from a diploid gamete or dispermy where the haploid ovum is fertilized by two spermatozoa. In this latter instance, similarity of the two parents for the major histocompatibility complex might predispose to the occurrence of this event. These investigators have shown that two or more antigens of the A and B series are shared between the parents in 18 % of couples who conceived a triploid conceptus compared with 11 % in normal couples. These differences are not significant but worthy of further study.

Reproductive disorders

Pre-eclampsia is a disorder of pregnancy characterised by hypertension, oedema and proteinuria. It occurs most commonly during first pregnancies and is less common during subsequent ones. Its cause is unknown but immunological mechanisms related to a hyperimmune response of the mother to the foetal allograft have been postulated. However, Jenkins et al. (15) have presented a contrary hypothesis in which they postulate that women with eclampsia are hyporesponsive to paternal histocompatibility antigens. They base this hypothesis on their study of 37 mothers with severe pre-eclampsia. They found that these women had a lower incidence of antibodies against HLA and were less reactive in the mixed-lymphocyte reaction against paternal lymphocytes, while

there was a greater degree of compatibility for HLA between couples in whom eclampsia occurred in the mother. This hypothesis is attractive in some respects, particularly as it would explain the decreased frequency of eclampsia with subsequent pregnancies. There has been another study of pre-eclampsia by Redman & Bodmer (16), and they have found an increased frequency of homozygosity for HLA in the mothers with an eclamptic history. They suggest that this might be due to homozygosity of a relevant recessive gene. There is a need for more extensive studies of eclampsia along the above lines, for it seems reasonable to suggest that eclampsia is related to either compatibility or incompatibility between mother and foetus for the major histocompatibility complex.

There are also reports of HLA in azospermy and infertility, but no impressive associations with HLA are noted.

Infection

This group of diseases is one of great potential interest in HLA-disease associations, as positive associations would provide an attractive explanation for the evolution of the extreme polymorphism of HLA in Caucasian populations compared with the restricted polymorphism of some isolated and primitive populations. Thus, this extreme polymorphism may have evolved due to the selective pressures exerted by the great killer disease of the past, e.g. plague, smallpox, cholera, tuberculosis, poliomyelitis, and malaria. The role of H2 in the mouse in determining susceptibility to Gross-virus and Friend-virus leukaemogenesis also lends support to this hypothesis. Nevertheless, studies of HLA in a number of infectious diseases have been disappointing. No association has been found with HLA in infectious mononu-

251

cleosis or tuberculosis, while possible associations have been reported in poliomyelitis, leprosy, haemophilus influenzae, recurrent urethritis, peridontitis, and Australian antigen-carrier state. However, the positive reports are either not in agreement or the numbers studied are too small to draw any firm conclusions.

Indirect evidence for a role for HLA in the determination of susceptibility to certain major infectious diseases has been presented by Piazza et al. (17) in their study of HLA in the highlands and lowlands of Sardinia. Until recently malaria was endemic in the lowlands and did not occur in the highlands. There was a much greater frequency of the two red-cell abnormalities, thalassaemia and G-6-PD deficiency in the lowlands than in the highlands. It is now commonly accepted that thalassaemia, G-6-PD deficiency, and sickle-cell anaemia are balanced polymorphisms maintained through the selective advantage of the heterozygote over the homozygote towards plasmodial infection. In these Sardinian studies there was also a significant difference between the frequencies of the HLA-B-locus antigens in the highlands and the lowlands which did not exist for 22 other genetic markers. Piazza et al. have suggested that differential selection, through the agency of malaria, was responsible for these differences in HLA. As malaria has been the most significant disease in mankind's history in terms of human wastage, it would certainly be expected to have exerted the greatest selective pressure on any polymorphism where the heterozygote received some advantage.

An interesting observation has been made by Honeyman et al. (18) in congenital rubella. They have shown a small increase in the frequency of A1 and B8 in patients with congenital ru-

bella, but have noted that the percentage of normal populations with positive serum reactions to rubella virus, indicating previous infection, falls with a decreasing frequency of A1 and B8. For example there is a very low seropositivity to rubella virus in the Japanese where A1 and B8 do not occur. They have suggested that A1 and B8 might act as favourable receptor sites for the rubella virus.

Vascular disorders

A large number of studies of HLA in various vascular disorders has now been reported. Perhaps the most interesting observations in this area are concerned with ischaemic heart disease and hypertension. Mathews (19) has previously reported that national death rates from ischaemic heart disease showed a significant correlation with population frequencies of B8 and the phenotype A1; B8, and that there was a trend for hypercholesterolaemia to show a similar correlation to the population frequency of B8. However, he now feels that this association of ischaemic heart disease with B8 can be explained by the increased frequency of B8 in diabetics who form a substantial proportion of patients with ischaemic heart disease. In their latest analysis of ischaemic heart disease (233 patients) and hypertension (144 patients), Mathews et al. (20) have failed to show any alteration in antigen distribution between the disease and control groups, but have shown a significant difference in haplotype frequencies in both disease groups compared with the normal population. They suggest that genetic factors linked to HLA contribute to the risk of hypertension and ischaemic heart disease in man. Two other studies of HLA in hypertension show an increased frequency of B8 and B12 in hypertensives

(21, 22), but it does not seem that any real association is likely to exist. However, the study of Mathews *et al.* needs to be enlarged and confirmed.

A possible association of HLA-B14 with temporal arthritis, a probable auto-immune disorder, has been noted by Seignalet *et al.* (23) in 61 well-defined patients (23 % in patients *versus* 9 % in control population), but further studies are needed for confirmation of this finding.

Professional diseases

There has not been a great number of studies in this area, but one condition which appears to be associated with HLA is asbestosis. Merchant *et al.* (24) first described an increase in the frequency of B27 in patients with asbestosis. Although this was not a dramatic increase in frequency, a similar finding has been reported by Matej *et al.* (25). (Table III). In this latter report, 134 workers in the same factory who had been in contact with asbestos for at least 20 years were studied. Of these 134 workers only 22 had developed asbestosis, and in this group there was a significant increase in frequency of B27 (Table III). The combined relative risk

TABLE III

Increased frequency of B27 in two groups of patients with asbestosis. The control population in the study of Matej et al. consists of workers exposed to asbestos who did not develop asbestosis. The combined relative risk of asbestosis for B27 is 3.5

| | Control population | | Asbestosis population | |
	No.	B27+	No.	B27+
Merchant *et al.*				
1975	153	5 %	56	18 %
Matej *et al.*				
1976	112	10 %	22	27 %

of asbestosis for B27 from the Polish and UK studies is 3.7. This finding does have important implications in industrial medicine, as it could provide help in determining the workers in contact with asbestos who are more likely to develop asbestosis. As the aetiology of asbestosis is no doubt based on an immunological mechanism, studies of D-locus antigens in this disease are likely to be relevant.

A rather similar disease, silicosis, which again probably has an immunological basis, has been studied by Gualde *et al.* (26). Although no significant deviation of antigen frequencies was noted when either a normal population or a population exposed to the pathogen but not developing silicosis were compared, there was a decreased frequency of A3 and B7 in the silicosis patients. This observation is worthy of further study.

Miscellaneous disorders

Several studies of HLA and the aged are important as it has been suggested in three of these studies that the elderly population show a greater heterozygosity for antigens of the A and B series than the younger population (27–30).

This supported a hypothesis that heterozygosity for HLA provided a post-natal selective advantage in immune-surveillance mechanisms directed particularly against cancer. However, further large and careful study by Bender *et al.* (31) has failed to show any difference in the frequency of heterozygotes in children under 10 and adults over 70 years of age. Nor were they able to confirm any of the apparently discrepant antigen frequencies between young and old people previously described.

References[1]

1. Tagawa, Y.. Sugiura, S., Yakura, H., Wakisaka, A., Aizawa, M. & Itakura, K. (1976) HLA and Vogt-Koyanagi-Harada Syndrone. *Proc. HLA and Disease Symp.*[1]
2. Shin, D. H., Becker, B. & Bell, C. E. (1976) HLA in primary open-angle glaucoma. *Proc. HLA and Disease Symp.*[1]
3. Becker, B. & Shin, D. H. (1976) Prognostic value of HLA-A3, BW35, B7 and B12 in ocular hypertension. *Proc. HLA and Disease Symp.*
4. Becker, B., Unger. H., Coleman, S. L., & Keates, E. U. (1963) Plasma cells and gamma-globulin in trabecular meshwork of eyes with primary open angle glaucoma. *Arch. Opthal.* **70**, 38.
5. Waltman, S. R. & Yarian, D. (1974) Antinuclear antibodies in Open-angle glaucoma. *Invest. Opthal.* **13**, 695.
6. Hoshino, K., Inouye, H., Unokuchi, T., Ito, M., Tamaoki, N. & Tsuji, K. (1976) HLA and Diseases in Japanese. *Proc. HLA and Disease Symp.*[1]
7. Kaiser, G., Lazlo, A., Gyurkovits, K. & Gyodi, E. (1976) HLA antigens in cystic fibrosis: a possible association of B18 with the disease. *Proc. HLA and Disease Symp.*[1]
8. Polymenidis, Z., Ludwig, H. & Gotz. M. (1973) Cystic fibrosis and HLA antigens. *Lancet ii,* 1452.
9. Lamm, L. U., Thorsen, I. L., Petersen, G. B., Jorgensen, J., Henningsen, B., Bech, B. & Kissmeyer-Nielsen, F. (1975) Data on the HLA-Linkage group. *Ann. Hum. Genetics* **38**, 383.
10. Goudemand, J., Mazurier, C. & Parquet-Gernez, A. (1976) HLA antigens and von Willebrand's disease. *Proc. HLA and Disease Symp.*[1]
11. Muller, N., Budde, U. & Etzel, F. (1976) von Willebrand's disease and HLA antigens. *Proc. HLA and Disease Symp.*[1]
12. Kissel, P., Raffoux, C.. Faure, G., Andre, J. M., Netter, P. & Streiff, F. (1976) HLA antigens and hereditary haemorrhagic telangiectasia. *Proc. HLA and Disease Symp.*[1]
13. Buc, M., Nyulassy, S., Stefanovic, J., Jakubcoua, I. & Bendekova, M. (1975) HLA2 and congenital heart malformations. *Tissue Antigens* **5**, 128.

[1] References marked with [1] were presented at 1st Int. Symp. on HLA and Disease, INSERM, Paris, June 1976.

14. Coullin, Ph., Bone, A., Bone, N., Ravise, N. & Hors, J. (1976) HLA markers in parents of triploid conceptuses. *Proc. HLA and Disease Symp.*[1]
15. Jenkins, D. M., Need, J. A., Pepper, M. & Scott, J. S. (1976) HLA in severe pre-eclampsia. *Proc. HLA and Disease Symp.*[1]
16. Redman, C. & Bodmer, W. "HLA types" in pre-eclampsia (Unpublished).
17. Piazza, A., Belvedere, M. C., Bernoco, D., Conighi, C., Conti, L., Curtoni, E. S., Mattiuz, P., Mayr, W., Richiardi, P., Scudeller, G. & Cepellini, R. (1973) HLA variation in four Sardinian villages under differential selective pressure by malaria. In: *Histocompatibility Testing* **1972**, eds. Dausset. J. & Bodmer, W., p. 73. Munksgaard, Copenhagen.
18. Honeyman, M. C., Dorman, D. C., Menser, M. A., Forrest, J. M., Guinan, J. J. & Clark, P. (1975) HL-A antigens in congenital rubella and the role of antigens 1 and 8 in the epidemiology of natural rubella. *Tissue Antigens* **5**, 12.
19. Mathews, J. D. (1975) Ischaemic heart disease: possible genetic markers. *Lancet ii,* 681.
20. Mathews, J. D., England, J., Shaw, J., Mathieson, I. D., Hunt, D., Cowling. D. C. & Tait, B. D. (1976) Antigen and haplotype frequencies in essential hypertension and ischaemic heart disease. *Proc. HLA and Disease Symp.*[1]
21. Low, B., Schersten, B., Santor, G., Thulin, T. & Mitelman, F. (1975) HL-A8 and W15 in diabetes mellitus and essential hypertension. *Lancet i,* 695.
22. Gelsthorpe, K., Doughty, R., Bing. R., O'Maltey, B., Smith, A. & Talbot, S. (1975) HL-A antigens in essential hypertension. *Lancet i,* 1039.
23. Seignalet, J., Janbon, C.. Sang, J., Janbon, F., Bidet, J., Brunel, M., Jourdan, J. & Bussiere. J, (1976) HLA in temporal arteritis. *Proc. HLA and Disease Symp.*[1]
24. Merchant, J. A., Klouda, P. T., Soutar, C. A., Parkes, W. R., Lawler, S. D. & Turner-Warwick, M. (1975) The HL-A system in asbestos workers. *Brit. Med. J.* **1**, 189.
25. Matej, H., Lange, A. & Smolik, R. (1976) HLA antigens in asbestosis. *Proc. HLA and Disease Symp.*[1]
26. Gualde, N., de Leobardy, J., Serizay, B. & Malinvaud, G. (1976) HLA and Silicosis. *Proc. HLA and Disease Symp.*[1]
27. Macurova. H., Ivanyi, P., Sajdlova, H. & Trojan, J. (1975) HLA antigens in aged

persons. *Tissue Antigens* **6**, 269.

28. Bender, K., Ruter, G., Mayerova, A. & Hiller, C. (1973) Studies on the heterozygosity at the HLA gene loci in children and old people. *Symp. Ser. Immunobiol. Stand.* S. Karger, Basel **18**, 287.

29. Gerkins, V. R., Ting, A., Menck, H. H., Cassagrande, J., Terasaki, P. I., Pike, M. C. & Henderson, B. E. (1974) HL-A heterozygosity as a genetic marker of long survival. *J. nat. Cancer. Inst.* **52**, 1909.

30. Wood, N. E. & Yunis, E. (1972) HL-A antigens and survival. *Fed. Proc.* **31**, 643.

31. Bender, K., Mayerova, A., Klotzbucker, B., Burckhardt. K. & Hiller, C. (1976) No indication of postnatal selection at the HL-A loci. *Tissue Antigens* **7**, 118.

Possible Mechanisms of Disease-Susceptibility Association with Major Transplantation Antigens

R. M. Zinkernagel[1] & P. C. Doherty[2]

Introduction

What mechanisms underlie the empirically found association between susceptibility to certain diseases and genes mapping at, or close to loci for the major transplantation (H) antigens? Speculation concerning this question or impinging on it, has been a central theme of immunobiology. The topic has been considered by Burnet & Fenner (1), Thomas (2), Burnet (3), Snell (4), Jerne (5), Bodmer (6), Amos et al (7), McDevitt & Bodmer (8), and many others (9–12). The concepts generated have obviously influenced the author's own hypothesis (13–16). Furthermore, many excellent reviews have been written on H antigens (4, 17–20) and their role in defining disease susceptibility (21–26). The authors do not, therefore, attempt to present a comprehensive and detailed account of the subject. The present discussion is confined to broad biological considerations and indications arising from experiments in mice. The experimental approach may prove ultimately to have provided the essential clues for analysis of mechanisms.

For this discussion, some general points should be kept in mind. First, among the many possible phenotypic markers, the major transplantation antigens seem to correlate best with disease susceptibility. Blood groups, for example, were screened intensely without revealing statistically impressive associations (4, 27). Thus, H antigens now appear to be important markers and seem well worth further investigation in this regard. Secondly, susceptibility to disease is a clinical definition. It therefore reflects the sum of a variety of causally related and unrelated factors and is rarely a clearly defined entity. As a direct consequence, associations of disease susceptibility with a certain phenotypic marker, for example H antigen, is rarely if ever absolute. This is particularly true for genetically heterogenous outbred populations such as man. Thirdly, the gene products which influence disease susceptibility may be identical with or linked in variable degrees to genes coding for the phenotypic marker, i.e. H antigen. The more distant such a linkage, the less clear is the association because of possible disruptions of linkage by crossing over. Fourthly,

[1] Scripps Clinic & Research Foundation, La Jolla, Calif. 92037.
[2] The Wistar Institute, Philadelphia, Pa. 19104. This is publication #1146 from the Department of Immunopathology, Scripps Clinic and Research Foundation, La Jolla, Calif. 92037 and publication #2 from the Unit of Immunovirology at the Wistar Institute. Part of this research has been supported by USPHS grant A1-07007.

256

nongenetic factors may play at least two roles. They can act directly or interact with certain genetic phenotypes. The most important ones which may set the stage for the genetically determined factors are environmental factors such as nutritional deficiencies, epidemiological conditions, atopies, basic hygiene and the influence of modern therapeutic medicine. Alternatively, genes influencing susceptibility patterns may map independently of the major H-gene complex (4, 22, 28).

It seems reasonable to assume that the immune system plays an important role in recovery from clinical disease and in disease susceptibility. The strong association between immune response and the H system is thus, perhaps, not unexpected. Strong transplantation antigens aroused immunological interests relatively early (17, 29). Graft rejection was a prominent phenomenon initiating, along with the necessity to develop inbred strains for cancer studies, development of transplantation immunology and of immunogenetics (4, 17–19). The net result is that the gene region coding for the major transplantation antigens is relatively well understood (17) and that current immunological thinking tends to be preoccupied with this region (15, 30–32).

Immunological mechanisms are probably decisive in determining disease susceptibility. However, it has to be kept in mind that immune responses may reflect interaction of complex but balanced contrasting systems. Essential components of this complex regulatory system are the helper and suppressor thymus-derived (T) lymphocytes which regulate generation of effector T cells or antibody formation (33, 34). Lymphokines, complement factors, blocking or enhancing antibodies, α-2-macroglobulin, histamine, slow reactive and C reactive substances may also be involved. Therefore, for example, increased susceptibility may be explained by lack of immune helper T cells or presence of excess suppressor T cells.

The immune response to lymphocytic choriomeningitis virus (LCMV) and perhaps to human hepatitis B virus may serve to illustrate clincally adverse consequences of immune mechanisms on disease (35, 36). If disease is caused by the intrinsic pathogenicity of, for example, a cytopathogenic virus, immune protection would decrease susceptibility to disease because immunity prevents virus from destroying host cells. However, under certain circumstances, for example, if the inherent cytopathogenicity of a virus is small, the immune response may cause pathology. The final result may be increased severity of the disease process as immune mechanisms destroy host cells which would not have been damaged by the virus itself, immunological autoaggression. Thus, for example, immunocompetent mice die of acute choriomeningitis when injected intracerebrally with LCMV (35, 37). Mice which have a deficient cell-mediated immune system survive. However, such mice do not eliminate LCMV because of lack of cellular immunity. Nevertheless, the host survives since the virus itself is poorly cytopathogenic, but the virus-carrier mice may later develop massive immune-complex disease (24, 38).

The complexity of the whole problem of associating disease susceptibility with genes in some degree of linkage disequilibrium with the H marker is great, especially in outbred populations and where multiple genetic and environmental factors can operate. Therefore, unless the associations are extraordinarily strong, only simplified experiments with genetically optimal systems will allow clear concepts to emerge. The mouse model may therefore contribute useful analogies to the analysis of associations between human disease and the human major histocompatibility (HLA) antigens.

Relevance of the mouse models

Most, but by no means all, of the observations which adequately demonstrated association between H antigens and susceptibility to tumor virus originated from experimental murine models. There are many reasons for this. The most crucial one is the availability of a wide range of different inbred, that is, genetically defined, uniform mouse strains. The existense of congenic-resistant strains of identical genetic background, allow comparison of the role of different alleles on a relatively small chromosomal segment (4, 9, 17–19). A considerable variety of congenic recombinant strains is also available to isolate particular genetic regions of the H-2-gene complex in this regard. Certain lines, the recombinant inbred strains, can also be used to give an estimate of the numbers of genes involved and of their relative significance. Unlike the derivation of congenic lines, in which the unwanted genetic contribution of the strain donating the desired characteristic (of H-2) is successively diluted out by repetitive crossing to the acceptor strain, the recombinant inbred lines are the inbred progeny of F1 parents. Two nonidentical strains are mated to produce a number of F1 hybrids which carry all the genes of both parents (except x and y). Pairs of F1 animals are then mated and their progeny successively sib-sib mated. Random contributions from both parents are thus retained and the chromosomal inheritance from parents can be determined (17). Certain human populations approach, to some extent, this type of model. With mice, experiments can be made in great numbers under standard conditions where environmental and other nongenetic factors can be optimally controlled. Many of these mouse strains have survived inbreeding in the laboratory for as long as 50 to 60 years, and have thus been shielded to some extent from some environmental factors such as infections, starvation and predation. This time interval corresponds to more than 150 generations which would represent more than 3000 years of human evolution. Domestication might be considered to have influenced mice in many ways. The lack of selective pressures may have allowed development of strains which are more susceptible to disease than would have been possible under natural conditions. Large-scale breeding may have produced resistance or susceptibility to certain epizootic diseases like ectromelia (mouse pox), Sendai, or lymphocytic choriomeningitis virus infections (39, 40). The selection of only a few H alleles out of the overall balanced polymorphism may enhance the chances of finding distinct different susceptibilities, for example, to one or the other defined infectious agents. Mouse pox in particular can have disastrous consequences when introduced into any mouse colony (40, 41). However, the A strain mouse is, for example, many orders of magnitude more susceptible to cutaneous infection with mouse pox than C57BL mice or mice of most other mouse strains (42).

Possible mechanisms

Mechanisms involving genes linked to the genes coding for the major transplantation antigens

Immune response genes

It is clear from the work of McDevitt and collaborators in mice, and of Benacerraf et al. in the guinea pig, that immune-response (Ir) genes regulate antibody production to certain antigens (43, 44). These Ir genes are linked to the loci coding for the H antigens. In the mouse, the I region is located next to the K region of H-2. Most of the antigens to which the antibody responses have been shown to be Ir dependent are small chemically defined synthetic antigens. However, many of the more common protein antigens, such as ovalbumin, are subject to Ir-gene control when administered in low doses.

The autosomally dominant Ir-gene functions are essentially mediated by T cells and are concerned mainly with the IgG rather than the IgM response. Possible mechanisms of operation of Ir-gene products have been discussed and summarized in various reviews (17, 19, 43, 44). The H-2 region of the mouse codes, in addition, for cell-surface structures present mainly on B cells (antibody-forming cell precursors) and macrophages and, for determinants which are involved in proliferative responses in mixed-lymphocyte reactions *in vitro*. In the HLA-gene complex these various functions are also closely linked together, although they map in a different position relative to the A and 4 loci (18–20, 45). It was thus to be expected in mice that associations would be found between certain I-region haplotypes and disease susceptibilities, that is, to viral or bacterial infections. However, no clear-cut association has yet emerged. Early work showing differential susceptibility for different mouse strains, has not been conclusively mapped as an Ir-gene function (24, 38, 46–48). Susceptibility to Gross virus is associated with the K end of H-2. However, it is not known whether the K region or the I region determines this trait (47). The report on a possible Ir effect on susceptibility to acute lymphocytic choriomeningitis virus infection (24) remains unconfirmed (38). However, some new evidence obtained with the LCMV model indicates, as will be discussed later, that a more direct association of cell-mediated immune response and H antigens may, in part, explain the small but statistically significant difference in the kinetics of occurrence of acute LCM (48).

Complement factors

Other immunologically important structures are coded for in the major histocompatibility complex. In both the murine and the human situation, certain complement (C') factors are coded for, or their serum concentration is determined by genes within or closely linked to this region (19). These C' factors could therefore influence C'-dependent immune mechanisms in an H-dependent fashion. However, a formal demonstration of an association of disease susceptibility with the examples of partial C' deficiencies is lacking.

Mechanisms involving genes coding for the major transplantation antigen

Virus receptor hypothesis

The early findings of an association between H-2 types and of susceptibility to certain tumors which are induced by the Gross virus (46), Friend virus (49), and polyoma virus (50) led Snell to postulate that H antigens, or products of genes closely linked to the H genes, might act as virus receptors (4). There is to date no direct evidence available to support this idea (22). Some data exist, however, which indicate that H antigens do not act as receptors, for example, the HLA or H-2 antigens are apparently not involved in virus absorption or penetration for measles virus (51), or for vesicular stomatitis virus (VSV) (52). More recently, it was shown that murine F9 teratoma cells, which lack detectable H antigens were fully susceptible to infection by lymphocytic choriomeningitis virus and vaccinia virus (53). The receptor model thus remains an unproven possibility.

The mimicry argument

This model postulates that antigenic determinants are shared between infectious agents or tumors and the host's H gene or phenotype or structures coded by genes closely linked to them (4). Accordingly, viruses, bacteria or parasites could in some hosts fail to induce any host response, whether immunological or not, because their antigens mimic self H antigens. The mimicry arguments could explain some increased disease susceptibility which seems to be dominant (e.g., Bittner mammary tumor virus, (54) rather than recessive (e.g., for Gross virus, 24, 46).

The serological crossreactivities between pneumococcal polysaccharides and H-2 antigens or the streptococcal M1 protein and human transplantation antigens (55, 56), although controversial (57), have been discussed as examples of mimicry. This mimicry hypothesis could explain how certain infectious agents in hosts of a particular H type escape immune-defense mechanisms. It also could explain resistance in others, where because of the high degree of

alloreactivity, such foreign "H-mimicking" antigens would induce a vigorous immune response.

The role of the H-2 gene complex in cell-mediated immunity

"Altered self" and dual recognition

The high degree of immune reactivity to foreign transplantation antigens and their polymorphism has been an unexplained phenomenon. Several hypotheses have been advanced to explain this empirical finding and they will be dealt with in the following chapter. Thomas (2) proposed that transplantation antigens may have two functions. First, alloantigen differences may be crucial in the feto-maternal relationship, preventing invasion of maternal tissue by fetal cells. Mammalian embryos, which are heterozygous with respect to their mothers, seem to possess larger placentas and a correspondingly higher birthweight than homozygotes. Second, transplantation antigens may prevent horizontal spread of tumors. There is to date no direct evidence available which would suggest that H antigens really fulfill such a function. Tumor incidence in inbred mouse or hamster colonies is, with the exception of some strains selected for this purpose, no higher than in randomly bred populations. Thomas' argument has been expanded by Burnet in the immunological surveillance concept against developing tumors (3) whereas Jerne and Bodmer separately proposed more general operational interpretations of the relationship of H antigens and immune system (5, 6). Recent findings described below have provided some experimental evidence in support of a generalized concept of immune surveillance of self, though not necessarily in the context of limiting oncogenic processes as stressed by Burnet (13).

260

It is now quite obvious that genes coding for major H antigens or genes mapping in close association play a fundamental role in cell-mediated immunity to virus. The initial crucial finding was that thymus-derived lymphocytes (T cells) from mice infected seven days previously with lymphocytic choriomeningitis virus (LCMV) were able to lyse LCMV-infected target cells *in vitro* (as measured in a ^{51}Cr-release assay) only when the donors of immune lymphocytes and the infected target cells were of the same H-2 type (15, 16, 48, 58). Similar evidence has been obtained independently for cytotoxicity mediated by T cells which were sensitized *in vitro* to trinitrophenol-coupled syngeneic spleen cells (59). Cytotoxic activity generated during ectromelia virus (60), vaccinia virus (61), Sendai virus (58), and some tumor virus infections, such as Friend virus (62), or murine sarcoma virus (63), have been subsequently shown to be H-2 restricted. The effector cells involved are specifically sensitized T cells. LCMV-immune lymphocytes do not lyse vaccinia-infected or Sendai-virus-infected target cells (48). Further analysis of the model (reviewed in 16, 58) revealed that: 1) only the H-2 genes but none of the non-H-2 genes are involved; 2) of the many genetic regions in the murine H-2-gene complex only the K and D regions which code for the major transplantation antigens are relevant; 3) compatibility at one out of the four (in H-2 heterozygotes) possibly different K or D alleles is sufficient; 4) the so-called private unique specificities, but not the public, (i.e. common) specificities are relevant; 5) the I region of H-2 which codes for immune-response (Ir) genes and other lymphocyte surface antigens (as Ia) is neither necessary nor alone sufficient for lytic interactions between virus-specific T cells and infected target cells; and 6) virus-immune T cells

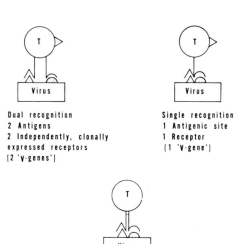

Figure 1.

from some mutant mice expressing a mutation in the K region of H-2 which cause skin-graft rejection when transplanted to wild-type recipients (16, 17, 58) cannot lyse infected H-2K wild-type target cells. These mutations, therefore, probably define the structure on the target, which is involved in cytotoxic T-cell interactions (16, 58, 64, 65).

There is no obvious trivial explanation, such as allogeneic inhibition or suppression for the H-2-restriction phenomenon (16). Two models have been proposed to explain the phenomenon (15, 16, 35, 48, 58, Figure 1).

Dual-recognition model

Virus-immune T cells are specific for viral antigens expressed on cell surfaces. For lysis to occur, a dual recognition has to take place. First, the immunologically specific receptor recognizes virally induced surface antigens. Secondly, for lysis a second independent clonally expressed recognitive structure for self is necessary. It could be envisaged that the two recognition structures both cod-

composite receptor which is specific for a complex of self and viral antigen. Self-recognitive structures are probably not identical to the products of H-2K or H-2D (16, 58, 64, 65). They recognize K or D structures for lytic interactions or I-region structures for helper-type functions. According to this model alloreactive cytotoxicity may be an exception requiring only a single recognition of the alloantigen (64, 65).

Altered-self hypothesis (single recognition)

Virus-specific cytotoxic T cells are specific for virally altered-self cell-surface structure coded for by the K and D regions of H-2, i.e. probably the major transplantation antigens or structures coded by genes which are very closely linked to them. Altered self can be envisaged as virus antigen complexed to K or D structures, as short- or long-range modifications of these structures, as a biochemical alteration, or as derepression of a genetic mechanism regulating expression of multigenically coded H antigens (66, 67). These possibilities have been discussed in more detail elsewhere (16, 58). Thus, cytotoxic T cells possess only one, and interact with an infected target cell only via one, immunologically specific receptor. A virus infection would trigger in homozygote mice the generation of two (four in heterozygotes) sets of T-cell specificities, each associated with one particular altered K- or D-gene product. This model explains cytotoxic T-cell activity against alloantigens as reactivity against one form of altered self.

If one proposes that the T-cell receptor consists of a composite receptor of two chains with distinct V-region equivalents, one for the viral antigen and one for self antigen, the distinction between the two models may become a matter of semantics (66, 67). This com-posite T-cell receptor model is so far functionally indistinguishable from the altered-self model. The following experimental evidence, which has been reviewed recently (16, 58), can be explained by either of the two extreme models. LCMV-infected mice of H-2^k-type generate two sets of cytotoxic virus-specific T cells are either specifically with H-$2K^k$ or alternatively with H-$2D^k$. Thus, in H-2 heterozygote F1 four separate sets of virus-immune T cells are present. According to the altered-self concept, distinct clones of T cells are specific for altered K or altered D structures. According to the dual-interaction model, T cells have two clonally expressed receptors, an immunologically specific one for viral antigens and one interaction structure for a particular K or D structure type (68, Figure 1).

Under conditions where tolerance to alloantigens is induced, as in irradiation, bone-marrow chimeras, virus-immune T cells are generated which can specifically lyse infected target cells of only the tolerated H-2 haplotype (16, 69, 70). Thus, some T cells from chimeras are either specific for altered alloantigen; or according to the dual-recognition model, some chimera T cells express besides the immunological receptor for viral antigen the recognizer for the tolerated alloantigens and therefore are lytic for infected allogeneic but tolerated targets. This and the fact that anti-H-2K or anti-H-2D antisera directed against the target specificities only can block virus-specific cytolytic interactions indicate that for virus-specific cytolysis the H-2K- and H-2D-coded surface structure are mandatory only on the target cell (71, 72). This notion is further supported by the finding that virus-infected target cells lacking H-2 antigens cannot be lysed by immune cytotoxic T cells although they express virus on their

262

surface since they are lysed by antiviral antisera plus complement or by antibody-dependent cell-mediated cytotoxicity (53). The important conclusion from these experiments is that in any case the variety of T-cell specificities is associated with the number and variety of major H-genes.

What is the *in vivo* function of virus-immune cytotoxic T cells? The LCMV model allows discussion of several aspects of virus immunity with respect to disease. In classical adoptive transfer models, it could be shown that LCMV-immune T cells can adoptively transfer the following capacities: first, antiviral protection, as measured by virus titer reduction in virus-infected syngeneic recipients; secondly, delayed-type hypersensitivity, as assessed by induction of footpad swelling in recipients infected acutely in the footpad; and thirdly, induction of acute lymphocytic choriomeningitis, a T-cell-mediated immunopathology leading to death. Kinetics of these *in vivo* functions are, in each case, the same as that of cytotoxic T cell activity *in* vitro. Furthermore, these three *in vivo* T-cell-mediated functions are subject to exactly the same H-2 restriction as demonstrated for *in vitro* cytotoxicity (16, 58).

T cells may, conceptually, exert their antiviral effects in two ways: first, T cells lyse newly infected cells before infectious virus progeny is assembled, and/or secondly, T cells do not actually lyse infected targets but release lymphokines upon contact with the relevant cell-surface antigen as immune interferon, migration inhibitory factor and others. These secreted factors may render surrounding cells resistant to infection by spreading virus. Direct evidence for the first mechanism has been produced. Target cells acutely infected with vaccinia virus can be lysed *in vitro* by virus-immune T cells before in-

fectious progeny is assembled (73). Evidence supporting the second effector mechanism mediated by lymphokines has been recently reviewed (74, 75). The relative importance of these two effector mechanisms probably varies between viruses. It must be emphasized that the role of T-cell-mediated or humoral immunity overall also varies with the virus or bacterium. It appears, however, that for viruses in general and for intracellular bacteria, cell-mediated immunity is a crucial early defense mechanism (40, 74, 75). Thus, the capacity of a particular agent to induce T help for the production of antibody may also be of major importance in recovery from infection. As the T-helper function is associated with structures coded in the H-2I region (31, 32, 76), it is only a speculation to propose that antigen associated with the structures probably trigger T helpers for B cells and possibly also for the generation of cytotoxic T cells (18, 20).

Thus, not only cytotoxic but also helper T-cell functions are associated with genes coding for major transplantation antigens or genes closely linked to them. These associations between immune-effector and regulatory mechanisms with the major H-gene complex may be the basis of at least one possible and likely reason for some of the empirically found associations between the H marker and disease susceptibility. A self-monitoring concept operating via the major H antigens thus proposes that the biological function of the major H-gene complex is to signal changes in self or in association with these self structures to the immune system (13, 15). The function of thymus-derived lymphocytes is to monitor the self markers coded for in the H-2-gene region to single out cells which show alterations on the cell surface in association with self structures. Cells bearing virus-induced, chemical modifications or alloantigens may thus be eliminated by these surveillance T cells.

This hypothesis has the following implications which could, mechanistically, explain at least some of the observed disease susceptibility associations with H systems. If different clones of virus-immune T cells are associated with each H-gene expressed then heterozygosity and gene duplication at the H-gene complex should be of selective advantage. In fact, H-2-heterozygous mice generate 140–200 % of the cell-mediated immune response of H-2-homozygous mice (14, 77). Furthermore, if one virus fails to associate with one particular H self marker immunogeneically, and if only one or a few H alleles existed, such an event could have disastrous consequences not only for an individual but for the whole species. H-gene duplication (19) and selection for heterozygosity could have given rise to polymorphism to avoid such an event. The multiplicity of potentially lethal infectious agents would prevent the positive selection of H types which would confer protection to only one virus, explaining the observed balanced polymorphism. However, the K and/or D types which happen to be »altered« less immunogeneically by one agent could be associated with increased susceptibilities, for example, to disease caused by cytopathogenic viruses. On the other hand, immunogeneic alteration in association with self markers would favor resistance. As pointed out previously, the reverse is true if immunopathological mechanisms determine disease. An extreme experimental example of such a T-cell-mediated immunopathology is acute fatal lymphocytic choriomeningitis developing after intracerebral infection of LCMV. A greater percentage of H-2 heterozygous mice die earlier than homozygous mice (14).

Whether the altered-self concept is generally applicable to, for example, all viruses which cause generation of cytotoxic T cells remains an open question. Also, whether such a concept can explain most of the examples of associations of H antigens and disease susceptibility remains to be seen. The H-restriction phenomenon has to be confirmed for many more antigens and has to be demonstrated (or disproven) in another species, particularly in man.

The lack of easy demonstration of such an HLA restriction in man may not be surprising since inbred strains do not exist. The following factors make it unlikely that the restriction will be as obvious as between inbred mouse strains. First, the great crossreactivity of various HLA types as defined today at least in serological terms (78), and secondly that some HLA alleles (which may be public antigens according to the H-2 terminology) are widely shared in some human populations (79) and, thirdly that compatibility at one out of four H-antigen loci is sufficient for T-cell interactions. This is also clear from a study in outbred mouse colonies of restricted heterogeneity, which showed that virus-immune cytotoxic T cells of individuals could lyse infected macrophage targets of other members. But, virus-specific cytotoxicity generated in different outbred strains of distinct origin were active only on target cells from the same strain (80). However, outbred mouse strains are derived from a much smaller gene pool than could be expected in any human population. The existing evidence failing to show HLA restriction in the Epstein-Barr killer-cell system may therefore be well explained (81). It seems quite likely from the evidence obtained in the mouse that in human studies of cellular immunity against conventional viruses or in tumor systems, the use of heterolo-

264

gous target cells (e.g. infected hamster-kidney cells) may only allow demonstration of antibody-dependent lymphocyte-mediated cytotoxicity (82, 83), rather than direct T-cell-mediated cytotoxicity. It would seem probable that cell-mediated immunity to viruses in humans is also strongly associated with the major transplantation antigens. Not only are the two murine and human H systems similar, even in molecular terms (84, 85), but it is also unlikely that their cell-mediated immune system should differ vastly.

References

1. Burnet, F. M. & Fenner, F. J. (1949) *The Production of Antibodies.* Monogr. Walter & Eliza Hall Inst., MacMillan, Melbourne.
2. Thomas, L. In: (1958) *Cellular and Humoral Aspects of the Hypersensitive States,* ed. Lawrence, H. S., p. 529, Hoeber, New York.
3. Burnet, F. M. (1970) *Immunological Surveillance,* Pergamon Press, Sidney, Australia.
4. Snell, G. D. (198) The H-2 locus of the mouse: Observations and speculations concerning its comparative genetics and its polymorphism. *Folia. Biol.* **14**, 335.
5. Jerne, N. K. (1971) The somatic generation of immune recognition. *Europ. J. Immunol.* **1**, 1.
6. Bodmer, W. F. (1972) Evolutionary significance of the HLA system. *Nature (Lond.)* **237**, 139.
7. Proceedings of Fogerty International Center, No. 15 (1972) Biological significance of histocompatibility antigens. *Fed. Proc.* **31**, 1087.
8. McDevitt, H. O. & Bodmer, W. F. (1974) HLA immune response gene and disease. *Lancet* **i**, 1269.
9. Klein, J. An attempt at an interpretation of the mouse H-2 complex. *Current Topics in Immunobiol.* **5**, (in press).
10. Allison, A. C. (1971) Unresponsiveness to self-antigens. *Lancet* **ii**, 1401.
11. Martin, W. J. (1975) Immune surveillance directed against depressed cellular and viral alloantigens. *Cell. Immunol.* **15**, 1.
12. Mitchison, N. A. (1954) Passive transfer of transplantation immunity. *Proc. roy. Soc. Lond. Ser. B* **142**, 72.
13. Doherty, P. C. & Zinkernagel, R. M. (1975) A biological role for the major histocompatibility antigens. *Lancet* **i**, 1406.
14. Doherty, P. C. & Zinkernagel, R. M. (1975) Immune surveillance and the role of major histocompatibility antigens. *Nature (Lond.)* **256**, 50.
15. Zinkernagel, R. M. & Doherty, P. C. (1974) Activity of sensitized thymus derived lymphocytes in lymphocytic choriomeningitis reflects immunological surveillance against altered self components. *Nature (Lond.)* **251**, 547.
16. Zinkernagel, R. M. & Doherty, P. C. Major transplantation antigens, virus and specificity of surveillance T cells: The altered self hypothesis. *Contemp. Topics Immunobiol.* **7**, (in press).
17. Klein, J. (1975) *Biology of the mouse histocompatibility-2 complex.* Springer-Verlag, New York.
18. Amos, D. B. & Ward, F. E. (1975) Immunogenetics of the HLA system. *Physiol. Rev.* **55**, 206.
19. Shreffler, D. C. & David, C. S. (1974) The H-2 major major histocompatibility complex and the I immune response region: Genetic variation, function and organization. *Adv. Immunol.* **20**, 125.
20. Bach, F. J., Bach, M. L. & Sondel, P. M. (1975) Differential function of major histocompatibility complex antigens in T lymphocyte activation. *Nature (Lond.)* **259**, 273.
21. Amos, D. B., Inou, T. & Rowland, D. T. (1973) Human histocompatibility and susceptibility to disease. *Science* **182**, 183.
22. Dausset, J. (1972) Correlation between histocompatibility antigens and susceptibility to illness. *Prog. Clin. Immunol.* **1**, 183.
23. Haverkorn, M. J., Hofman, B., Masurel, N. & van Kood, J. (1975) HLA linked genetic control of immune response in man. *Transplant. Rev.* **22**, 120.
24. McDevitt, H. O., Oldstone, M. B. A. & Pincus, T. (1974) Histocompatibility-linked genetic control of specific immune responses to viral infection. *Transplant. Rev.* **19**, 209.
25. Vladutiu, A. O. & Rose, N. R. (1974) HLA antigens: Association with disease. *Immunogenetics* **1**, 305.

26. Morris, P. J. (1974) Histocompatibility systems immune response and disease in man. *Contemp. Topics Immunobiol.* **3**, 141.

27. Muschel, L. H. (1966) Blood groups, disease and selection. *Bact. Rev.* **30**, 427.

28. Goodman, G. T. & Koprowski, H. (1962) Macrophages as a cellular expression of inherited natural resistance. *Proc. nat. Acad. Sci. (Wash.)* **48**, 160.

29. Gorer, P. A. (1937) The genetic and antigenic basis of tumor transplantation. *J. Pathol. Bacteriol.* **44**, 691.

30. Lennox, E. (1975) Viruses and histocompatibility antigens: An unexpected interaction. *Nature (Lond.)* **256**, 7.

31. Katz, D. H. & Benacerraf, B. (1975) The function and interrelationship of T cell receptors, Ir genes and other histocompatibility gene products. *Transplant. Rev.* **22**, 175.

32. Katz, D. H. & Benacerraf, B. (1976) *The Role of Products of the Histocompatibility Gene Complex in Immune Responses.* Academic Press, New York, (in press).

33. Bretscher, P. A. (1974) On the control between cell-mediated IgM and IgG immunity. *Cell. Immunol.* **13**, 171.

34. Gershon, R. K. (1974) T cell control of antibody production. *Contemp. Topics Immunol.* **3**, 1.

35. Doherty, P. C. & Zinkernagel, R. M. (1974) T cell-mediated immunopathology in viral infections. *Transplant. Rev.* **19**, 89.

36. Mackayy, I. R. & Morris, P. J. (1972) Association of auto-immune active chronic hepatitis with HLA 1, 8. *Lancet* **ii**, 793.

37. Hotchin, J. (1971) Persistent and slow virus infections. *Monog. Virol.* **3**, 1.

38. Oldstone, M. B. A. Relationship between major histocompatibility antigens and disease: Possible associations to human arenavirus diseases. Int. Symp. on Arenaviral Infections of Public Health Importance, *W.H.O. Bulletin,* (in press).

39. Fenner, F. J. (1968) *The Biology of Animal Viruses,* vol. III. Academic Press, New York.

40. Blanden, R. V. (1974) T cell response to viral and bacterial infection. *Transplant. Rev.* **19**, 5.

41. Anslow, R. O., Ewald, B. H., Paknes, S. P., Small, J. D. & Whitney, R. A. (1975) Control of infectious diseases among rodent stocks. *Science* **189**. 248.

42. Blanden, R. V., Deak, B. & McDevitt, H. O. (unpublished observation).

43. Benacerraf, B. & McDevitt, H. O. (1972) Histocompatibility-linked immune response genes. *Science* **175**, 273.

44. Benacerraf, B. (1975) Immune response genes. *Scand. J. Immunol.* **4**, 381.

45. Yunis, E. J. & Amos, D. B. (1971) Three closely linked genetic syystems relevant to transplantation. *Proc. nat. Acad. Sci. (Wash.)* **68**, 3031.

46. Lilly, F., Boyse, E. A. & Old, L. J. (1964) Genetic basis of susceptibility to viral leukemogenesis. *Lancet* **ii**, 1207.

47. Vladutiu, A. O. & Rose, N. R. (1971) Autoimmune murine thyroiditis relation to histocompatibility (H-2) type. *Science* **174**, 1137.

48. Zinkernagel, R. M. & Doherty, P. C. (1974) Restriction of *in vitro* T cell-mediated cytotoxicity in lymphocytic choriomeningitis within a syngeneic or semiallogeneic system. *Nature (Lond.)* **248**, 701.

49. Lilly, F. (198) The influence of histocompatibility-2 type on response to the Friend leukemia virus in mice. *J. exp. Med.* **127**, 665.

50. Sjögren, H. O. & Ringertz, N. (1961) Histopathology and transplantability of polyoma-induced tumors in strain A/Sn and three coisogeneic resistant substrains. *J. nat. Cancer Inst.* **28**, 859.

51. Joseph, B. & Oldstone, M. B. A. (1975) Replication and persistence of measles virus in defined subpopulations of human leukocytes. *J. Virol.* **16**, 1638.

52. Hecht, T. & Summers, D. (1972) Effect of vesicular stomatitis virus infection on the histocompatibility antigen of L-cells. *J. Virol.* **10**, 578.

53. Zinkernagel, R. M. & Oldstone, M. B. A. (1976) F9 mouse teratoma cells lacking H-2K and H-2D are permissive for virus and are lysed by antibody dependent but not by T-cell mediated virus-specific immune attack. *Proc. nat. Acad. Sci. (Wash.),* **13**, 3666.

54. Nandi, S. (1967) The histocompatibility-2 locus and susceptibility to red blood cell-borne Bittner virus in mice. *Proc. nat. Acad. Sci. (Wash.)* **58**, 485.

55. Rapaport, F. T., Chase, R. M. & Soloway, D. C. (1966) Transplantation antigen activity of bacterial cells in different animal species and intracellular localization. *Ann. N.Y. Acad. Sci.* **129**, 102.

56. Hirata, A. A. & Terasaki, P. I. (1970) Cross reactions between streptococcal glycoproteins and human transplantation antigens. *Science* **168**, 1095.

266

57. Fox, E. N. & Peterson, R. D. (1970) Streptococcal M protein, vaccines, rheumatic fever and human histocompatibility antigens. *J. Immunol.* **105**, 1031.

58. Doherty, P. C., Blanden, R. V. & Zinkernagel, R. M. (1976) Specificity of virus-immune effector T cells for H-2K or H-2D compatible interactions. Implications for H-antigen diversity. *Transplant. Rev.* **29**, 89.

59. Shearer, G. M. (1974) Cell-mediated cytotoxicity to trinitrophenyl-modified syngeneic lymphocytes. *Europ. J. Immunol.* **4**, 527.

60. Blanden, R. V., Doherty, P. C., Dunlop, M. B. C., Gardner, I. D., Zinkernagel, R. M. & David, C. S. (1975) Genes required for T cell-mediated cytotoxicity against virus infected target cells are in the K or D region of the H-2 gene complex. *Nature (Lond.)* **254**, 269.

61. Koszinowski, H. & Ertl, H. (1975) Lysis mediated by T cells and restricted by H-2 antigen of target cells infected with vaccinia virus. *Nature (Lond.)* **255**, 552.

62. Blank, K. J., Freedman, H. A. & Lilly, F. T. (1976) T lymphocyte response to Friend virus-induced tumor cell lines in mice of strains congeneic at H-2. *Nature (Lond.)* **260**, 250.

63. Gomard, E., Duprez, V., Henin, Y. & Levy, J. P. (1976) H-2 region products as determinants in immune cytolysis of syngeneic tumor cells by anti-MSV T lymphocytes. *Nature (Lond).* **260**, 707.

64. Doherty, P. C., Gotze, D., Trinchieri, G. & Zinkernagel, R. M. (1976) Models for recognition of virally modified cells by immune thymus derived lymphocytes. *Immunogenetics* **3**, 517.

65. Zinkernagel, R. M. & Doherty, P. C. The concept that T cell recognition of virally modified cells is mediated via the same V gene subset that determines alloreactivity. *Cold Spring Harbor Symp. Quant. Biol.* **42**, (in press).

66. Invernitzi, G. & Parmiani, G. (1975) Tumor-associated transplantation antigens of chemically induced sarcoma cross reacting with alloantigeneic histocompatibility antigens. *Nature (Lond.)* **254**, 713.

67. Garrido, F., Schirmacher, V. & Festenstein, H. (1976) H-2-like specificity of foreign haplotypes appearing on a mouse sarcoma vaccinia virus infection. *Nature (Lond.)* **259**, 228.

68. Zinkernagel, R. M. & Doherty, P. C. (1975) H-2 compatibility requirement with lymphocytic-choriomeningitis virus.

Different cytotoxic T cell specificities are associated with structures coded in H-2K or H-2D. *J. exp. Med.* **141**, 1427.

69. Pfizenmaier, K., Starzinski-Powitz, A., Rodt, H., Rollinghoff, M. & Wagner, H. (1976) Virus and TNP-hapten specific T cell mediated cytotoxicity against H-2 incompatible target cells. *J. exp. Med.* **143**, 999.

70. Zinkernagel, R. M. (1976) Virus specific T cell mediated cytotoxicity across the H-2 barrier to "virus-altered alloantigens". *Nature (Lond.)* **261**, 139.

71. Germain, R. M., Dorf, M. E. & Benacerraf, B. (1975) Inhibition of T-lymphocyte mediated tumor-specific lysis by alloantisera directed against the H-2 serological specificities of the tumor. *J. exp. Med.* **142**, 1023.

72. Schrader, J. W., Cunningham, B. A. & Edelman, G. M. (1975) Functional interactions of viral and histocompatibility antigens at tumor cell surfaces. *Proc. nat. Acad. Sci. (Wash.)* **72**, 5066.

73. Zinkernagel, R. M. (1977) Anti-viral protection by virus-immune cytotoxic T cells: Infected target cells are lysed before infectious virus progency is assembled. *J. exp. Med.,* (in press).

74. Bloom, B. R. & Rager-Zisman, B. (1976) Cell-mediated immunity in viral infections. *Viral Immunology and Immunopathology,* ed. Notkins, A. L. p. 113, Academic Press, New York.

75. Notkins, A. L. (1976) Interferon as a mediator of cellular immunity in viral infections. *Viral Immunology and Immunopathology,* ed. Notkins, A. L., p. 149, Academic Press, New York.

76. Kindred, B. & Shreffler, D. C. (1972) H-2 dependence or cooperation between T and B cells *in vivo. J. Immunol.* **109**, 940.

77. Degos, L., Colombani, J., Chavente, A., Bengtson, B. & Jacquard, A. (1974) Selective pressure on HLA polymorphism. *Nature (Lond.)* **249**, 62.

78. Mittal, K. K. & Terasaki, P. I. (1972) Cross-reactivity in the HLA system. *Tissue Antigens* **2**, 94.

79. Dausset, J., Colombani, J., Legrand, L., Lepage, V., Marcelli-Barge, A. & Dehay, C. (1972) Population and family studies in a French population with special reference to non-HLA antibodies. *Histocompatibility Testing 1972,* p. 107, Munksgaard, Copenhagen.

80. Zinkernagel, R. M., Dunlop, M. B. C. & Doherty, P. C. (1975) Cytotoxic T cell

activity is strain specific in outbred mice infected with lymphocytic choriomeningitis virus. *J. Immunol.* **115**, 1613.

81. Jöndal, M., Svedmyr, E., Klein, E. & Singh, S. (1975) Killer T cells in a Burkitt's lymphoma biopsy. *Nature (Lond.)* **255**, 404.

82. Steele, R. W., Hensen, S. A., Vincent, M. M., Faccillo, D. A. & Bellanti, J. A. (1973) A ^{51}Cr microassay technique for cell-mediated immunity to viruses. *J. Immunol.* **110**, 1502.

83. Ramshaw, I. A. (1975) Lysis of herpes virus-infected target cells by immune spleen cells. *Infect. Immunol.* **11**, 767.

84. Terhorst, C., Parham, P., Mann, D. L. & Strominger, J. (1976) Structure of HLA antigens: Amino acid and carbohydrate composition and NH$_2$-terminal sequences of 4 antigen preparations. *Proc. nat. Acad. Sci. (Wash.)* **73**, 910.

85. Vitetta, E. S., Capra, J. D., Klapper, D. G., Klein, J. & Uhr, J. W. (1976) The partial amino acid sequence of an H-2K molecule. *Proc. nat. Acad. Sci. (Wash.)* **73**, 905.

Theoretical Consideration in the Association Between HLA and Disease[1]

D. B. Amos[2] & F. E. Ward[3]

Introduction

The original disease association reported in man, between Hodgkin's disease and the specificity originally described as 4c, was not a close one and indeed has not been fully substantiated in later studies (1, 2). This attempt, however, was the forerunner of many subsequent searches for correlations between leukocyte-antigen markers and diseases. Several different correlations have emerged; some are detectable at the population level while some are detectable only at the haplotype level within families. Most of the associations were first detected using the HLA-A and HLA-B markers of the HLA system; more recently better correlations have been found with HLA-D and with antigens restricted to B lymphocytes. Most of the associations are much stronger than those reported with any red-cell marker except perhaps the association between resistance to malaria and the Duffy blood group.

However, susceptibility to disease is a clinical definition. It is an interesting finding that diseases associated with HLA are often not easily categorized; a precise diagnosis is often difficult and some of the criteria for defining them are probably inadequate. What is presently classified as a single disease or disease syndrome may result from phenotypic similarity between the expression of two or more underlying processes. The splitting process, so familiar to HLA serologists, may be contagious and may soon extend to the classification of diseases. Also, many of the diseases appear to be dependent upon the coincidental presence of more than one gene, and environmental factors may be very marked depending upon the degree of access to the agent (allergen, pathogen, etc.) and also to the gene or genes affected.

[1] The authors were originally asked by Dr. Dausset to collaborate with Drs. Zinkernagel and Doherty on the preceeding manuscript. As writing progressed, however, it became apparent that much of the detailed knowledge from the mouse was simply not available for man, and may indeed not be applicable. It was also apparent that disease associations with HLA are much more varied than those known for the mouse. The authors, therefore, decided to write a coda for the Zinkernagel & Doherty paper.

[2] Division of Immunology and Veterans Administration Hospital. Supported in part by USPHS funds # GM-10356 and K06 AI-18399.

[3] Duke University Medical Center, Division of Immunology, Durham N. C. 27710.

269

The nature of an H system

It appears that each species has a major H system, a collection of genetic loci involved in immunologic processes. Each major H system (the HLA region in man and the H-2 region in the mouse) includes one or more genetic loci coding for glycoproteins which are expressed on all lymphoid tissues, on epidermal cells, and on most somatic tissues (3). These glycoproteins or H antigens resemble immunoglobulins in that some sequences are highly mutable, while other portions of the molecule are conserved. Consequently, there is considerable sequence homology between the H antigens of widely separated species such as the mouse and man. This similarity was first shown for the antigens of the D and K loci of H-2 and the A- or B-locus antigens of HLA, but evidence to date also suggests great similarities between the Ia antigens of the mouse and the B-cell antigens of man (4). The major H system also includes genes regulating cellular and humoral responsiveness. The products of the H system are critical for recognition processes, particularly at the T-cell level, and different T subsets are highly sensitive to differences between haplotypes, especially within the species (5). Regulation of complement component levels is another attribute of an H system. It is believed that there are at least 10 genetic loci, relevant to the immunological system, in the HLA region. To the three HLA loci, A, B, and C, must be added at least two structural loci for antigens expressed on B cells. There appear to be at least four loci controlling complement and regulating the level of immune responsiveness, though it is not completely clear which of these are structural and which are regulatory. HLA-D requires one and more probably two loci, and the MLR also requires a response gene, although this could be an ancillary function of one of the known Ir genes. It is usually concluded that the structural H antigens serve as the targets for cellular immunity in allograft reactions in the same way that they stimulate a humoral response. This has not been unequivocally proven, and soluble H products lack much of the immunogenicity of the intact cell. To overcome some of the problems of relating cellular responsiveness to HLA, Yunis & Amos presented an hypothesis that placed a separate gene evoking cellular immune responses close to but outside HLA-B (6). Preliminary evidence of CML in the recombinant Schl. family suggest this location was correct (7). It still seems fair to state now, as the authors did in 1971, that although much is known of the individual components of the region and of the biological properties of the region as a whole, detailed information about the precise number of genetic loci, the activities of the individual loci, and of the collaboration between genes in cis (and even possibly in trans) relationship still need further intensive investigation.

For many reasons, studies in man have followed different pathways from studies in mice and other laboratory animals, and the types of diseases studied are often different. The classic example of a disease associated with HLA in man is ankylosing spondylitis (AS) and HLA-B27, but as yet no such disease as AS has been described in the mouse. Susceptibility to Gross, FMR group, and Tennant viruses are firmly established for specific alleles of the mouse (8). Human leukemia viruses are not yet known for man (despite intensive searching, no particular haplotype or A, B or C specificity appears to be assoc-

270

iated with human leukemia), and the only leukemia association appears to be between chronic lymphocytic leukemia and the Merritt system of B-cell antigens (9). However, the Merritt system has many alleles and at least some of the antigens are detectable on normal B lymphocytes (10). Any of a number of alleles can be found on cells from a leukemic individual, so either there are a dozen human leukemia viruses each associated with a different Merritt allele or the analogy between the mouse and man breaks down.

There are other differences between the H system of the mouse and man. Position of the genes on the chromosome is one of them. Strong MLC stimulation has been mapped to the I region of H-2, i.e., between D and K, with D and K being almost universally recognized as the outer limits of the H-2 region. Strong MLC stimulation in man has been located in the D region of HLA and this locus maps outside the A and B regions. HLA thus appears to be open ended. The designation HL-í has been proposed for this loosely defined complex of H genes which includes Ir, the A, B, and C loci of HLA, HLA-D and the genes for B-cell antigens. However, there are some ambiguities in both systems. Of the many intra-H-2 recombinations, only two place I inside K, and the possibility that these represent double recombinants cannot be ignored (11). Genes with products similar to those of the D and K loci have been reported outside D. Serologic and transplantation studies have established at least two and possibly four H loci lying between D and *Tla* and at least one (and probably at least two) H loci have been located between K and *tf,* five crossover units away (12, 13). There is presumptive evidence for an Ia-like antigen outside the limits of D and K (14), and a search is being made for Ir function outside the limits of H-2. In man, the map distance between HLA-B and HLA-D has been estimated to be approximately 0.5 units. This is not a firm figure and is largely based on the incidence of stimulation between HLA-identical sibs. By analogy with the mouse, at least some of the "recombinants" are likely to be mutants. In the mouse, mutants are detected in inbred lines and in F_1-hybrid animals from crosses of two inbred strains, so recombination at the gametic level can be excluded. Mutants may be serologically indistinguishable from the parental type but MLR and skin or tumor rejection reveals the immunologic difference. Mutants of this type appear to reflect an unusually high mutation rate at a locus or loci within the H-2 system. The distinction between mutation and recombination in man can only be made if, (a) a sibling sharing both HLA-D alleles of the recombinant is available, or (b) the recombinant HLA-D allele can be identified by typing with the appropriate homozygous typing cell.

Human model systems

Whereas the laboratory mouse has been selected for adaptation to domestication for at least a century, and further selected and made more homogeneous by successive inbreeding for up to 100 generations, the human population is outbred to very varying degrees. It is easily possible to select mice of any desired characteristic, whether this be high incidence of a particular tumor, renal disease, retinal degeneration, or an enzymatic or immunological defect, and to repeat an observation changing one variable at a time if desired. By contrast, human experimentation is quite different, and the methods of study must be adapted accordingly. Except for monozygotic twins, human individuals are genotypically and phenotypically unique. Even monozygotic twins show phenotypic differences. Ethical considerations, (some of legal sanction and some imposed by the beliefs of the investigator), the size of the usual human family, and the impossibility of exactly repeating any *in vivo* determination are all additional factors to be dealt with.

To obtain direct evidence for an H-linked disease gene by simple association analysis using population data, there must be significant genetic disequilibrium between the pertinent "disease-gene" allele and a specific HLA allele. Otherwise, genetic recombination between the HLA gene and the disease gene would soon eliminate any initial allelic association in the population. Furthermore, it should be noted that even in the case where significant population association can be demonstrated, one cannot conclude that this association is due to the activities of linked genes. An alternative explanation might be a common precursor substance. It is obvious, also, that variant expression of the "disease-gene" allele because of incomplete penetrance, modifying genes, and the effects of a host of environmental factors, etc., could reduce the measure of association.

Fortunately, many of the problems inherent in any study of man can be circumvented. In some instances where they cannot, animal experimentation can supplement human experimentation. Genetic studies may be carried out in two, three and occasionally four generation families. Detection of an H-linked gene by family studies does not require genetic disequilibrium between

alleles of the two genes, a possible advantage over population studies. In many populations, "super families" of over 100 members can be identified, thus some features such as the attributes of certain haplotypes can be determined against a variety of genetic backgrounds. Within large families, sibs sharing the same haplotypes can be contrasted with sibs or parents sharing one of the haplotypes, and with other sibs sharing neither. Covariate and other forms of statistical analysis can reduce the background "noise" from multigenic inheritance and variability of environmental factors, etc.

While the majority of populations is outbred, certain groups have considerable degrees of consanguinity. Religious, geographic, ethnic, and cultural isolates are found in all areas of the world and some, such as the Hutterites, the Amish, Bedouins, inhabitants of formerly isolated areas such as the Outer Banks of North Carolina etc., have given valuable information about the frequency of HLA haplotypes in closed populations and are now being used especially profitably for linkage studies for immune-response genes. From studies of antibody levels to eight common pathogenic viruses in Amish families, at least two genetic systems of Ir are found to segregate together, one linked and one not linked to HLA (15).

Recombination within the HLA system itself is not uncommon and families with two recombinant members are known. Whether clustering of recombinants in H-2 or HLA is purely fortuitious remains to be determined, but the suspicion can be entertained that it is not. Recombinants also seem to be more common in families contacted through hospitals than those found in the field. Whether this reflects population fitness also remains to be determined and must await the establishment of a registry of recombinants. However, despite the relatively short interval since the description of the first HLA recombinants, more recombinants have already been described within the HLA region than within H-2. By comparing intraregional recombination and recombinants between HLA and outside markers, fine genetic mapping can be accomplished.

One other feature of the HLA haplotype that is too recently described to have found extensive use as yet, is the rich variety of biochemical and red-cell polymorphisms showing varying degrees of linkage to HLA, some apparently very loosely linked and others at 10 or less crossover units distant (16). Linkage studies will show if linkage disequilibrium is a result of hybridization between antigenically distinct population groups or if it has some selective advantage. Some of the theoretical ways in which the HLA haplotype could express a selective advantage have recently been presented and will not be discussed here (17). It does appear to the authors, however, that the conservation of so many diverse genes together on a short chromosomal segment in species as diverse as the mouse and man cannot possibly be fortuitous. These genes must be clustered together in order to subserve a series of integrated functions, many of which are probably still unrecognized and which contribute to health or disease. The possibility that linkage disequilibrium is not fortuitous must be borne in mind.

Maintenance of the extreme linkage disequilibrium seen between various alleles of genes within the HLA complex may also "trap" other genetic loci within this chromosomal region. Enzyme deficiencies or variants could possibly be candidates for such "trapped" genes, and an apparent association between HLA and the resulting clinical state would be expected.

Genes controlling factors in the complement system might be an integral part of the HLA complex, actively maintained within it, or they might be examples of trapped genes. The first complement-related gene to be linked to HLA, Bf, maps within the HLA region, defined by HLA-A and HLA-D (18). This pro-activator gene for C_3 may be analogous to a gene in the Ss-Slp region of the H-2 system (19). A gene involved in the alternate pathway, such as Bf, could be expected to influence disease resistance and/or susceptibility, but this may be of a general nature and, hence, not associated with a particular disease state. Deficiencies for and/or electrophoretic variants of complement factors C_1, C_2, C_3, C_4, C_5, C_6, and C_8 have been identified, and their association with the HLA complex has been examined by family studies. Deficiencies for $C_1{}^r$, C_5, and C_6 apparently do not segregate with HLA haplotypes (20, 21, 22) and do not appear to be closely linked to HLA. The gene for electrophoretic variants of C_3 and C_6 does not segregate with HLA either (23, 24). C_2, C_4, and C_8 deficiencies, on the other hand, do segregate with HLA haplotypes (25, 26, 27), and attempts are now being made to map these genes on chromosome 6. Deficiency for C_2 is most common, and consequently best studied. It is often associated with the A10-B18 haplotype (28), possibly because of linkage disequilibrium, but associations with other HLA alleles have been described (29).

The genetic control for C_6 appears to be somewhat ambiguous. A family showing apparent non-linkage of C_6 to HLA was a small one (22). Recombination cannot be excluded as a cause of apparent independent segregation.

Other information places a structural gene in linkage with HLA and several map units from it. The placing of a structural gene for C_6 outside the HLA- A and -D loci indicates, as in the mouse, that genes relevant to immunological function may be scattered along a considerable segment of chromosome.

Mechanisms

Possible mechanisms to explain the association between particular components of the HLA system, or an HLA haplotype, and disease can be listed as follows:

1) Immune-response genes linked to HLA
2) Molecular mimicry
3) Receptors
4) Abnormal expression of a differentiation antigen
5) Interaction of environmental factors with the genome
6) Modified self
7) Complement factors
8) Enzymatic modifications
9) Common precursor.

Immune-response genes

The possible importance of immune-response genes in the etiology of disease has been stressed by many investigators. Supporting evidence for this comes from studies with ragweed hypersensitivity, from an examination of viral antibody titers, and a response to cutaneous allergens, including pollens and microbial and fish proteins (30, 31). The original observation of Levine *et al.* (32) indicates linkage of ragweed antigen E hypersensitivity to the HLA haplotype in families. This was confirmed by Blumenthal *et al.* (33), and although challenged by Bias & Marsh (34) who instead reported an association with an HLA-7 crossreacting group of specificities (35), evidence is accumulating of linkage to the haplotype rather than to

the specificity. Studies of antibody levels to ragweed antigens are in progress. Antibody levels to many common viruses are HLA-haplotype associated within Amish families (15). Cellular responsiveness to streptococcal nuclease is associated with the presence of HLA-B5 (36), and is now known to segregate with the HLA haplotype in families (37). The authors would like to introduce one additional concept into the discussion of the relevance of Ir genes to disease. It is usually assumed that the functions of the Ir genes are regulatory, since different alleles control the level of antibody synthesis to a given antigen. Variations in complement component levels are also taken as evidence for regulatory genes. It is possible that neither of these assumptions is right, and certainly it should be pointed out that the usual conceptions *are* based on assumptions. It is quite interesting to speculate what might happen if some of the Ir genes coded for structural products on B cells or T cells that acted as receptors for antigens.

Molecular mimicry

An infectious or other environmental agent having a similarity to a normal tissue antigen is likely to elicit a weaker immune response than an agent which is clearly different. While crossreactivity to streptococcal M protein has been reported, the nature of the shared determinant, if any, is not known (38). Attempts have been made to demonstrate crossreactivity with a variety of bacterial antigens, but the only positive finding was weak crossreactivity with Salmonella (39).

Receptor

The clearest example of the importance of a receptor and the outcome of a disease producing infection relates to the Duffy (40) rather than the HLA system, but it is indicative of the type of association being sought. Duffy-null individuals are rare; however, a high concentration of such individuals has been found in Nigeria. Infants of this phenotype resist malarial infection because they lack the receptor for the malarial parasite. A similar phenomenon may exist in gluten-sensitive enteropathy (41). Diseased individuals appear to possess a receptor for gliadin. Some antisera also react with this receptor and can block the attachment of the antigen. While this receptor itself is not under control of the HLA system, GSE patients frequently possess the specificity HLA-B8 and even more frequently type as HLA-Dw3, indicating a possible link between genes of the HLA region and the development of the receptor. Since receptors for virus and the ability of the cell to transport virus across the membrane play a large part in the susceptibility of individuals to a variety of viral diseases too, epidemiologic opportunities during a pandemic of influenza could perhaps be informative.

Abnormal differentiation antigens

In this section the authors will examine the possibility that genes important for normal differentiation are expressed on the same chromosome and possibly on the same haplotype. The mouse 17th chromosome carries several loci which are active during embryogenesis. These include genes of the T region, the gene for hairpin tail (Hp), and also genes of the Fused-Kinky system. In their mildest form, the T alleles produce tail abnormalities; in a more severe form they produce anencephaly and spina bifida; and in their extreme expression they block development of the embryo at several stages specific for the particular allele represented. Boyse et al. have speculated that T and H-2 are alternatively effective in differentiation, T in embryogenesis, and H-2 in later life (42). While the evidence is not yet conclusive, a previous report of possible loose linkage between spina bifida occulta and HLA suggests a similar chromosomal arrangement (43). Interestingly, Hp, which like T produces a variety of skeletal abnormalities, produces different effects depending upon the sex of the heterozygous parent (44). If the Hp allele is inherited from the mother the effects are apt to be severe; if the abnormality is carried by the sperm, they are mild. This is very reminiscent of human spina bifida where female transmission has been a notable feature of the disease and male transmission much less frequent. This would lead us to suppose that spina bifida, which has, until now, been thought to be an analogue of T, might be the analogue of Hp. In any event, developmental abnormalities giving rise to a disease state could be attributed to differentiation loci linked to HLA.

Interaction between environmental factors and the genome

The interaction between environmental factors with a particular genome is frequently suspected but is often difficult to prove. For example, in the preceeding section spina bifida occulta was discussed briefly. Spina bifida cystica is the overt form of the disease. Spina bifida occulta depends upon a radiological diagnosis and gives little disability. There has been a series of papers on the causal role of infected food, notably potatoes, in spina bifida cystica. One pedigree included several individuals with the clinical form of spina bifida and environmental factors could well result in the transition of the minor to the major defect. A very specific example of interaction between environment and gene is provided by cleft palate in the mouse. Bonner & Slavkin administered cortisone to pregnant mice of different strains (45). The A strain and its H-2-congenic partner B10.A had an extremely high incidence of cleft palate while B10 mice which differ from B10.A at H-2 had a low incidence. Further, in reciprocal hybrids, high B10.A mothers produced 64 % affected offspring while low B10 mothers produced only 31 % affected offspring ($p \leq .05$). While the study does in itself not prove linkage between cleft palate and the H system, the suggestion is very clear.

Modified self

This has been expertly discussed for H-2 in the companion paper by Zinkernagel & Doherty. H-2 is clearly implicated in the response to LCM and ectromelia. Presumptive supportive evidence from man comes from studies in which T cells and B cells are separated and recombined, or are neuraminidase treated and then incubated with unmodified autologous cells. The response that is observed may be an effect of altered self from environmental exposure (as postulated by Uphoff in bone-marrow-transfer experiments in mice (46)). One classic example of a response to modified self in man is Sedormid purpura (47). Hypersensitive patients react

against their own platelets exposed *in vitro* to the drug but not to their unmodified platelets. There has been, to the authors knowledge, no attempt to test HLA association in this disease. The involvement of HLA in many autoimmune diseases in suspected and may fit the model of modified self. At present, information is lacking as to the inciting antigen in these diseases, and all autoimmune diseases cannot be expected to fit one model. Antibodies in lupus, for example, tend to be panreactive rather than autoreactive.

Since genes in the HLA system do control differentiation antigens, e.g. those of B cells and of vascular endothelium, it is possible that other HLA-associated differentiation antigens are expressed on other tissues, e.g. renal tissues, synovial membranes, thyroid cells. It would, therefore, be of interest to test for autoimmunity using as targets tissues from the patients as well as from other individuals. Further, T-cell immunity, as in the Zinkernagel-Doherty or Shearer models, and B-cell autoreactivity could appear independently of each other.

Complement factors

Effects of complement deficiency have been mentioned earlier. However, the authors would also like to suggest that the complement-controlling genes usually regarded as regulatory, could in some instances be deficient or deleted structural genes; the net result would be the same as from repressive regulation. In man, complement-deficient individuals generally lack the gene product, and homozygous individuals have half the quantity of the component. These observations would be consistent with complete suppression by a regulatory gene in the cis position or with failure of a structural gene.

276

Enzymatic modifications

Many diseases are known to result from single enzyme deficiencies. While the linkage relationship of many of these is known, it is not known for others. It would seem to be worthwhile surveying enzyme-deficiency states to see if reduced enzyme levels in sibs and parents are HLA-haplotype associated.

Common precursor

The possibility of a common precursor has been mentioned earlier. A mutation in a shared pathway leading to an excess or a deficiency of a particular metabolite could have many consequences. The products of a genetic locus can subserve more than one function at different stages of development. For example, the recognition of differences between cells from different mouse strains can be exerted as early as the primitive streak stage (48). Pigmented and non-pigmented hair follicle cells separate as segments in tetraparental mice; the genes for hair pigment do not express this function until neonatal life, yet they are distinguishable in the embryo. A gene product can also be used to regulate or contribute to more than one process. This might be true of a protein but perhaps even more so for a glycoprotein. Deficiencies in β_2 microglobulin are known for some cell lines, but to the authors' knowledge they have not been sought at the level of the individual and neither have abnormal carbohydrates. The carbohydrates of HLA have received virtually no attention, since no serologic reactivity has been attributed to them. However, it is premature to dismiss the possibility of a biologic function for the carbohydrates, and abnormal glycoslyation of products of the haplotype could be a cause of disease.

References

1. Amiel, J. L. (1967) Study of the leukocyte phenotypes in Hodgkin's disease. In: *Histocompatibility Testing 1967*, p. 79, Munksgaard, Copenhagen.
2. Morris, P. J., Lawler, S. & Oliver, R. T. (1973) HL-A and Hodgkin's disease. In: *Histocompatibility Testing 1972*, p. 669, Munksgaard, Copenhagen.
3. Amos, D. B. & Ward, F. E. (1975) Immunogenetics of the HL-A system. *Phys. Rev.* **55**, 206.
4. Springer, T. (1976) The biochemistry of H-2 and HLA antigens. *Transplant. Proc.* (in press).
5. Zinkernagel, R. M. & Doherty, P. C. (1975) H-2 compatibility requirement for T-cell-mediated lysis of target cells infected with lymphocytic choriomeningitis virus. Different cytotoxic T-cell specificities are associated with structures coded for in H-2K or H-2D. *J. exp. Med.* **141**, 1427.
6. Yunis, E. J. & Amos, B. (1971) Three closely linked genetic systems relevant to transplantation. *Proc. nat. Acad. Sci. (Wash.)* **68**, 3031.
7. Long, M. A., Handwerger, B. S., Amos, D. B. & Yunis, E. J. (1976) The genetics of Cell-Mediated lympholysis. *J. Immol.* **117**, 2092.
8. Lilly, F. & Pincus, T. (1973) Genetic control of murine viral leukemogenesis. *Adv. Cancer Res.* **17**, 231.
9. Walford, R. L., Gossett, T., Troup, G. M., Gatti, R. A., Mittal, K. K., Robbins, A., Ferrara, G. B. & Zeller, E. (1976) The Merrit alloantigenic system of human B-lymphocytes: Evidence for thirteen possible factors including one six-member segregant series. *J. Immunol.* **116**, 1704.
10. Johnson, A. H., Pool, P. A., McKeown, P. T., Bigelow, R. A. Kovarsky, D. B., Ward, F. E. & Amos, D. B. (1977) Analysis of sera specific for human B cells. *Transplant. Proc.*, (in press).
11. Plate, J. M. D. (1974) Mixed lymphocyte culture reactions of mice. Genetic analysis of the responses to H-2D^d specificities. *J. exp. Med.* **139**, 851.
12. Flaherty, L. & Wachtel, S. S. (1975) H(T1a) system: Identification of two new loci, H-31 and H-32, and alleles. *Immunogenetics* **2**, 81.
13. Flaherty, L. (1975) H-33 – A histocompatibility locus to the left of the H-2 complex. *Immunogenetics* **2**, 325.

277

14. Flaherty, L., Stanton, T. & Boyse, E. A. (1977) Contamination of Ia antisera with antibodies related to the Tla-region. *Immunogenetics,* (in press).

15. Buckley, C. E. III & Roseman, J. M. (1976) Immunity and Survival. *J. Amer. Geriatrics Soc.* **24,** 241.

16. McKusick, V. A. (1976) The human gene map. *The Gene Mapping Newsletter.*

17. Amos, D. B. (1974) HL-A, Fertility and natural selection. In: *Karolinska Symposia on Research Methods in Reproductive Endocrinology,* 7th Symposium, Immunological Approaches to Fertility Control, July 29–31, p. 318.

18. Allen, F .H., Jr. (1974) Linkage of HL-A and GBG. *Vox Sand.* **27,** 382.

19. Demant, P., Capkova, J., Hinzova, E. & Vozacova, B. (1973) The role of the histocompatibility-2-linked Ss–S1p region in the control of mouse complement. *Proc. nat. Acad Sci. (Wash.)* **70,** 863.

20. Day, N. K., Rubinstein, P., de Bracco, M., Moncada, B., Hansen, J. A., Dupont, B., Thomsen, M., Svejgaard, A, & Jersild, C. (1975) Hereditary C1r deficiency: Lack of linkage to the HL-A region in two families. In: *Histocompatibility Testing 1975,* p. 960, Munksgaard, Copenhagen.

21. Weitkamp, L. R. Personal communication.

22. Mittal, K. K., Wolshi, K. P., Lim, D., Gerwurz, A., Gewurz, H. & Schmid, F. R. (1976) Genetic independence between the HL-A system and deficits in the first and sixth components of complement. *Tissue Antigens* **7,** 97.

23. Lamm, L. V., Thorsen, I., Peterson, G. B., Jørgensen, J., Henningsen, B. & Kissmeyer-Nielsen, F. (1975) Data on the HL-A linkage group. *Ann. Human Genetics* **38,** 383.

24. Hobart, M. J., Lachmann, P. J. & Alper, C. A. (1975) Polymorphism of human C6. In: *Protides Biological Fluids,* ed. Peters, H., Pergamon Press, New York, **22,** 575.

25. Fu, S. M., Kunkel, H. G., Brusman, H. P., Allen, F. H. Jr. & Fotino, M. (1974) Evidence for linkage between HL-A histocompatibility genes and those involved in the synthesis of the second component of complement. *J. exp. Med.* **140,** 1108.

26. Rittner, C., Hauptmann, G., Grosse-Wilde, H., Grosshans, G., Tongio, M. M. & Mayer, S. (1975) Linkage between HLA (major histocompatibility complex) and genes controlling the synthesis of the fourth component of complement. In: *Histocompatibility Testing 1975,* p. 945, Munksgaard, Copenhagen.

27. Merrit, A. D., Petersen, G. H., Biegel, A. A., Meyers, D. A., Brooks, G. F. & Hodes, M. E. (1976) Chromosome 6: Linkage of the eighth component of complement (C8) to the histocompatibility region (HLA). *The National Foundation March of Dimes. Birth Defects original series. Human Gene mapping III from the Baltimore Conference 1975,* Vol. **12,** Book 7, 331.

28. Friend, P. S., Handwerger, B. S., Kim, Y., Michael, A. F. & Yunis, E. J (1975) C2 deficiency in man. Genetic relationship to a mixed lymphocyte reactions determinant (7a*). *Immunogenetics* **2,** 569.

29. Gibson, D. J., Glass, D., Carpenter, C. B. & Schur, P. H. (1976) Hereditary C2 deficiency: Diagnosis and HLA gene complex associations. *J. Immunol.* **116,** 1065.

30. Stephens, C., Haysman, M. L., Sullivan, J. B. & Buckley, C. E. III (1976) A comparison of antigenic polymorphisms among fish allergens in two mouse strains. *Fed. Proc.* **35,** 824.

31. Buckley, C. E. III, Dorsey, F. C., Corley, R. B., Ralph, W. B., Woodbury, M. A. & Amos, D. B (1973) HL-A linked human immune-response genes. *Proc. nat. Acad. Sci. (Wash.)* **70,** 2157.

32. Levine, B. B., Stember, R. H. & Fotino, M. (1972) Ragweed hay fever: Genetic control and linkage to HL-A haplotypes. *Science* **178,** 1201.

33. Blumenthal, N. M., Amos, D. B., Noreen, N., Mendell, N. R. & Yunis, E. J. (1974) Genetic mapping of Ir locus in man: Linkage to second locus of HL-A. *Science* **184,** 1301.

34. Bias, W. B. & Marsh, D. G. (1975) HL-A linked antigen E immune response genes: An improved hypothesis. *Science* **188,** 375.

35. Marsh, D. G., Bias, W. B., Hsia, S. H. & Goodfriend, L. (1973) Association of the HL-A7 cross-reacting group with a specific reagenic antibody response in allergic man. *Science* **179,** 691.

36. Greenberg, L. J., Grey, E. D. & Yunis, E. J. (1975) Association of HL-A5 and immune responsiveness *in vitro* to streptococcal antigens. *J. exp. Med.* **141,** 935.

37. Greenberg, L. J. & Yunis, E. J. Personal communication.

38. Hirata, A. A. & Yunis, E. J. (1970) Cross-reactions between streptococcal M and human transplantation antigens. *Science* **168,** 1095.

278

39. Brede, D. Personal communication.
40. Miller, L. H., Mason, S. J., Clyde, D. F. & McGinniss, M. Personal communication.
41. Mann, D. L., Katz, S. I., Melson, D. L., Abelson, L. D. & Strober, W. (1976) Specific B-cell antigens associated with gluten-sensitive enteropathy and dermatitis herpetiformis. *Lancet* **i**, 110.
42. Bennett, D., Boyse, E. A. & Old, L. J. (1972) Cell surface immunogenetics in the study of morphogenesis. In: *Cell Interactions,* Third Lepetit Coloquium, p. 247.
43. Amos, D. B., Ruderman, R., Mendell, N. R. & Johnson, A. H. (1975) Linkage between HL-A and spinal development. *Transplant. Proc.* **7**, 93.
44. Johnson, D. R. (1972) Private communication. *Mouse Newsletter* **47**, 52.
45. Bonner, J. J. & Slavkin, H. C. (1975) Cleft palate susceptibility linked to histocompatibility-2 (H-2) in the mouse. *Immunogenetics* **2**, 213.
46. Uphoff, D. E. (1969) Immunological considerations of bone marrow transplantation. *Transplant. Proc.* **1**, 39.
47. Ackroyd, J. F. (1958) Thrombocytopenic purpura due to drug hypersensitivity. In: *Sensitivity Reactions to Drugs,* eds. Rosenheim, M. L. & Moulton, R., Blackwell, Oxford.
48. Mintz, B. (1974) Gene control of mammalian differentiation. *Ann. Rev. Genet.* **8**, 411.

Population Genetics and Evolution of the HLA System

Walter Bodmer & Glenys Thomson[1]

Extraordinary variability and clustering of many genes are among the most striking features of the HLA system. More than 300 million genetically different individuals can be generated by the known alleles of the HLA-A, -B, -C and -D loci, and of these more than 30 million have distinguishable combinations of antigens. With respect to just the HLA-A and -B loci, more than 75 percent of typical caucasoid individuals have four different antigens, that is, are heterozygous at both loci, while less than 2 percent have only two antigens, being homozygous at both loci. Some further data on HLA variability are summarized in Table I.

The genetic region between the A and B loci is about 1/3,000th of the total human genome, and so the HLA region as a whole, which clearly extends to some extent on either side of these two loci, probably represents only around 1/1,000th of the human genetic material. This however is likely to include at least several hundred, if not a thousand or more genes, even allowing for the fact that much of the DNA may be functionally redundant. The genes identified so far in the HLA and H-2 systems have a variety of functions connected with the immune system and the cell surface, as discussed in earlier chapters. Some cell-surface functions connected with cell-cell interaction outside the immune system may also, as suggested by Bodmer (1), be controlled by genes in this region. It is, of course, these various functions, including especially the control of immune response, which underlie the mechanisms proposed for HLA and disease associations as

TABLE I

Some data on HLA Variability (in caucasoid populaitons based on the VIth Histocompatibility Testing Workshop, 1975)

Locus	HLA-A	HLA-B	HLA-C	HLA-D
Number of alleles (incl. blank)	19	26	6	8
Average heterozygosity (percent)	88	92	44	76
Maximum possible number of phenotypes	172	326	16	37

For all four loci together:

Maximum possible total:		
Haplotypes:		26,676
Genotypes:		355,817,826
Phenotypes:		33,194,624

[1] Genetics Laboratory, Dept. of Biochemistry, University of Oxford, South Parks Road, Oxford, OX1 3QU, England.

TABLE II

A summary of possible mechanisms for HLA and disease associations

1. Molecular mimicry between pathogen and antigen
2. Interaction with pathogen receptors
3. Membrane-antigen pick-up by pathogen
4. Interaction between antigen and pathogen to form "altered" determinant as proposed by Zinkernagel & Doherty
5. Linked immune-response genes
6. Linked complement genes
7. Disturbance of cell-cell interaction

summarized in Table II.

It seems likely that many, if not most, of these associations are not due to the direct effects of the products of the HLA-A, -B, -C or even -D loci, but to those of other closely linked genes within the HLA region. The observed associations must then, as discussed in previous chapters, arise from linkage disequilibrium between alleles at the so-far undetected disease-spsceptibility loci and those at the A, B, C or D loci. Linkage disequilibrium, which is the tendency for alleles at different loci to occur together more often on the same haplotype than expected by chance, tends to occur especially between closely linked loci, such as those of the HLA system. Thus, an understanding of the population genetics and evolution of the HLA system and of its association with disease depends on an understanding of the population genetics of linked loci, and so of the forces that tend to produce and maintain linkage disequilibrium. In this chapter, some of the possible explanations for the extensive polymorphism of the HLA system will be discussed as well as the types of forces which lead to linkage disequilibrium, and then there will be a discussion of the evolution of the region and the relationship between its constituent genes.

Polymorphism through advantage of new variants

The work of Lewontin & Hubby (2) in Drosophila and Harris (3, 4) in man, and subsequently many others, has shown that at least 30 percent and probably many more, of all gene loci are polymorphic. The overall average frequency of heterozygotes per locus in man is probably about 15 percent (4, 5). This is much lower than that for any of the known HLA loci, for which the overall level of heterozygosity is higher than that for any other known human polymorphism including all the complex red-cell blood groups. Even if the HLA-A, -B, -C and -D products each reflected the contribution of a small cluster of loci, as suggested by Bodmer (6), it seems unlikely that such a high overall level of polymorphism would be maintained in the absence of some distinguishing feature of the HLA system.

There is currently much argument among population geneticists about the extent to which observed overall levels of polymorphism can be accounted for assuming the absence of natural selection, that is, complete neutrality of the polymorphic differences (see e.g. Lewontin, 5). On the assumption of neutrality, differences between systems, would have to be due to differing mutation rates, which would imply that the explanation for the relatively high level of HLA polymorphism lay in a correspondingly high mutation rate. There is, however, no shortage of possible mechanisms by which natural selection could act on the loci of the HLA system, including any of the mechanisms suggested in Table II for HLA and disease associations. Though most of the diseases whose HLA association is established are unlikely themselves to be of much selective significance, because they are very rare, occur late in life, or have little effect on viability or fertility, it seems quite possible that associations will be found with important infectious diseases, such as smallpox, malaria, cholera, or tuberculosis, and these would be of considerable selective significance. Natural selection therefore seems, as already emphasized by Snell (7), Bodmer (1), Bodmer et al. (8), Thomson et al. (9) and others, to be the most likely explanation for polymorphism, at least in the case of the HLA and H-2 systems. In this case, mutation-rate differences are not relevant and one is led to postulate whether there is any particular feature of the way that selection acts on the HLA system which might account for the observed high overall levels of polymorphism. One possible answer the authors would like to emphasize is that the system may tend to give an advantage to new variants, (1).

At least four of the mechanisms for resistance to pathogens listed in Table II (numbers 1, 2, 4 and 5) imply that a pathogen has to adapt to the antigenic or immune-response status of the host. The phenomenon of co-evolution of host and pathogen is, of course, quite familiar to epidemiologists. Thus, for example, a change in a host antigen mimicked by a pathogen or used by it as a receptor, may necessitate a corresponding change in the pathogen for it to be successful on the altered host. Similarly, an improved immune response of the host, due either to a change in an immune-response gene or to an antigen change which leads to a better interaction between antigen and pathogen (à la Zinkernagel and Doherty 10)

with respect to immune response, will confer increased resistance to the pathogen. In all these cases the host with the new form of antigen or immune response has a selective advantage over other unchanged individuals with respect to resistance to the particular pathogen. The selective advantage remains until the pathogen adapts, presumably by mutation and selection, to the new type of host.

These mechanisms of resistance to pathogens associated with the HLA system therefore tend to confer a selective advantage on appropriate new variants. This is a form of frequency-dependent selection that is well known as a mechanism for giving rise to polymorphism (Lewontin 5). In other words, these arguments imply that the functions of at least some of the HLA-region genes are such as to lead naturally to an advantage for certain new mutations, and so to a continuing accumulation of polymorphic variants.

In general, one might expect that the greater the population heterogeneity with respect to the relevant antigens and immune-response genes, the more difficult it would be for a pathogen to adapt successfully to infect a significant fraction of the population. Conversely, a population which lacks the appropriate immune response or other form of genetically determined protection against a highly virulent variety of pathogen is in danger of extinction. A striking example of this problem in another context is the extreme disease susceptibility of some of the new varieties of cultivated cereals, grown as uniform stocks or so-called 'monocultures'. Such uniform cereal cultures can be completely wiped out by a new adapted variety of fungus or other pathogen. A human example of this could be the relatively restricted distribution of HLA types found amongst American Indians, which might, as suggested by Bodmer *et al.* (8), have cost them their resistance to infections brought from the Old World, such as measles to which they were especially susceptible.

Linkage disequilibrium and its causes

The *HLA-A1, B8* haplotype in caucasoid populations is, perhaps, the best known case of linkage disequilibrium and it will be used as an example to describe the phenomenon. In a typical Northern European population, the frequency of the antigen A1 is about 0.31 and that of B8 about 0.21. If there were no association between A1 and B8 then the expected frequency of individuals with both A1 and B8 would simply be the product of the two separate frequencies, namely $0.31 \times 0.21 = 0.065$. The observed frequency of A1 + B8 + individuals is, however, 0.172, which is nearly three times as high as that expected in the absence of any association. In fact, if B8 were a disease, and A1 the associated antigen, the relative risk of A1 among the B8s would be 21.4, a highly significant increase. This association of the antigenic types actually reflects an association at the genetic level between the alleles *A1* and *B8* as illustrated in Table III. Thus, the frequency of allele *A1* is 0.17 and that of *B8* is 0.11 so that, on the assumption of no association between the alleles, the expected frequency of the *A1, B8* haplotype would be $0.17 \times 0.11 = 0.019$. The observed frequency of this haplotype is actually 0.088 and so more than four times the expectation on the assumption of indepence. The difference between the observed and expected is the measure of linkage disequilibrium,

$$D = 0.088 - 0.019 = 0.069.$$

The phenotypic association between antigens A1 and B8 depends entirely on this linkage disequilibrium and disappears if D is zero (11).

Thus, an association between traits controlled by linked genes such as *A1* and *B8*, or a B-locus allele and an allele of an HLA-linked immune-response gene, depends entirely on the existence of linkage disequilibrium.

The mathematical definition of linkage disequilibrium in terms of haplotype frequencies and gene frequencies is outlined in Table IV in terms of a two-locus two-allele model. The alleles *A* and *B* at the two separate loci control say, antigens A and B, and *a, b* represent the corresponding complementary alleles with respective frequencies p_x, p_B, p_a and p_b. There are four possible haplotypes *AB, Ab, aB, ab* with corresponding frequencies f(*AB*), etc. The equations given in Table IV show the relationships between the haplotype and gene frequencies and the linkage disequilibrium,

TABLE III
The HLA-A1, B8 association in caucasoids

Phenotypes

Observed antigen
frequencies	A1 +	B8 +	A1 + B8 +
	0.31	0.21	0.172

Expected frequency of
A1 + B8 + if independent $0.31 \times 0.21 = 0.065$
'relative risk' of A1 among B8 $= 21.4$

Genotypes

Observed gene and
haplotype frequencies	A1	B8	A1, B8
	0.17	0.11	0.088

Expected *A1, B8* haplotype
frequency if independent $0.17 \times 0.11 = 0.019$

Linkage Disequilibrium
$$D = 0.088 - 0.17 \times 0.11 = 0.069$$

TABLE IV

Definition of linkage disequilibrium in terms of haplotype and gene frequencies

Alleles	$A \quad a \quad ; \quad B \quad b$
Frequencies	$p_A \quad p_a \quad ; \quad p_B \quad p_b$
	$p_A + p_a = 1 \quad ; \quad p_B + p_b = 1$
Haplotypes	$AB \quad Ab \quad ; \quad aB \quad ab$
Frequencies	$f(AB) \quad f(Ab) \quad f(aB) \quad f(ab)$
	$f(AB) + f(Ab) + f(aB) + f(ab) = 1$
Linkage disequilibrium is defined as	$D = f(AB)f(ab) - f(Ab)f(aB)$
and	$f(AB) = p_A\, p_B + D$
	$f(Ab) = p_A\, p_b - D$
	$f(aB) = p_a\, p_B - D$
	$f(ab) = p_a\, p_b + D$

Note: When D = O, the haplotype frequencies f(*AB*) etc. are just equal to the products of the gene frequencies $p_A\, p_B$, etc.

$$D = f(AB)f(ab) - f(Ab)f(aB).$$

From the first of these equations we can see that the linkage disequilibrium can also be calculated as

$$D = f(AB) - p_A\, p_B,$$

which was the form used in discussing the association between A1 and B8. D is really a measure of the extent of non-random association between the alleles in haplotypes. The important point to note is that the haplotype frequencies (f(*AB*), etc.) are only equal to the products of the gene frequencies ($p_A\, p_B$, etc.) when the linkage disequilibrium D = O, and it is, as already emphasized, only in this case that there is no population association between antigens A and B.

Out of the more than 150 pairwise combinations of HLA-A- and -B-locus alleles, on average six to eight show detectable linkage disequilibrium in any given population (see e.g. Bodmer & Bodmer 12). Each group of populations tends to have its characteristic pairs such as *A1,B8, A3,B7* and *A29,B12* in Northern European populations. Linkage disequilibrium between the HLA-B and -C, or B- and D-locus alleles on the other hand seems to be more common, with each C- or D-locus allele having a B-locus partner (see Histocompatibility Testing, 1975 ref. 13).

A number of the diseases associated with B-locus alleles show stronger associations with D-locus alleles and, in some cases, even stronger ones with the emerging Ia types (see Chapter III and later Chapters). The most striking example of this is multiple sclerosis, where the association with *A3* and *B7* is relatively weak, while that with *DW2* and, apparently, Ia is much stronger. The associations with at least *A3,B7* and *DW2* all seem to be secondary to the real association with the disease locus, which must be in stronger linkage disequilibrium with *DW2* than with either *B7* or *A3*. Certainly, in this case at least, it seems very hard to explain the pattern of associations in any other way than by linkage disequilibrium between an HLA-linked disease gene and the detectable alleles at the A, B and D loci. Another line of evidence from population data which favours this explanation for HLA and disease associations comes from studies which show that Graves' disease is associated with *B8* in caucasoids, but with *BW35* in Japanese. If the same disease susceptibility is involved in both populations, then these results can only be explained by different patterns of linkage disequilibrium with the disease gene in different populations, just as is found for the A- and B-locus combinations. Graves' disease in caucasoids provides, incidentally, another example of an association that is stronger with the D locus (DW3) than with the B locus.

Even in the case of ankylosing spondylitis (AS) where the association with B27 is so strong that some have suggested the susceptibility might in this case be due to the B27 product itself, family data suggest otherwise. Thus Ceppellini and co-workers (Chapter IV) have shown that the proportion of B27-positive relatives of B27 individuals with AS who get the disease is more than twice that of individuals who get it amongst a random sample of B27-positive individuals. As Thomson *et al.* (9) and Thomson & Bodmer (14) have discussed, this difference is most easily explained by assuming the existence of a linked disease gene which is carried by only a fraction of the *B27*-carrying haplotypes. In the case of AS, the D-locus association is not stronger than that with B27, but it remains to be seen whether an Ia type might be found which is shared by B27-negative and B27-positive cases of AS.

Given that linkage disequilibrium among alleles of the HLA-region loci is a relative common though by no means universal phenomenon and, in particular, underlies many if not most of the HLA and disease associations, it is important to ask: what are the possible explanations for linkage disequilibrium and why is it such a variable phenomenon? It is a classic result of population genetics, originally due to Jennings (15) and Robbins (16), that in a truly random-mating population and in the absence of selection, the linkage disequilibrium D should always be zero at equilibrium. Thus, D = O

is the normal expected condition and the question really is, what are the factors that can give rise to non-zero D?

Jennings and Robbins showed that if in such a random-mating population, D were for any reason not zero, it would approach zero at a rate $(1 - r)$ per generation where r is the recombination fraction between the two loci. Thus the smaller r is, that is, the more tightly linked the loci, the longer it will take for D to approach zero. Linkage disequilibrium may therefore exist for very closely linked loci in a random-mating population even in the absence of selection, simply because equilibrium has not yet been reached. As an illustration, consider the number of generations, n, needed to reduce the linkage disequilibrium between a pair of alleles of the HLA-A or -B loci by say a factor of 5, (for example, from 0.05 to 0.01). In this case r = 0.008 and so n must be such that

$$(1 - 0.008)^n = 1/5$$

This gives n = 200 which is about 5,000 years in humans, allowing 25 years per generation. If for example r = 0.001, the time would be 40,000 years, while if r = 0.0001, it would be 400,000 years, emphasizing the extent to which small values of r can lead to a persistence of linkage disequilibrium in the absence of any other factors, such as natural selection.

What factors can lead to persistence of linkage disequilibrium even when a stable state equilibrium has been reached (or should have been on the assumption of random mating and no selection). Fisher (17) in 1930, was the first to suggest how certain types of natural selection in random-mating populations, in which pairwise combinations of alleles at different loci were favoured, could be particularly advantageous if the genes were closely linked and so might form a basis for the evolution of a cluster of linked genes such as the HLA system. Such selective interactions are one explanation for the persistence of linkage disequilibrium in a random-mating population.

Other possible mechanisms all involve some form of departure from random mating. They include effects of migration and population admixture, inbreeding, and random fluctuations in frequencies in relatively small populations, or what is commonly called "random genetic drift". Each of these mechanisms for generating linkage disequilibrium is discussed in somewhat more detail below.

Selection

Using a two-locus two-allele model, such as has already been discussed in defining D, Fisher (17) pointed out that under certain circumstances selection in favour of the combination of alleles *AB* could give rise to persistent linkage disequilibrium. Since then, many theoretical studies on two (and more) loci have confirmed and extended this result (see e.g. Lewontin 5, Bodmer & Felsenstein 18, Karlin & Feldman 19), and have shown that linkage and selection can interact both to favour new haplotype combinations and to produce stable situations in which one or more haplotypes are in linkage disequilibrium. There is, in general, a balance between the magnitude of the recombination fraction and of the selective interactions which is such that if linkage between the genes involved is sufficiently tight, then particular haplotype combinations will be maintained in linkage disequilibrium in the presence of appropriate selective advantages.

Even if selection is not such as to maintain D ≠ O at equilibrium, it may nevertheless considerably slow down

the rate at which D approaches zero relative to (1 − r), the rate in the absence of selection. This can lead to a transient persistence of linkage disequilibrium that in human populations may be hard to distinguish from a stable maintenance of D ≠ O (see Thomson *et al.* 9). In some cases one can show that as a single allele increases in frequency because of a selective advantage, quite large linkage disequilibrium can be created with alleles at closely linked loci even if these are completely neutral. These levels of linkage disequilibrium may persist for considerable lengths of time. It is even possible to maintain linkage disequilibrium in this way between two neutral alleles sitting on either side of a selectively advantageous allele that is increasing in frequency. Consider for example, a locus X situated halfway between A and B, where the recombination fraction between A and B is r = 0.01 (about the same as that between HLA-A and -B) and alleles at loci A and B are selectively neutral. It can be shown that an allele at the intermediate locus X which arose in the haplotype *AB* and is increasing in frequency from an initially low value of say 1 % with a selective advantage of 5 % over its alternative, can maintain a D between *A* and *B* of about 0.05 for 100 generations and 0.02 for 200 generations (20).

This occurs for the following reason. When a selectively favourable mutation occurs in a population and increases in frequency to an equilibrium value or to fixation, the frequencies of alleles at closely linked loci will also alter. Alleles present on the chromosome on which the original mutation occurred will tend to increase in frequency, being pulled along with the selected gene, that is they "hitch-hike" along. It is this pulling along together of the gene frequencies that increases the linkage disequilibrium, both between the selected locus and closely linked neutral loci, and also between pairs of closely linked neutral loci. The relevance of this result is that selection could, for example, be acting on the immune-response genes within the HLA region and not on the HLA-A, -B and -C loci themselves, and through this, linkage disequilibrium between alleles at HLA-A and -B could be generated.

Migration and admixture

Linkage disequilibrium can be generated by mixing two populations which are genetically different, even if there is no linkage disequilibrium in either population to start with. As an illustration, consider the extreme case where there are two populations, in the first only alleles A and B occur, while in the second only alleles a and b are found. When these two populations are mixed, it is obvious that linkage disequilibrium is created since the alleles are not associated at random, as A always occurs with $B,$ and a with b. If the two loci are closely linked it will take some time for this association to break down, essentially at the usual rate $(1 - r)$ if there is no selection. This is clearly a very simplistic static model of migration that does not take into account the more realistic situation where in each generation there is a small amount of mixing or migration between a set of populations. However, it does serve to illustrate the general principle involved. This latter case, involving continual migration between populations has, for example, been considered by Nei & Li (21) and Feldman & Christiansen (22). Feldman & Christiansen studied the effects of population subdivision on the evolution of two linked loci without selection and showed that gradients in gene frequencies and significant linkage

disequilibrium can be maintained for relatively long periods of time.

Closely related to the study of migration patterns is the question of admixture, such as occurs from American Whites into the American Black population. It has, for example, been shown by Thomson et al. (9) that the existence of linkage disequilibrium for the haplotype *HLA-A1, B8* in the American Black population appears to be quite adequately explained by admixture from the white population, taking into account both the lack of linkage disequilibrium between *A1* and *B8* and the low frequency of these alleles in African Black populations. This, of course, gives no explanation for the existence of persistent linkage disequilibrium for the haplotype *HLA-A1, B8* in caucasian populations.

Are migration and admixture strong enough forces to create significant values of D, comparable to those observed in the HLA system, for sufficiently long periods of time, as suggested by Degos & Dausset (23)? The magnitude of the linkage disequilibrium generated by migration or admixture is very dependent on the gene-frequency differences between the initial populations, the rate of migration or mixing, and the recombination fraction between the loci. The initial D following mixing is approximately the product of the rates of mixing and the two gene-frequency differences. If, for example, both gene frequencies differed by 0.2 in the populations being mixed, then even a 1:1 mixture of the population only generates an initial D of $(0.5) \times (0.5) \times (0.2) \times (0.2) = 0.01$, which, in the absence of selection, decreases steadily at a rate of at least $(1 - r)$ following the initial mixing. World-wide data on HLA-gene frequencies (Bodmer et al. (24)), show that few gene frequencies even approach values as high as 0.2. Moreover, admixture could only be a significant factor if it involved populations that are relatively close to each other as within Europe or at most say covering the range from Northern Europe to the Middle East. The maximum gene-frequency differences over this range are about 0.05 and rates of admixture, even between adjacent populations, are unlikely to be much above five to ten percent. It thus seems very unlikely that any significant proportion of the linkage disequilibrium seen for the HLA system could be due to migration and admixture, except for special cases involving recent mixing between widely differing groups, such as the American Blacks.

Inbreeding

Inbreeding is another potential cause of linkage disequilibrium. However, very high levels of inbreeding, similar in magnitude to D itself, are necessary to give rise to significant values of D, and even then these will tend to be negative rather than positive (Degos & Bodmer 25). Inbreeding levels in most human populations are sufficiently low, generally less than 2 per 1,000 population, to make this an insignificant factor as a cause of linkage disequilibrium.

Random drift

If the population size is very small or the linkage between the two loci extremely tight, significant disequilibrium may be created by chance, that is random-drift effects. The population sizes involved in most studies of the HLA system and the recombination fractions between the HLA-A, -B, -C and -D loci are sufficiently large that drift can also, in general, be eliminated as a significant factor causing linkage disequilibrium between these loci (26).

It seems likely, therefore, that for most populations, selection is the only one of the above mechanisms for generating persistent linkage disequilibrium that could give rise to some of the high D values observed for combinations of alleles at the HLA-A, -B, -C and -D loci. The main question to answer is whether there has been sufficient time since the origin of the haplotypes involving high values of D for it to be expected that equilibrium would have been reached in the absence of selection. As pointed out by Bodmer in 1972 (9, 27), several HLA haplotypes including *A1 B8 A3 B7 A1 BW17* and *A1 B5* show gradients in frequency among caucasoids across Europe from the North (high *A1 B8 A3 B7,* low *A1 BW17 A11 B5)* to the Middle East and Far East (low *A1 B8 A3 B7,* high *A1 BW17 A11 B5)* as illustrated in Table V. It seems likely that these gradients may be correlated with the advance of the neolithic peoples from their centre

TABLE V

Some caucasoid HLA-A, B haplotype frequencies (frequency x 10³)

Populations	A1, B8	A3, B7	A1, BW17	A11, B5
N. Scots (Hebrides)	121	36	22	–
English	87	55	12	2
French	46	53	11	7
Italians (Ferrara)	42	20	7	–
Basques	31	23	51	5
Turks	10	–	16	13
Lebanese	4	6	17	24
Arabs (Israel)	28	6	9	45
Pakistanis	–	8	43	80
Indians	7	11	34	45

Data are based on Bodmer *et al.* (24). The populations are arranged in approximate geographical sequence from North to South. Italicized values are those which are significant at least at a five percent level: – means negligible estimated frequency.

of origin in the Middle East, starting some 9,000 years ago, as suggested by Cavalli-Sforza (28). The gradients presumably have their origin in gradual admixture between the genes of the advancing neolithic peoples and those of the populations indigenous to the regions where they were settling. The constituent haplotypes of the original populations, which may be close to those of Northern Europe and the Middle East respectively, must already, therefore, have been in linkage disequilibrium, for as has already been emphasized, migration and admixture are most unlikely themselves to be adequate explanations for the observed levels of D. This implies that significant linkage disequilibrium between *A1* and *B8,* and probably also between the other three pairs of A- and B-locus alleles, has persisted for at least 5,000 years, which is the time since the neolithic revolution reached northernmost Europe. As discussed above, D values for loci separated by a recombination fraction of 0.8 percent would decrease by a factor of 5 in this period of time in the absence of selection, and so would undoubtedly have become insignificant. Thus, in these cases at least, the persistence of the linkage disequilibrium seems most likely to be due to some sort of natural selection acting on the alleles *A1* and *B8* themselves, or on one or more alleles at closely linked loci. It is, of course, not possible to say just from data on the persistence of the haplotype whether interactive selection of the sort originally proposed by Fisher (17) is involved, or whether the alleles *A1* and *B8* are just "hitchhiking" along with a selected allele at a locus somewhere nearby.

The distinction between time and selection as causes of linkage disequilibrium is not so easy to establish for the putative disease alleles at loci linked to the HLA-B or -D loci. Thus, a rare disease-susceptibility allele which arose by mutation or recombination comparatively recently may still, of course, reflect its origins by linkage disequilibrium with those alleles that were present in the haplotype that carried the original mutation. This linkage disequilibrium could persist for some time by the hitchhiking effect if favourable selection is acting to increase the frequency of the disease allele or an allele at a linked locus. This is certainly one possible explanation for the extraordinary linkage disequilibrium between the C2 deficiency allele, *AW25* and *BW18* (29). It could also underlie the association between B27 and AS and other related diseases. In this case, however, the presence of the same association in widely differing populations would have to be explained by admixture into different populations from a common original population, presumably most likely that in which it is most frequent. The group of populations which appear to have the highest frequency of the B27-associated diseases are however the North American Indians (30), whose first contact with the caucasoids came with the conquest of the Americas a few hundred years ago. It is surely impossible to believe that B27-associated AS in Europeans has its origins from that source. It seems equally unlikely that the flow has been in the other direction from Europeans to American Indians. Thus, if the association with B27 is due to an allele at a linked locus, and if this is the same in different populations, it would appear that the disease allele and *B27* haplotype has been around for a long time, perhaps even before the separation of the major human races some 50,000 to 100,000 years ago. In this case, there could be little doubt of the need for selection to maintain persistence of the linkage disequilibrium between *B27* and its linked disease allele unless the two loci were extremely closely linked. In general, it seems likely that when a disease association occurs with the same allele at roughly comparable frequencies in widely differing populations, selection underlies the maintenance of the corresponding linkage disequilibrium. When, as in the case of Graves' disease, the association is with different alleles in different populations, it is of course possible that the disease-susceptibility alleles are not the same in the two populations. If they are, however, then again this suggests persistence of linkage disequilibrium due to selection, since lack of time could not readily account for a persistence of linkage disequilibrium with two alleles at the same locus. The only situation that is readily compatible with a comparatively recent origin as the explanation for an HLA and disease association is if the association is found mainly in one, or one group of populations, and in particular if the associated HLA-A, -B, -C or -D allele is not connected with an increase in the frequency of the disease in other populations.

Evolutionary homologies and gene duplication

It has often been suggested that the genes of the H-2 and HLA systems originated by a series of duplications, (Klein & Shreffler 31, Stimpfling 32, Bodmer 1, 33). Recent biochemical evidence, especially from preliminary amino acid sequence data, provides strong support for this notion, at least in the case of the HLA-A and -B and H-2K and D loci (Henning et al. 34, Vitetta et al. 35, Silver & Hood 36, Terhorst et al. 37 and Bridgen et al. 38). Thus, at least 10 of the first 16 amino acids of the HLA-A- and -B-locus products are the same, as might be expected if the A and B loci, or clusters of loci had a common origin by duplication. However, even among these first 16 amino acids (out of a total of nearly 400 for a molecular weight of 43,000), there are at least one or two differences which seem to be allele specific. If this extent of difference for the first 16 amino acids is representative of the whole molecule, then apparent alleles may differ from each other at a number of amino-acid positions, as has been suggested for H-2 by Nathensen et al. (39). This is not unexpected if, as suggested by Bodmer (6), the A and B loci are actually small clusters of closely linked loci and at least some of the polymorphism is for the control of which gene in the cluster is expressed. In this case, cross-reacting specificities, such as A2 and A28, may be true alleles, while specificities that differ to a greater extent such as A1 and A2 and which show no cross-reaction, may be products of different genes within the cluster. It will be interesting to delineate the evolutionary relationship between the various products as more amino acid sequence data become available.

Recent work in man has shown that the HLA-linked Ia antigens have a two-chain structure consisting of a non-covalently linked complex of one 28,000 and one 33,000 mol. wt. glycosylated polypeptide chain (Snary et al. 40). Studies with somatic cell hybrids (Barnstable et al (41)) have shown that it is the 33,000 mol. wt. chain which carries the polymorphic determinants and is coded for by a gene in the HLA region, while the 28,000 mol. wt. chain may be coded for by a gene on another chromosome. This is analogous to the situation involving the HLA-A, -B and -C-locus products that are associated with β_2 microglobulin (β_2m), which is coded for by a gene on chromosome 15. The relationship between immunoglobulins and products of the HLA region that was suggested by Bodmer (1) and Gally & Edelman (42) was encouraged by the finding that β_2m, which has an homology with immunoglobulins, was associated with HLA products. None of the (admittedly limited) amino acid data so far available lends much support to this suggestion, but much more data are needed to answer this question properly.

The difference in molecular weights between the Ia chains and those of the A, B and C loci rules out a simple common origin by duplication. However, if Edelman's concept of dominans for the immunoglobulins (see e.g. Gally & Edelman 42) applies to the HLA region, then homologies between Ia chains (either 33,000 or 28,000) and the 43,000 mol. wt. products of the A, B and C loci may nevertheless be found. Data in the mouse, and to some extent in man, clearly suggest the existence of several Ia genes (*Transplant. Rev.*, vol. 30), and so an Ia region which may have some analogies with the immunoglobulin constant heavy chain regions. The relationship of these products to the complement components (C2, Bf, C4 and possibly some part of C8) controlled by genes in the HLA region also remains to be established. The HLA-A, -B, -C and -D and Ia products may, as suggested by Barnstable *et al.* (41), perform complement-like functions on the cell surface which might then explain why they occur close to some of the complement genes. This, of course, again raises the possibility of common origins through gene duplication. It is worth noting that the smallest of the three chains of C4 has a molecular weight of about 30,000 (Schreiber & Muller-Eberhart 44), similar to that of the Ia chain coded for in the HLA

region. This suggests that it may be this part of C4 which is controlled by the major histocompatibility region and so, at least, that there may be evolutionary homology between this C4 chain and the I-region products, a possibility which can easily be checked. There is, indeed, some evidence that C4, or at least a part of it, is on the lymphocyte surface (Ferrone *et al.* 45). There is also evidence that Bf, another of the HLA-coded complement components, is on lymphocyte surfaces (Lachman *et al.* 46). C2, which is thought to be closely homologous to Bf and is also controlled by an HLA-linked gene, is, of course, the component that complexes with C4 in the early stages of the complement pathway. Is this a model for interactions between other pairs of products of the HLA and H-2 regions? Such functional interactions could certainly provide the basis for the sort of selective interaction that Fisher first pointed out could maintain linkage disequilibrium and might indeed account for some of the high observed D values. It is also possible that recombination between particular haplotypes might disrupt favourable combinations of genes and so bring together poorly interacting gene products which are associated with disease susceptibility. The C2 deficiency, *AW25, B18* haplotype, associated with systemic lupus erythematosus might be such an example. In this case, the association of the alleles in the haplotype would be due to linkage disequilibrium, but would simply reflect the bringing together on one haplotype of an unfavourable combination of genes. This would be a likely explanation if it turned out that diseased individuals tended to show this association of C2 deficiency with *AW25, B18,* while clinically normal individuals did not.

A comparison of the limited amino

acid sequence data so far available for H-2K and H-2D and HLA-A and -B, while clearly suggesting homology between the two systems (Howard 47), also show a contrasting and puzzling phenomenon. This is that the HLA-A and -B products appear to be more similar to each other than either is to H-2K or H-2D. Now, the two 'gene' structure for these serological determinants clearly suggests that the duplication and separation of the two loci occurred before the evolutionary separation of the species. Thus if, as is often suggested, H-2K is homologous with HLA-B, and H-2D with HLA-A, then one would expect the K products, for example, to be more like those of locus B than A. The fact that this is not so, but that on the contrary similarity between A and B has been maintained

during evolution, suggests that selection tends to favour new alleles at one locus only if they somehow fit with the products of the other locus. The evolution of the two loci within a species would then proceed in parallel, maintaining some similarity of their products, while the loci of different species which do not have to fit together would tend to diverge by the normal processes of evolution. This is again, of course, just the sort of selective interaction which would favour linkage disequilibrium and might arise because of interaction between the gene products on the cell surface, or more likely because of their need to act with a common intermediary product, such as β_2m, or perhaps in relation to their role in T-cell recognition, following Zinkernagel & Doherty (10).

Summary and conclusions

The four established loci of the HLA region are remarkably polymorphic. The genetic region they encompass may include at least several hundred loci, many of which could be as polymorphic as those so far known, creating an almost infinite variety of individuals with respect to the HLA system. The functions so far known to be controlled by genes in the HLA region, including immune-response and cell-surface interactions, provide ample opportunities for explaining the observed variety of HLA and disease associations. In so far as these associations are not due to the detected products of the HLA-A, -B, -C or -D loci, they must reflect linkage disequilibrium between alleles at these loci and those at closely linked disease-susceptibility loci.

One possible explanation for the relatively high level of polymorphism of HLA loci is that their functions may be

such as to tend to give a temporary advantage to new variants. This is consistent with mechanisms of resistance to infectious diseases via molecular mimicry, interaction with pathogen receptors or with pathogen determinants themselves, and with effects of linked immune-response genes.

Linkage disequilibrium is the tendency for alleles at different loci to occur together more often on the same haplotype than expected by chance. Its magnitude D is measured by the difference between the haplotype frequency and the products of the frequencies of the alleles it includes. Most pairs of alleles at the HLA-A and -B loci are not associated, but some, such as *A1* and *B8*, provide notable examples of linkage disequilibrium. There are more associations between alleles of the B and C, and B and D loci and perhaps more still between the B and D loci and those di-

rectly responsible for disease susceptibility.

In the absence of differential natural selection, a random-mating population should end up with $D = O$ at equilibrium for any pair of loci, however closely linked. On the other hand, the rate at which D approaches zero is $1 - r$, where r is the recombination fraction between the loci and this decreases as r becomes smaller. One reason for having $D \neq O$ is, therefore, that there has not yet been enough time to reach equilibrium. A major explanation for having $D \neq O$ even at equilibrium is, as was first suggested by Fisher, that there is interactive selection favouring certain combinations of alleles over others. Selection acting on a single locus can lead to significant levels of D for substantial periods of time even though D may eventually reach zero. This happens because a favoured allele while increasing in frequency may pull along with it linked alleles even if these are neutral, a phenomenon known as "hitch-hiking". Other possible causes of linkage disequilibrium, which include migration and admixture, inbreeding and chance or random-drift effects, do not seem likely to be important as explanations for the observed levels of linkage disequilibrium in the HLA system. All these mechanisms, including selection especially, are more likely to lead to larger D values the smaller the recombination fraction between the loci.

The patterns of frequency distribution of some haplotypes such as *A1, B8* in different populations suggest a persistence which could only reasonably be be explained by some sort of natural selection. Disease associations due to linkage disequilibrium may also, unless they are mainly restricted to one group of populations, reflect the action of natural selection.

The genes of the HLA region are likely to have originated by a series of duplications. Limited amino acid sequence data already clearly indicate a striking homology between the HLA-A- and -B-locus products, while supporting the suggestion that some alleles may nevertheless differ for a substantial number of amino acids. The Ia antigens consist of two chains of which one, with a mol. wt. of 33,000, is coded for in the HLA region, while the other, with a mol. wt. of 28,000, may be coded for elsewhere. The relationship of the A, B, C, D and Ia products to the complement components (C2, Bf, C4 and possibly C8) coded for by genes in the HLA region remains to be established, but could also involve some evolutionary homologies. Many of the products of the region, including those so-far detected only by serological techniques, may perform complement-like functions on the cell surface which would be in line with such postulated evolutionary relationships. Products of the region may interact with each other functionally, as do C2 and C4 in the complement cascade, thus providing some basis for the sorts of selective interactions that can maintain persistent linkage disequilibrium. Some disease associations, such as that between C2 deficiency and systemic lupus erythematosus, could be due to disruptive recombinant haplotypes, which carry alleles whose products interact poorly.

The answer to the many questions raised concerning the functional and evolutionary interrelationships between the genes of the HLA region will only come from further detailed cellular, genetic, and molecular studies. This fascinating region provides a fine example, through its association with disease and its obvious fundamental biological significance, of the interaction between basic biological research and the practical needs of the clinicians.

Acknowledgements

This work was supported in part by a grant from the U.K. Medical Research Council.

References

1. Bodmer, W. F. (1972) Evolutionary significance of the HL-A system. *Nature (Lond.)* **237**, 139.
2. Lewontin, R. C. & Hubby, J. L. (1966) A molecular approach to the study of genic heterozygosity in natural populations. II. Amount of Variation and degree of heterozygosity in natural populations of *Drosophila pseudoobscura. Genetics*, **54**, 595–609.
3. Harris, H. (1966) Enzyme polymorphisms in man. *Proc. roy. Soc. B.*, **164**, 298.
4. Harris, H. (1975) *The Principles of Human Biochemical Genetics*. 2nd revised and enlarged edition. North-Holland Publishing Co.
5. Lewontin, R. C. (1974) *The Genetic Basis of Evolutionary Change*. Columbia University Press.
6. Bodmer, W. F. (1973) A new genetic model for allelism at histocompatibility and other complex loci: Polymorphism for control of gene expression. *Transplant. Proc.*, **5**, 1471–1476.
7. Snell, G. D. (1968) The H-2 locus of the mouse: Observations and speculations concerning its comparative genetics and its polymorphism. *Folia Biol. Prague*, **10**, 335–358.
8. Bodmer, W. F., Cann, H. & Piazza, A. (1973) Differential genetic variability among polymorphisms as an indicator of natural selection. In: *Histocompatibility Testing, 1972*, eds. Dausset, J. & Colombani, J., p. 753, Munksgaard, Copenhagen.
9. Thomson, G., Bodmer, W. F. & Bodmer, J. (1976) The HL-A system as a model for studying the interaction between selection, migration and linkage. In: *Population Genetics and Ecology*, eds. Karlin, S. & Nero, E., p. 465. Academic Press Inc., New York.
10. Zinkernagel, R. M. & Doherty, P. C. (1974b) Restriction of *in vitro* T cell-mediated cytotoxicity in lymphocytic choriomeningitis virus within a syngeneic or semi-allogeneic system. *Nature (Lond.)*, **248**, 701.
11. Bodmer, W. F. & Payne, R. (1965) Theoretical consideration of leukocyte grouping using multispecific sera. In: *Histocompatibility Testing 1965*, eds. Balner, H., Cleton, S. G. & Eernisse, J. G., p. 141. Munksgaard, Copenhagen.
12. Bodmer, J. & Bodmer, W. F. (1973) Population genetics of the HL-A system. A summary of data from the 5th International Histocompatibility Testing Workshop. *Isr. J. Med. Sci.*, **9**, 1257.
13. Kissmeyer-Nielsen, F. (ed.) (1975) *Histocompatibility Testing, 1975*, Munksgaard, Copenhagen.
14. Thomson, G. & Bodmer, W. (1976) The genetic analysis of HLA and disease associations, (this volume).
15. Jennings, H. S. (1917) The numerical results of diverse systems of breeding, with respect to two pairs of characters, linked or independent, with special relation to the effects of linkage. *Genetics*, **2**, 97.
16. Robbins, R. B. (1918) Some applications of mathematics to breeding problems. II. *Genetics*, **3**, 73–92.
17. Fisher, R. A. (1958) *The Genetical Theory of Natural Selection*. 2nd Edition, New York, Dover.
18. Bodmer, W. F. & Felsenstein, J. (1967) Linkage and selection. Theoretical analysis of the deterministic two locus random mating model. *Genetics*, **57**, 237.
19. Karlin, S. & Feldman, M. W. (1970) Linkage and selection: Two locus symmetric viability model *Theoret. Population Biol.*, **1**, 39.
20. Thomson, G. (1977) The effect of a selected locus on closely linked neutral loci. *Genetics*, (in press).
21. Nei, W. & Li, W. H. (1973) Linkage disequilibrium in subdivided populations. *Genetics*, **75**, 213–219.
22. Feldman, M. W. & Christiansen, T. B. (1975) The effect of population subdivision on two loci without selection. *Genet. Res.*, **24**, 151–162.
23. Degos, L. & Dausset, L. (1974) Human migrations and linkage disequilibrium of HL-A system. *Immunogenetics*, **3**, 195–210.
24. Bodmer, J. G., Rocques, P., Bodmer, W. F., Colombani, J., Degos, L., Dausset, J. & Piazza, A. (1973) Joint report of the fifth International Histocompatibility Workshop. In: *Histocompatibility Testing, 1972*, eds. Dausset, J. & Colombani, J., p. 619. Munksgaard, Copenhagen.
25. Degos, L. & Bodmer, W. F. (1973) The effects of inbreeding on a two locus

system. In: *Histocompatibility Testing 1972*, eds. Dausset, J. & Colombani, J., p. 545. Munksgaard, Copenhagen.

26. Bodmer, W. F. (1973) Population Genetics of the HL-A System: Retrospect and Prospect. In: *Histocompatibility Testing, 1972*, eds. Dausset, J. & Colombani, J., p. 611, Munksgaard, Copenhagen.

27. Bodmer, W. F. (1973) In: *Histocompatibility Testing 1972*, eds. Dausset, J. & Colombani, J., p. 667, Munksgaard, Copenhagen.

28. Cavalli-Sforza, L. L. (1972) Pygmies, an example of hunters-gatherers, and genetic consequences for man of domestication of plants and animals. In: *Human Genetics, Proc. IVth Int. Congr. Human Genetics 1971*, eds. de Grouchy, J., Ebling, F. J. G. & Henderson, I. W., p. 79. Excerpta Medica, Amsterdam.

29. Gibson, D. J., Glass, D., Carpenter, C. B. & Schur, P. H. (1976) Hereditary C2 deficiency, diagnosis and HLA gene complex associations. *J. Immunol.* **116**, 1065.

30. Gofton, J. P., Chalmers, A., Price, G. E. & Reeve, C. E. (1975) HL-A 27 and ankylosing spondylitis in B.C. Indians. *J. Rheumatol.*, **2**, 3.

31. Klein, J. & Shreffler, D. C. (1971) The H-2 model for the major histocompatibility systems. *Transplant. Rev.*, **6**, 3–29.

32. Stimpfling, J. H. (1971) Recombinations within a histocompatibility locus. *Ann. Rev. Genet.*, **5**, 121–142.

33. Bodmer, W. F. (1975) Evolution of HL-A and other major histocompatibility systems. *Genetics, 79*, 293.

34. Henning, R, Milner, R. J., Reske, K., Cunningham, B. A. & Edelman, G. M. (1976) Subunit structure, cell surface orientation and partial amino-acid sequences of murine histocompatibility antigens. *Proc. nat. Acad. Sci. (Wash.)*, **73**, 118.

35. Vitetta, E. S., Capra, J. D., Klapper, D. G., Klein, J. & Uhr, J. W. (1976) The partial amino acid sequence of an H-2K molecule. *Proc. nat. Acad. Sci. (Wash.)*, **73**, 980.

36. Silver, J. & Hood, L. (1976) Structure and evolution of transplantation antigens: Partial amino acid sequences of H-2K and H-2D alloantigens. *Proc. nat. Acad. Sci. (Wash.)*, **73**, 599.

37. Terhorst, C., Parham, P., Mann, D. L. & Strominger, P. L. (1976) Structure of HLA antigens: Amino acid and carbohydrate compositions and N-terminal sequences as four antigen preparations. *Proc. nat. Acad. Sci. (Wash.)*, **73**, 910.

38. Bridgen, J., Snary, D., Crumpton, M. J., Barnstable, C., Goodfellow, P. & Bodmer, W. F. (1976) Isolation and N-terminal amino acid sequence of membrane-bound human HLA-A and HLA-B antigens. *Nature (Lond.)*, **261**, 200.

39. Nathenson, S. G., Brown, J. K., Ewenstein, B. M., Rajan, T V., Freed, J. H., Sears, D. W., Mole, L. E. & Scharff, M. D. (1976) Studies of the chemical basis of variability and the complex cellular expression of the H-2K and H-2D products. In: *The role of Products of the Histocompatibility Gene Complex in Immune Responses*, eds. Katz, D. H. & Benacerraf, B., p. 647. Academic Press Inc., New York.

40. Snary, D., Barnstable, C. J., Bodmer, W. F., Goodfellow, P. N. & Crumpton, M. J. (1976) Cellular distribution purification and molecular nature of human Ia antigens. *Scand. J. Immunol*, (in press).

41. Barnstable, C. J., Jones, E. A., Bodmer, W. F., Bodmer, J. G., Arce-Gomez, B., Snary, D. & Crumpton, M. (1976) Genetics and serology of HLA linked human Ia antigens. *Cold Spring Harbor Symp. on Quantitative Biology*, vol. **41**, (in press).

42. Gally, J. A. & Edelman, G. M. (1972) The genetic control of immunoglobulin synthesis. *Ann. Rev. Genet.*, **6**, 1.

43. Moller, G. (ed.) (1976) *Transplant. Rev.*, **30**.

44. Schreiber, R. D. & Muller-Ebehard, H. J. (1974) Fourth component of human complement: Description of a three polypeptide chain structure. *J. exp. Med.*, **140** 1324.

45. Ferrone, S., Pellegrino, M. A. & Cooper, N. R. (1974) Expression of C4 on human lymphoid cells and possible involvement in immune recognition phenomena. *Science*, **193**, 53–55.

46. Lachman, P. J. & McDonnell, I. (1976) Complement and cell membranes. *Transplant. Rev.* **32**, 72.

47 Howard, J. C. (1976) H-2 and HLA sequences. *Nature (Lond.)*, **261**, 189.

295

Clinical Implications (Nosology, Diagnosis, Prognosis and Preventive Therapy)

J. Dausset

It is not necessary to emphasize the extreme importance of the numerous association of HLA with diseases and the perspectives which they open up, not only in the understanding of the normal function of the genes of the HLA complex and of the physiopathology of numerous diseases which up till now have remained a mystery, but also in the daily practice of medicine. It is especially to these clinical implications that this chapter is devoted. It will deal successively with epidemiological implications, nosological, diagnostic, prognostic, and finally therapeutic and social aspects.

It is remarkable to consider that these different associated diseases have certain general features in common which enable us to draw a type of "identikit picture" (Table 1). They are all of unknown physiopathogeny. For none of them is there a causal agent known to exist for certain, although often nonidentified viruses can be suspected. They are most often hereditary diseases but with weak polyfactorial and very likely polygenic penetrance. Susceptibility to disease is transmitted within families, but the segregation does not follow simple Mendelian laws. We note the

Institut de Recherches sur les maladies du Sang, Hôpital Saint-Louis 2, Paris – Xe.

frequent immunological abnormalities which sometimes concern cellular infiltrations in the tissue lesions, or else anti-virus circulating antibodies, or very often anti-organ antibodies which have autoantibody characteristics.

The evolution is sub-acute or even chronic, and only seldom concerns a vital prognosis before adult age, so consequently has little or no impact on reproduction and selection.

In spite of these common features, it is possible to classify the diseases in three broad categories according to their degree of association with one or another locus or gene in the HLA complex. In the first category, there is a very strong association with an HLA-B locus antigen, as in the case of ankylos-

TABLE I

"Identikit picture" of an HLA-associated disease

- Unknown physiopathogenicity
- No known agent (viral?)
- Very often hereditary but weak penetrance (polyfactorial or polygenic?)
- Not simple mendelian segregation
- Many immunological abnormalities:
    - Cellular infiltration
    - Anti-virus antibodies
    - Anti-organ autoantibodies
- Subacute or chronic course
- Weak or no effect on reproduction (weak or no selective effect)

ing spondylitis. In the second category, the association is stronger with HLA-D than with HLA-B. This is the case with a number of auto-immune diseases, diabetes and coeliac disease. In the third category, the linkage occurs owing to a defect in a gene present in the HLA complex but not belonging to the HLA loci. This is the case for the genes controlling C2 or C4 and perhaps IgE. Finally, there is the possibility of a fourth type, where the association is found especially with an HLA-A locus antigen, as in idiopathic hemochromatosis.

In the first category, typified by ankylosing spondylitis and associated syndromes, the disease is usually familial and of incomplete penetrance. There is male predominance, and the disease appears to be dominant. The presence of B27 in only one dose is apparently sufficient. There is no known causal agent; however, certain bacterial infec-

tions evidently play a role in the initiation of Reiter's syndrome. There is no major immunological disorder.

In all the world's populations, the disease is associated with B27. Particularly in the Japanese, in spite of a very low frequency of B27, this antigen is, however, present in 66 per cent of patients (Figure 1). There is also a smaller percentage of patients with B27 among the American Blacks, suggesting that the susceptibility is not monogenic (1–5). The strange distribution of B27 in the northern hemisphere, which could not be pure chance, may be noted in passing.

The characteristics of diseases in the first category are in contrast to those of the second category, where the diseases are especially associated with HLA-D or even more strongly with a gene coding for the B-lymphocyte specificities (analogous to Ia in the mouse). There is often a marked familial cha-

B27 AND ANKYLOSING SPONDYLITIS

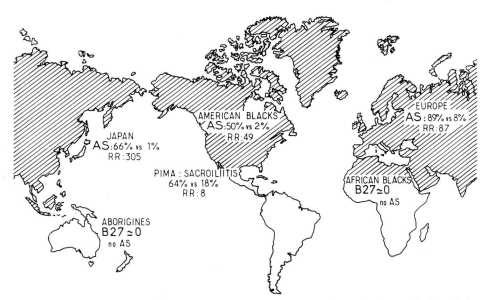

Figure 1. Distribution of B27 in the world. B27 is practically absent in the population of the southern hemisphere. The frequencies of B27 in ankylosing spondylitis (AS) or sacroiliitis patients *versus* controls are given for some populations, as well as the relative risk (RR).

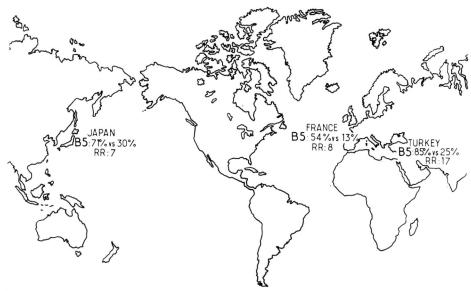

Figure 2. B5 is found in all populations of the world already tested. Behçet's disease is common in Turkey, but is not rare in other populations. The B5 frequencies in patients *versus* controls are given, as well as the relative risk (RR).

racteristic. Their penetrance is, however, incomplete. In this case it is often the woman who is diseased. Sometimes a clear dosage effect can be observed with a tendency to recessivity. Here again there is no known causal agent but rather a viral agent is more strongly suggested, and there are numerous immunological abnormalities of an autoimmune character.

Indeed, this category includes many so-called autoimmune diseases, such as myasthenia gravis, Graves' disease, Addison's disease, Sjögren's syndrome, chronic active hepatitis, and possibly lupus erythematosus. However, truly autoimmune diseases, such as Hashimoto's disease or autoimmune hemolytic anemia are not included in this list. In coeliac disease, diabetes, and multiple sclerosis, autoimmune processes are strongly suspected. The cellular infiltration of psoriasis could also perhaps be interpreted in this light.

When the HLA-B marker is distributed throughout the world, as is the case with B5, the same association is found in Japan as in Europe (Figure 2). This is the case for Behçet's disease (6, 7, 8), for which the relative risk is about the same everywhere. When the distribution of the antigen is very different, as is the case with B8, then a different association exists. In the Japanese (Figure 3) Graves' disease is associated with BW35 and not B8, which does not exist in this population (9). If multiple sclerosis is taken as an example, it can be seen that this disease is very rare in the Japanese, as is B7, which is a Caucasoid gene. It is interesting to note that the incidence of multiple sclerosis diminishes as one goes from the north to the south of Europe, which corresponds to the decreasing frequency of B7 (Figure 4).

Finally, the third category depends on non-HLA genes, but only those

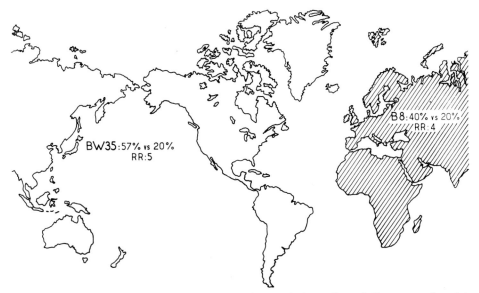

B8:40% vs 20%
RR:4

BW35:57% vs 20%
RR:5

Figure 3. B8 is practically absent from Mongoloid populations. Graves' disease was found to be associated with B8 in Caucasoids, and with BW35 in Japanese. Frequencies of the corresponding antigens are given in patients *versus* controls, as well as the relative risk (RR).

B7, DW2 AND MULTIPLE SCLEROSIS

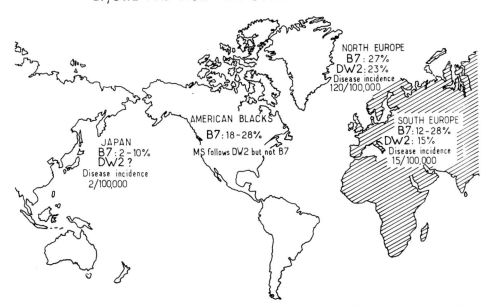

NORTH EUROPE
B7: 27%
DW2: 23%
Disease incidence
120/100,000

AMERICAN BLACKS
B7: 18-28%
MS follows DW2 but not B7

JAPAN
B7: 2-10%
DW2 ?
Disease incidence
2/100,000

SOUTH EUROPE
B7: 12-28%
DW2: 15%
Disease incidence
15/100,000

Figure 4. B7 is practically absent from Mongoloid populations. The incidence of multiple sclerosis roughly follows the frequency of B7 in the various populations. Multiple sclerosis is even more closely associated with DW2 than with B7.

299

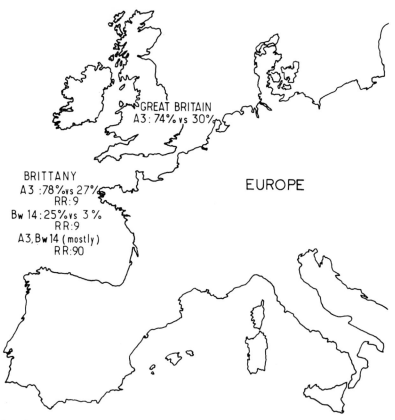

GREAT BRITAIN
A3 : 74% vs 30%

BRITTANY
A3 :78% vs 27%
RR:9
Bw 14:25% vs 3%
RR:9
A3,Bw14 (mostly)
RR:90

EUROPE

Figure 5. Idiopathic hemochromatosis is common in Brittany. It has been found to be associated with A3 and BW14, and mostly with the haplotype A3, BW14. The same association with A3 has been found in Great Britain. Frequencies in patients *versus* controls are given, as well as the relative risk (RR).

strongly linked to HLA. Here the familial transmission of disease is obvious. There is almost total penetrance, no predominance in either sex, and a very strong dosage effect, sometimes reaching recessivity. There is no known agent, but pathological mutation of a gene of the region is highly likely, the typical example being the C2 deficiency which leads to immunological disorders.

It is likely that the linkage described in some allergic families belongs to this third category. Then the disease follows a certain haplotype in a family, without there being any special association in the population with an HLA gene.

It is possible that a localized mutation is responsible for hemochromatosis, which is found in Brittany and England, associated with A3 (10–12, Figure 5). A remarkable observation is that these broad categories correspond so closely to three major mechanisms which will be discussed later in this volume.

– in Category 1, very close to HLA-

TABLE II
Nosological clustering around B27 (see text)

B27 associated diseases		B27 nonassociated diseases	
	%	Chronic	Acute
AS	89	Crohn's disease	Dysentery { Yersinia
Sacroilitis	25–70	Ulcerative colitis	Shigella
Reiter's	78	Psoriasis	Salmonella
Anterior uveitis	43		
Frozen shoulder	42		Nonspecific urethritis
JRA	31		Nonspecific conjunctivitis
		50 %	70 %
		of B27 among patients who developed AS or Reiter's	
Asbestosis	18–27		

B, there is a possibility that the direct intervention of the HLA molecule itself may be modified by an external agent; this is the theory of the altered self;

– in Category 2, closer to HLA-D, there is a possible disorder to the immune-response gene, leading to an abnormality in the immunological response;

– in Category 3, there is a pathological alteration of a metabolic gene linked to HLA.

One of the benefits already acquired from the discovery of the associations between HLA and disease is in the field of *nosology*. Already the clustering, or sometimes on the contrary, subdivision of diseases or syndromes has been made possible.

Among the more obvious clusterings is that of arthritis associated with B27. Indeed, it has been known for a long time that there was a close link between Reiter's syndrome, anterior uveitis, and ankylosing spondylitis, but there were no more than clinical observations to support this statement. It is now known that a common genetic denominator exists. There is at least one common gene which involves a susceptibility to this family of diseases. On the left of Table II are listed the diseases which are definitely associated with B27, and on the right, the symptoms or diseases which are frequently encountered in the same patient although B27 is not prevalent. In the left-hand list, the frequency of B27 among the patients goes in decreasing order from ankylosing spondylitis to juvenile rheumatoid arthritis. Anterior uveitis is frequently observed with the disorders. All these diseases concern sacro-spinal articulation, with one particularly interesting exception, frozen shoulder (13), situated outside the spinal zone. This disease could be singularly instructive in the understanding of the underlying mechanisms. The diseases given on the right are not associated with B27, at least when they are primitive and isolated, but when they occur by chance in a B27 individual, they favor or reveal sacro-spinal lesion. Some of these are chronic, namely Crohn's disease, ulcerative colitis, and psoriasis, which favors ankylosing spondylitis in particular. Others are acute, such as dysentery due to yersinia, shigella or salmonella, or such as nonspecific urethritis or conjunctivits, which

301

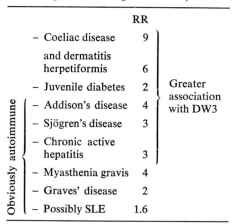

TABLE III		
Nosological clustering around B8, DW3		
	RR	
– Coeliac disease	9	
and dermatitis herpetiformis	6	
– Juvenile diabetes	2	Greater association with DW3
– Addison's disease	4	
– Sjögren's disease	3	
– Chronic active hepatitis	3	
– Myasthenia gravis	4	
– Graves' disease	2	
– Possibly SLE	1.6	

(Obviously autoimmune brace spanning Addison's through Chronic active hepatitis; Myasthenia gravis through Possibly SLE bracketed as obviously autoimmune)

B8 is common to all these diseases. However, in a given family the disease is often the same.

TABLE IV
Nosological clustering around C2 gene defect
Mostly associated with BW18 and frequently with AW25, BW18, DW2 haplotypes
– Failure to clear immune complexes
– Familial, recessive C2 deficiency
– SLE-like syndrome
– Some forms of multiple sclerosis

mostly enhance Reiter's syndrome. One should also mention here the strange observation of the association of B27 with asbestosis (14, 15), which, however, has no apparent relationship with rheumatology.

The second large clustering is formed around B8 and DW3 (Table III). Here, almost all the diseases of the second category are assembled. The relative risk is given for each of them. The risk is particularly high for coeliac disease and dermatitis herpetiformis; there is a lesser risk, around three of four, for the other diseases. It is doubtful for systemic lupus erythematosus. For most of these diseases, except the latter three, it has already been shown that the association is stronger with the DW3 gene than with B8. Nevertheless, if the association with B8 is common to all these diseases in a given family, the same disease will be observed. This is, however, not always the case. In diabetic families autoimmune diseases like Graves' disease sometimes appear.

Another clustering is becoming apparent, that of diseases with C2 defi-

ciency, mostly associated with the haplotypes AW25, B18, DW2 (Table IV). The most obvious is the recessive disease, or lupic syndrome, with or without nephopathy, due to a partial C2 deficiency or even to certain forms of multiple sclerosis (16–21).

More practical perhaps are the subdivisions which have been established through HLA associations. In this way, possibly recessive juvenile familial diabetes is distinguished from the adult diabetes which is not associated with HLA. It is also distinguishable from the dominant juvenile form for which onset is as in the mature form. This particular form may segregate with the HLA haplotypes. Myasthenia is divided into two distinct forms: one with hyperplasia associated with B8, the other with thymoma and anti-muscular antibody. Juvenile rheumatoid arthritis could include particular forms: one associated with B27 which might evolve into ankylosing spondylitis, the other which might rather be compared with chronic arthritis, not associated with B27 but possibly with DW4, like chronic arthritis. In the same way, psoriasis has two forms: one without arthritis, the other with arthritis, either peripheral or axial. The distribution of the HLA antigens is not the same in these two forms, There is a predominance of B27 in the axial form. The impact of these clusterings or subdivisions is obvious.

The interest of the clinician is also attracted towards the *diagnostic aspects*.

Already, in some specific cases, determination of the HLA types helps the clinician.

By virtue of its exceptional strength, it is the B27 association which contributes most to the rheumatologists for sero-negative arthritis, and more especially for the early diagnosis of Reiter's syndrome in its peripheral or oligoarticular forms and in the assymmetrical forms (22); for the diagnosis of the incomplete forms of ankylosing spondylitis or Reiter's syndrome in the presence of back pain of an inflammatory type sensitive to phenyl butazone; and for the radiological diagnosis between spondylitis and Forestier's disease. It must be emphasized, however, that the value of B27 is not absolute, since there are five per cent false negative results among the patients and eight to ten per cent false positive results among the healthy population (23–26). The next in order of interest is the determination of B5 for the diagnosis of Behçet's disease, especially in its forms masked by corticotherapy or its incomplete forms. Furthermore, the presence of B8 and especially of DW3 could help the diagnosis of difficult forms of Addison's disease, coeliac disease, or other autoimmune diseases. The presence of B7, DW2 will assist diagnosis of atypical forms of multiple sclerosis, and the presence of BW35 will perhaps enable the investigator to distinguish between Quervain's thyroiditis and Hashimoto's disease. The presence of B18, DW2 will be useful for the heterozygous C2 deficiency. Lastly, the presence of A3 could help diagnose early or incomplete forms of hemochromatosis.

In addition to these few examples, the associations with the HLA-A or -B locus antigens are still too weak to be a definite aid to the clinician faced with an isolated non-familial case.

On the other hand, the diagnostic interest becomes considerable in families already afflicted by a particular disease. Thus, susceptible children can be detected early. Conversely, by calculating the risk, a distressed family could be reassured.

On the *prognostic* level, it is interesting to observe that it is often the earliest forms which are most strongly associated with HLA (27–32). In juvenile diabetes, more than 80 per cent of patients possess either B8, B15 or B18 when the onset of the disease is between birth and ten years (32). This percentage decreases with increasing age at onset (Figure 6). The presence of one of the antigenic markers seems, therefore, to favour early development of the illness.

However, the most important concept on the prognostic level is given by the determination of the HLA type of a patient with an accompanying syndrome which favors the development of the disease. It is of prime importance in isolated anterior uveitis. Crohn's disease, isolated ulcerative colitis or isolated optic neuritis, to determine the HLA type of the patient. The presence of B27 indicates an increased risk of ankylosing spondylitis or Reiter's syndrome. The presence of B7, DW2 raises the frightening prospect of multiple sclerosis (33).

The third element of prognosis is to be found in the genotype, and no longer in the simple HLA phenotype. Indeed, the homozygosity for the predisposing antigen seems to indicate a more severe form. This has been noted in myasthenia gravis (34) and chronic active hepatitis (35). In the case of diabetes, for example, where two antigens B8 and B15 (or B8 and B18, personal observation) are involved, the coexistence of these two genes in the same individual increases the risk (36). Finally, this notion of dosage effect is also shown in the diabetic by the excess pairs of HLA-identical sibs, both diseased, compared

B8, BW15 and B18 in 90 diabetic patients according to age at onset of the disease.

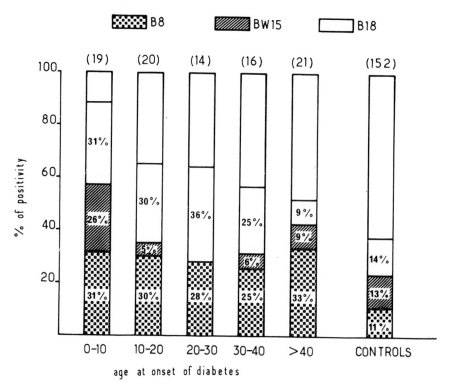

Figure 6. Correlation between age of onset of insulin-dependent diabetes and HLA associations. The association is stronger in early onset cases, especially for BW15. The difference between the first and fifth columns is statistically significant (p < 0.01) (32).

with other pairs of sibs (HLA-semi-identical or different sibs). Thus in one sibship the HLA-identical brothers or sisters of a child already suffering from diabetes have a much greater risk than the other sibs.

Are all these observations and considerations purely speculative or do they have immediate *therapeutic* and useful consequences for patients? A certain number of therapeutic measures, while certainly still limited, have come out of these studies. The systematic detection of ankylosing spondylitis could allow the choice of a sedentary profession and the initiation of early treatment in order to avoid disabilities. Similarly, the

detection of individuals susceptible to diabetes could avoid the major causes of onset or deterioration of the disorder, such as obesity, corticotherapy, the taking of oral contraceptives, and so on. In Behçet's disease, corticotherapy could be prescribed at the appearance of the first symptoms and before the appearance of serious symptoms. In myasthenia gravis, the indication of thymectomy could be facilitated.

It is certainly in *pediatrics* that the interest is greatest, since it will be possible from now on to distinguish the susceptible children in a sibship, and even those who are most susceptible. The children susceptible to diabetes and coeliac disease will be especially watched, and an appropriate diet will be given to them. It can thus be hoped that a normal structural development will be possible and a balanced life assured. The care of familial hemochromatosis will allow the initiation of early treatment by bleeding and chelators.

The diagnostic and therapeutic consequences are still as yet of modest proportions, but one can predict with certainty that they will be extended according to future discoveries. The service that biologists will be able to render to patients will be more and more evident when the gene marker is more closely associated to the susceptibility gene. The trail has already been blazed in multiple sclerosis. For example, the first association found was with HLA-A3. It was weak. With B7 it was much stronger, and with DW2 stronger still. Perhaps with a gene coding for a B-lymphocyte specificity, it will be even more closely associated with the susceptibility gene (37).

It is also probable that in polygenic illness, biologists will discover markers of several suceptibility genes in the same disease. The coexistence of two markers in the same individual will then have a high prognostic value. It is therefore in the future, but most probably in the near future, that these discoveries will find all their practical importance, and that collective treatments of *preventive medicine* will be put into practice.

For serious hereditary diseases like multiple sclerosis or even diabetes, the doctor will be able to help parents with wise *eugenic counselling*. In the most dramatic cases, *abortion* could even be accepted for fetuses carrying the antigen marker. In veterinary practice, one could use the haploid expression of the histocompatibility antigen on spermatozoa to practice *artificial insemination* after elimination of spermatozoa carrying a defect, in order to avoid, for example, big bovine epizoties, and why should this not also be applied to human beings, in the case of severe associated diseases (38)?

Lastly, if in the future it may be possible to *vaccinate* a population against an infectious agent whose susceptibility is associated with HLA, one can visualize the priority vaccination of susceptible individuals.

The social impact of these studies can be easily seen, and could lead to a *specific and personalized preventive medicine,* when it is known that out of 100,000 men, 4,000 will contract ankylosing spondylitis, and that at least 20 per cent of those who have no apparent trouble are nevertheless diseased, and that three per cent of the population is susceptible to diabetes.

However, it is clear that true progress will come with a better knowledge of the *etiology* of diseases.

Table V contains a list of germs which are involved in the different diseases associated with HLA (39, 40, 41). In the first category, closely linked with HLA-B, three germs are related to Reiter's syndrome, yersinia enterolitica, shigella and salmonella. All three are gram-negative bacteria but produce no crossreactions among themselves. They cause intestinal infection without having any association with HLA. However, those patients with B27 run a greater risk of developing a spinal disease. The histories of intoxication by shigella are very informative (42, 43). One which occurred in Finland and caused 1,500 cases of dysentery is especially instructive in this regard. A retrospective study has shown that among those intoxicated who have survived and developed ankylosing spondylitis, 39 out of 50 were B27.

Should it then be concluded that these germs are fully responsible for

TABLE V

Associated agents		Possible agents
Reiter's	Yersinia Shigella Salmonella Chlamydia?	(Inclusion in urethritis and conjunctivitis)
Multiple sclerosis	Measles	Paramyxovirus
Diabetes	Rubella	Coxsakie B (type 4)
	Mumps	
CA Hepatitis	Hepatitis virus B	
Psoriasis	Streptococcus	
Graves'	Yersinia?	

ankylosing spondylitis? Should it be thought that the intestinal infection was the door letting in the germ responsible? This conclusion would be premature, but there is no doubt about the existence of a link between these bacterial infections and the appearance of articular symptoms. Could it be assumed that in other case, a nonapparent infection has actually occurred?

By contrast, in the diseases of Category 2, strongly associated with HLA-D, one can only suscept viral agents, the coxsackie B type 4 in diabetes, a paramyxovirus in multiple sclerosis. There is no precise data for man. However, on the contrary in NZB mice (the model for autoimmunization), there is almost certainly a viral etiology, a copy of viral DNA being incorporated in the genome. It is not impossible that this model could be applied to man.

Another approach to the same problem consists of studying the *antibodies* which develop in the patients and their correlations with HLA types. Table VI summarizes the present data on this subject. The main fact is the great ability of individuals carrying B8 for humoral immunological response (44–49).

Among diabetics, the B8 individuals respond well against insulin and pancreatic islets. In Addison's disease they possess a high titer of anti-adrenal antibodies. Among polytransfused dialyzed patients, B8 individuals are more capable than others of rapid disposal of virus particles of the hepatitis B virus (50). The same B8-positive individuals pre-

TABLE VI

Humoral antibodies correlated with HLA antigens. Possible assimilation of B8 as high responders and B7 as low responders

B8 are high responders
- rapidly clear HbsAg
- high titer
  - anti-rubella, measles muscle and nuclear } Hepatitis
  - anti-insulin
  - anti-pancreatic islet } Diabetes
  - anti-adrenal   Addison
  - anti-gluten   Coeliac d.

B7 are low responders
- low titer
  - anti-thyroglobulin
  - anti-microsome } Grave
  - anti-insulin   Diabetes

Possible protective effect of B7 in diabetes, coeliac disease

ferentially develop autoimmune diseases, and a link probably exists between these two facts. If this were the case, the humoral hyperimmune response of the B8 individuals would not be favorable, on the contrary, detrimental. This reminds one, remarkably, of the observation made by Biozzi *et al.* (51) with the help of their mouse strains selected for their high or low humoral response. It is known that among Biozzi's mice, the high reponders are, paradoxically, very susceptible to the endocellular gram-negative germs, while the low responders are amazingly resistant. On the other hand, the high responders could easily be vaccinated against the *exocellular* germs which are not hidden in the cells. Biozzi interprets this phenomenon by talking of an enhancing antibody which protects the endocellular agent. Likewise, in man, besides the B8 high responders, the B7 individuals seem to constitute the group of low responders (52, 53). The B7 diabetic patients have a low titer of anti-insulin antibody and, curiously, the B7 antigen seems to protect against diabetes and also against coeliac disease, myasthenia gravis, psoriasis and even ankylosing spondylitis. It has still to be demonstrated that this decreased frequency in these patients is not merely due to the compensatory effect of the increase of another HLA-B antigen with a negative linkage disequilibrium.

Many links in the chain are missing. Very little is known of the quality of the cellular immune response in these patients. Is there a defect of cellular immunity in these B8 individuals (54, 55) or a hyperresponse? This information would help choose between two hypotheses:

– first, that the disease is due to the inability of the organism to clear a latent virus which is thus directly responsible for the trouble;

– secondly, that the potential virus serves only to initiate a self-maintained autoimmune process in a particularly predisposed genetic background.

It is certain that there is not just one single *mechanism*. The number of genes contained in the HLA complex is considerable, and they govern multiple and subtle immunological and nonimmunological processes. It is thus conceivable that the genetic defect may be very varied.

In conclusion, one can, from now on, state that the discovery of numerous associations between HLA and disease is on the verge of revolutionizing the understanding of certain physiological mechanisms and of a great number of pathological states.

These diseases are indeed true *natural experiments* which will enable biologists and clinicians to analyze the function of many genes of the human major histocompatibility complex, man's central immunological unit. In the first place, one can reasonably hope that the delicate mechanism of the normal human immune response may thus be studied with greater precision, and furthermore, that the means of defence against external aggression and somatic mutation leading to tumors, in particular, will be better understood. When a physiological mechanism is dismantled, the treatment of the corresponding disorders is within reach.

A second consequence is the genetic definition of these various diseases whose mystery was hidden, out of decency, under names like degenerative diseases, systemic diseases, collagen diseases, or even autoimmune diseases. The full benefit of such a precise genetic definition on a practical level have yet to be grasped. These new markers make it possible to detect susceptible individuals, calculate with accuracy the risks run by any one population of patients or any one individual, and thus initiate indispensable preventive measures.

Like all discoveries, this one introduces new limitations, wherein lies its greatness. The calculated knowledge of the personal risk run could perhaps develop a certain anxiety in the population; but this would probably be largely compensated for by a definitely increased efficiency in preventive medicine. Indeed, preventive medicine, which until now has been blind indiscriminative medicine, will henceforth be specific and, if it may be said, personalized, less expensive, and considerably more efficient.

References

1. Schlosstein, L., Terasaki, P. I., Bluestone, R. & Pearson, G. M. (1973) High association of an HL-A antigen, W27, with ankylosing spondylitis. *New Eng. J. Med.* **288**, 14, 704.
2. Shirakura, R., Mori, T., Shichikawa, K., Tsujimoto, M. & Manabe, H. (1976) Genetic significance of HLA B27 in AS. A study of 27 families. Abstract N° I–39, *HLA and Disease,* INSERM, Paris, vol 58.
3. Good, A. E., Kawanishi, H. & Schultz, J. (1976) HLA B27 in Blacks with ankylosing spondylitis or Reiter's disease. *New. Eng. J. Med.* **294**, 3, 166.
4. Khan, M. A., Kushner, I. & Braun, W. E. (1976) Low incidence of HLA-27 in American Blacks with AS. *Lancet* **i**, 483.
5. Calin, A., Bennett, P. H., Jupiter, J. & Terasaki, P. I. (1976) HLA B27 and sacroiliitis in Pima Indians. Abstract N° I–6, *HLA and Disease,* INSERM, Paris, vol. 58.
6. Ohno, S., Aoki, K., Sugiura, S., Nakayama, E., Itakura, K. & Aizawa, M. (1973) HL-A5 and Behçet's disease. *Lancet* **ii**, 1383.
7. Godeau, P., Torre, D., Campinchi, R., Bloch-Michel, E., Schmid, M., Nunez-Roldan, A., Hors, J. & Dausset, J. (1976)

8. Ersoy, F., Berkel, A. I., Firat, T. & Kazokoglu, H. (1976) HLA antigens associated with Behçet's disease. Abstract N° III–6, *HLA and Disease,* INSERM, Paris, vol. 58.
9. Grumet, F. C., Payne, R. O., Konishi, J., Mori, J. & Kriss, J. P. (1975) HLA antigens in Japanese patients with Graves' disease. *Tissue Antigens* **6**, 347.
10. Simon, M., Pawlotsky, Y., Bourel, M., Fauchet, R. & Genetet, B. (1975) Hémochromatose idiopathique, maladie associée à l'antigène tissulaire HLA-3? *Nouv. Presse Méd.* **4**, 1432.
11. Fauchet, R., Simon, M., Bourel, M., Genetet, B., Genetet, N. & Alexandre, J. L. (1976) Idiopathic haemochromatosis and HLA antigens. Abstract N° V–5, *HLA and Disease,* INSERM, Paris, vol. 58.
12. Kennedy, L. & Batchelor, J. R. (1976) HLA-A3 and idiopathic haemochromatosis. Abstract N° V–1, *HLA and Disease,* INSERM, Paris, vol. 58.
13. Bulgen, D. Y., Hazleman, B. L. & Voak, D. (197) HLA-B27 and frozen shoulder. *Lancet* **i**, 1042.
14. Merchant, J. A., Klouda, P. T., Soutar, C. A., Park, R., Lawler, S. D. & Turner-Warwick, M. (1975) The HL-A system in asbestos workers. *Brit. Med. J.* **1**, 5951, 189.
15. Matej, H. & Lange, A. (1976) HLA antigens in asbestosis. Abstract N° IX–16, *HLA and Disease,* INSERM, Paris, vol. 58.
16. Fu, S. M., Stern, R., Kunkel, H. G., Dupont, B., Hansen, J. A., Day, N. K, Good, R. A., Jersild, C. & Fotino, M. (1975) Mixed lymphocyte culture determinants and C2 deficiency: LD-7a associated with C2 deficiency in four families. *J. exp. Med.* **142**, 2, 495.
17. Gibson, D. J., Glass, D., Carpenter, C. B. & Schur, P. M. (1976) Hereditary C2 deficiency: diagnosis and HLA gene complex association *J. Immunol.* **116**, 1065.
18. Wolski, K. P., Schmid, F. R. & Mittal, K. K. (1975) Genetic linkage between the HL-A system and a deficit of the second component (C2) of complement. *Science* **188**, 4192, 1020.
19. Agnello, V. (1976) Association of C2 deficiency (C2D) and HLA genes with systemic and discoid lupus erythematosus (SLE, DLE). Abstract N° A–8, *HLA and Disease,* INSERM, Paris, vol. 58.

HLA-B5 and Behçet's disease. Abstract N° III–7, *HLA and Disease,* INSERM, Paris, vol. 58.

20. Noel, L. H., Descamps, B., Jungers, P., Bach, J. F., Busson, M., Guillet, J. & Hors, J. (1976) HLA serotyping in five well defined kidney diseases. Abstract N° VII–14, *HLA and Disease,* INSERM, Paris, vol. 58, and personal communication.

21. Bertrams, J., Opferkuch, W., Grosse-Wilde, H., Netzel, B., Rittner, Ch., Kuwert, E. & Schuppien, W. (1976) HLA linked C2 deficiency in multiple sclerosis (MS). Abstract N° A–7, *HLA and Disease,* INSERM, Paris, vol. 58.

22. Arnett, F. C., McClusky, O. E., Schacter, B. Z. & Lordon, R. E. (1976) Incomplete Reiter's syndrome: discriminating features and HL-A W27 in diagnosis. *Ann. Int. Med.* 84, 1, 8.

23. Calin, A. & Fries, J. F. (1975) Striking prevalence of ankylosing spondylitis in "healthy" W27 positive males and females. A controlled study. *New Eng. J. Med* 293, 17, 835.

24. Möller, E. & Olhagen, B. (1975) Studies on the major histocompatibility system in patients with ankylosing spondylitis. *Tissue Antigens* 6, 237.

25. Cohen, L. M., Mittal, K. K., Schmid, F. R., Rogers, L. F. & Cohen, K. L. (1976) Increased risk for spondylitis stigmata in apparently healthy HL-AW27 men. *Ann. Intern. Med.* 84, 1, 1.

26. Ceppellini, R. & Carbonara A. O. (1976) See Chapter 5 in this volume.

27. Fritze, D., Herman, C., Naeim, F., Smith, G. S. & Walford, R. L. (1974) HLA antigens in myasthenia gravis. *Lancet* i, 240.

28. van den Berg-Loonen, E. M., Dekker-Saeys, E. J., Meuwissen, S. G. M., Nijenhuis, L. E. & Engelfriet, C. P. (1976) Histocompatibility antigens and other genetic markers in ankylosing spondylitis and inflammatory bowel diseases. Abstract N° I–41, *HLA and Disease,* INSERM, Paris, vol. 58.

29. Svejgaard, A., Svejgaard, E., Staub-Nielsen, L. & Jacobsen, B. (1973) Some speculations on the associations between HLA and disease based on studies of psoriasis patients and their families. *Transplant. Proc.* 5, 1797.

30. Krulig, L., Farber, E. M., Grumet, F. G. & Payne, R. O. (1975) Histocompatibility (HL-A) antigens in psoriasis. *Arch. Dermatol.* 111, 857.

31. Shulman, L. E., Goldberg, M. A., Arnett, F. C. & Bias, W. B. (1973) Histocompatibility antigens (HL-A) in systemic lupus erythematosus (SLE). *Excerpta Medica* 229, 95.

32. Cathelineau, G., Cathelineau, L., Hors, J., Schmid, M. & Dausset, J. (1976) Les groupes HLA dans le diabète à début précoce. *Nouv. Presse Méd.* 9, 586.

33. Arnason, B. G. W., Fuller, T. C., Lehrich, J. R. Wray, S. M. (1974) Histocompatibility typing and measles antibodies in MS and optic neuritis. *J. Neurol. Sci.* 22, 419.

34. Feltkamp, T. E. W., van den Berg-Loonen, E. M., Nijenhuis, L. E., Engelfriet, C. P., van Rossum, A. L., van Loghem, J. J. & Oosterhuis, H. J. G. H. (1974) Myasthenia gravis, autoantibodies, and HL-A antigent. *Brit. Med. J.* 1, 131.

35. Page, A. R., Sharp, H. L., Greenberg, J. & Yunis, E J. (1975) Genetic analysis of patients with chronic active hepatitis. *J. Clin. Inv.* 56, 530.

36. Thomsen, M., Platz, P., Ortved Andersen, O., Christy, M., Lyngsøe, J., Nerup, J., Rasmussen, K., Ryder, L. P., Staub Nielsen, L. & Svejgaard, A. (1975) MLC typing in juvenile diabetes mellitus and idiopathic Addison's disease. *Transplant. Rev.* 22, 125.

37. Terasaki, P. I. & Mickey, M. R. (1976) A single mutation hypothesis for multiple sclerosis based on the HLA system. US/Japan Conference on Multiple Sclerosis, *Neurology* 2, 56.

38. Dausset, J., Colombani, J., Legrand, L. & Fellous, M. (1970) Genetics of the HL-A system. Deduction of 480 lymphocytes. *Histocompatibility Testing 1970,* p. 53. Munksgaard, Copenhagen.

39. Aho, K., Ahvonen, P., Lassus, A., Sievers, K. & Tiilikainen, A. (1973) HL-A antigen 27 and reactive arthritis. *Lancet* ii, 157.

40. Hakansson, U., Löw, B., Eitrem, R. & Winblad, S. (1975) HLA-27 and reactive arthritis in an outbreak of salmonellosis. *Tissue Antigens* 6, 366.

41. Leirisalo, M., Tiilikainen, A. & Laitinen, O. (1976) HLA phenotypes in rheumatic fever and yersinia arthritis. Abstract N° I–29, *HLA and Disease,* INSERM, Paris, vol. 58.

42. Sairanen, E. & Tiilikainen, A. (1975) HL-A27 in Reiter's disease following shigellosis. *Scand. J. Rheumat. suppl.* 8, Abstract N° 30–11.

43. Calin, A. & Fries, J. F. (1976) B27 and post-shigella Reiter's syndrome, an epidemic revisited. Abstract N° I–7, *HLA and Disease,* INSERM, Paris, vol. 58.

44. Schernthaner, G., Mayr, W. R. & Ludwig, H. (1976) HLA-antigens and autoimmunity in idiopathic Addison's disease. Abstract N° IV–24, *HLA and Disease,* INSERM, Paris, vol. 58.

45. Thorsby, E., Seegaard, E., Solem, J. M. & Kornstad, L. (1975) The frequency of major histocompatibility antigens (SD and LD) in thyrotoxicosis. *Tissue Antigens* **6**, 54.

46. Galbraith, R. M. & Batchelor, J. R. (1976) Enchanced antibody response in active chronic hepatitis in relation to HLA-B8 and HLA-B12 and porto-systemic shunting. *Lancet* **i**, 930.

47. Scott, B. B., Rajah, S. M., Swinburne, M. L. & Losowsky, M. S. (1974) HL-A8 and the immune response to gluten. *Lancet* **ii**, 374.

48. Eddleston, A. L. W F., Galbraith, R. M., Williams, R., Pattison, J., Doniach, D., Kennedy, L. A. & Batchelor, J. R. (1976) HLA-B8 and B12 and enhanced antibody responses in chronic active hepatitis. Abstract N° V–4, *HLA and Disease,* INSERM, Paris, vol. 58.

49. Bertrams, J., Jansen, F. L., Gruneklee, D., Reis, H. E., Drost, H., Beyer, J., Gries, F. A. & Kuwert, E. (1976) HLA antigens and immune responsiveness to insulin in juvenile onset insulin-dependent diabetes mellitus. *Tissue Antigens* **8**, 13.

50. Bach, J. F, Zingraff, J., Descamps, B., Naret, C. & Jungers, P. (1975) HLA 1,8 phenotype and HBs antigenaemia in haemodialysis patients. *Lancet* **i**, 707.

51. Biozzi, G., Stiffel, G., Mouton, D. & Bouthillier, I. (1975) Selection of lines of mice with high and low antibody responsiveness to complex immunogenes. In: *Immunogenetics and Immunodeficiensy,* ed. Benacerraf, B., Medical and Technical Publications, Lancaster, England.

52. Ludwig, H., Schernthanen, G. & Mayr, W. R. (1976) Is HLA-B7 a marker associated with a protective gene in juvenile onset diabetes mellitus. *New Eng. J. Med.* **294**, 19, 1066

53. van de Putte, I., Vermylen, C., Decraene, P., Vlietinck, R. & van den Berghe, H. (1976) Segregation of HLA-B7 in juvenile onset diabetes mellitus. *Lancet* **ii**, 251.

54. Ciongoli, A. K., Platz, P., Dupont, B., Svejgaard, A., Fog, T. & Jersild, C. (1973) Lack of antigen response to myxoviruses in multiple sclerosis. *Lancet* **ii**, 1147.

55. Finkelstein, S., Walford, R. L., Myers, L. W. & Ellison, G. W. (1974) HL-A antigens and hypersensitivity to brain tissue in multiple sclerosis. *Lancet* **i**, 736.

Conclusions and Prospects

H. O. McDevitt*

Conclusions

As this volume indicates, the last few years have brought an extraordinarily rapid growth in knowledge of the role of the HLA system in disease susceptibility, and in the number and diversity of diseases which are associated with the HLA system [1, 2]. As the number of associations increases, a pattern emerges which permits some generalization. In most instances it seems clear that genes of the HLA system are only one of several genetic factors predisposing to a particular disease, and for the most part, the other genetic factors have not yet been identified. Apart from a few possible exceptions (e.g., ankylosing spondylitis) there are no instances in which the HLA or MLC type associated with the disease is found in all of the patients with that disease. Because knowledge of the genes in the HLA complex is so incomplete, it is not yet possible to determine whether these exceptions also reflect polygenic inheritance, or an inability to type for a rare disease susceptibility allele which is detected only through its linkage disequilibrium with an *HLA-B* or an *HLA-D* allele. Even if the latter possibility proves to be the case, it seems unlikely that all individuals bearing the disease-susceptibility gene will manifest the disease, because other genetic and environmental factors are required to permit the development of clinical detectable disease.

Almost all of the HLA and disease associations exhibit a dominant susceptibility effect. Since all of the genes in the HLA system are codominantly expressed, and all of the current theoretical mechanisms for association between HLA and disease would result in dominant inheritance, this generalization has been of little value in understanding the nature of these associations.

The most striking generalization to emerge from a survey of HLA and disease associations is that many, if not most, of the HLA and disease associations appear to be due to genes in the *HLA-D* region, or alternatively, to genes which show the strongest linkage disequilibrium with genes in this region [1, 2]. Frequently, as was the case with multiple sclerosis [3], a disease has initially been reported to be associated with an *HLA-A* or *-B* locus antigen. Further study has usually shown that the association with the HLA-B antigen is stronger, and where MLC typing has been performed, the disease association has frequently been shown to be strongest with an *HLA-D* allele.

* Division of Immunology. Department of Medicine. Stanford University School of Medicine, Stanford, California 94305. Supported in part by NIH Grants A1 07757 and A1 11313.

311

TABLE I

HLA and Disease Associations

Disease	B-Locus Association	B and D Association	D-Locus Assoc. Only
Rheumatoid arthritis			x
Ankylosing spondylitis	x		
Reiter's disease	x		
Diabetes mellitus		x	
Addison's disease		x	
Hyperthyroidism		x	
Multiple sclerosis		x	
Myasthenia gravis		x	
Gluten-sens. enteropathy		x	
Dermatitis herpetiformis		x	
Psoriasis	x	?	
Chronic active hepatitis		x	
Sjögren's syndrome		x	

Table I classifies some of the major HLA and disease associations with respect to the locus showing the strongest association. A few diseases, such as ankylosing spondylitis, Reiter's disease, and hemochromatosis (not listed) appear to be associated primarily with the HLA-B or -A allele (e.g., hemochromatosis [2]). A number of diseases show a definite association with an HLA-B locus allele, but an even stronger association with an HLA-D locus allele. This category includes multiple sclerosis, Addison's disease, and several others, and exemplifies the most rapidly expanding category of associations. Many of the diseases which are listed in this table as being associated with the B locus have not yet been tested for association with HLA-D alleles (as indicated with a question mark). At present, rheumatoid arthritis is the only disease which is associated with an HLA-D allele and shows no association with HLA-A or -B.

If most of these associations are due to the effect of genes in the HLA-D region, or to genes showing the strongest linkage disequilibrium with genes in the HLA-D region, it must first be assumed that the function of genes in the HLA-D region will provide clues to the mechanism of the association. However, knowledge of the function of genes in the HLA-D region is limited. Because genes in the D region determine the structure of antigens which elicit the mixed-lymphocyte culture reaction, it has been assumed that the HLA-D region is analogous to the I (immune-response) region in the mouse. In the mouse, it seems clear that the Ia antigens encoded by the I region are responsible for electing the mixed-lymphocyte culture reaction [4]. It is equally clear that the genes determining the structure of the Ia antigens are at present genetically inseparable from genes determining immune responsiveness (Ir genes) [4, 5], and immune suppression (Is genes) [6]. There is, in addition, considerable evidence that the Ia antigens are a part of antigen-specific T-cell-derived "receptor" molecules [7, 8].

The analogy between the HLA-D region and the I region in the mouse has led to the hypothesis that HLA-D locus disease associations are due to the effects of immune-response (Ir) or immune-suppression (Is) genes regulating the immune response to specific antigens. Since many of the HLA-D-associated diseases appear "autoimmune" in nature, this is an attractive and reasonable hypothesis. However, while it is probable that immune-response and immune-suppression genes underlie many HLA and disease associations, it should be noted that Ir genes have not yet been conclusively demonstrated in man. No real evidence on the function of genes in the HLA-D region has been produced, beyond their demonstrated role in determining the structure of cell-surface antigens eliciting the mixed-lymphocyte culture reaction. There is no information on the number of genes in the *HLA-D* region, on the genetic organization of this region, and on the relationship of genes in this region to genes determining the structure of complement components. Until disease susceptibility can be shown to be due to the effect of an HLA-linked *Ir* or *Is* gene, this mechanism must be regarded as likely, but unproven.

Such proof may be difficult to obtain, because it is already apparent from the murine model that *I*-region genes can mediate both help and suppression, and that for a number of antigens, two interacting genes are required to develop immune responsiveness or immune suppression [9–13]. Complete understanding of the system will probably require identification of the antigen (or agent, for example a virus) inducing disease, as well as typing reagents premitting detection of allelic variance at the several genetic loci which are presumed to exist within the human counterpart of the *I* region in the mouse. The techniques are presently not available for such studies.

While it is likely that genes controlling the immune response are a major cause of HLA and disease associations, it seems equally likely that many other mechanisms for HLA and disease associations will be found and proven to result in susceptibility to specific diseases. The association of idiopathic hemochromatosis with *HLA-A3* [2], and primary open-angle glaucoma with *HLA-B12* [2] provides examples in which it is difficult to postulate an effect due to genetic control of immune responsiveness. The demonstration by Zinkernagel, Shearer and others that the gene products of the *HLA-A* and -*B* loci are intimately involved in the specificity of T-cell-mediated cytotoxicity [2]; and by Chesebro and others that particular alleles of *H-2D* can have direct effects on viral replication which appear to be independent of the immune response [2], indicate the variety of effects of genes in the HLA system. There is evidence that intracellular cyclic-AMP levels [14], and testosterone levels [15] are correlated with *H-2* type in the mouse. These effects might be due to *H-2*-linked genes, or to the effects of different forms of the *H-2K* and *D* cell-surface proteins on other surface-receptor molecules. It therefore seems likely that the major histocompatibility system has a variety of other functions which have not yet been documented, but which might predispose to disease. It is certainly probable that there will be multiple mechanisms underlying HLA and disease associations.

Prospects

If the present situation is confusing, future prospects seem bright. In the very near future, one can expect rapid progress in clinical studies designed to resolve the question of whether particular HLA and disease associations are due to the effect of *HLA-A, -B, -C* or -*D* gene products, or to the effects of linked genes in linkage disequilibrium. While this information will be of considerable value, more precise typing techniques will be required to resolve many of these questions. It is clear from an examination of the recent progress in the functional and genetic analysis of the *H-2* system that one of the most exciting prospects for understanding HLA and disease associations lies in carrying out a similar analysis of the HLA system.

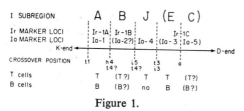

Figure 1.

Figure 1 is a schematic diagram of the postulated genetic organization of the *I* region of the *H-2* complex [16]. Analysis of standard inbred strains and congenic strains bearing recombinant *H-2* chromosomes have permitted a subdivision of the *I* region into five subregions. Four of these *(I-A, I-J, I-E, and I-C)* are known to code for Ia antigenic specificities. Three of these loci *(Ir-1A, Ir-1B,* and *Ir-1C)* are known to control immune responsiveness. Recent studies have indicated that two complementing genes in the *I* region, for example, in the *I-A* and *I-C* region, are required for immune responsiveness to a specific antigen [9]. Genes determining the development of immune suppression have also been localized to the *I* region [6]. In addition, it has also been found that two complementing genes are required for the development of immune suppression to certain antigens [13]. Recently it has become apparent that Ia antisera detect antigens found on the surface of suppressor T cells and on suppressor factors [16]. Analysis of strains bearing *H-2*-recombinant chromosomes indicate that these latter Ia specificities must lie between the *I-B* and *I-C* regions, and this has led to the definition of a new region, the *I-J* region. The *I-J* region determines the selective expression of Ia specificities on suppressor T lymphocytes. It is now clear that the *I* region is made up of several, and perhaps many genes, at least some of which are selectively expressed on functionally distinct lymphocyte subpopulations. *I-A-* and perhaps

I-C-region gene products appear to function in T-cell help, while *I-J*-region gene products function in T-cell immune suppression [16, 17].

Based on the *H-2* system, there is every reason to believe that the *HLA-D* locus or region in man is genetically as complex as the *I* region in the mouse. The next major step in analyzing the HLA system and its disease associations must therefore involve development of methods for subdividing the *HLA-D* region in a manner analogous to the genetic subdivision of the *I* region, and for identifying allelic variance of the multiple genes which must be included within the *D* region. It seems clear that some pregnancy sera contain antibodies which react with the human analogue of the murine Ia antigens [2]. We can therefore hope that analysis of this alloantigenic system will permit subdivision of the *HLA-D* region and identification of allelic variance at the component loci. The ability to type for *HLA-D* genes, coupled with studies of immune responsiveness, should permit conclusive demonstration and mapping of human *Ir* and *Is* genes and the assignment of specific functions to specific subregions of the *HLA-D* region.

The availability of such typing techniques will probably result in the detection of very strong associations between particular alleles of genes in the *HLA-D* region and particular diseases. At the same time, the availability of these methods should also permit the detection of association of particular alleles of genes within the *HLA-D* region with several diseases which are not yet known to be associated with the HLA system, because of the requirement in MLC typing that stimulator and responder cells share the same alleles for most of the genes in the *HLA-D* region.

If stronger associations, as well as

new associations, are discovered with *HLA-D*-typing techniques, this approach may well become extremely important in diagnosis and prognosis. In addition, the demonstration that genes known to be associated with genetic control of immune responsiveness are also associated with specific diseases should lead to a search for the environmental agent, whether it be a virus or toxin or other foreign antigen which is responsible for initiating the disease process.

Studies of the structure of the *HLA-A* and *-B* and, hopefully, of the *HLA-D* [18] gene products should deepen understanding of the nature of the extreme polymorphism in the HLA system, and might lead to new understanding of the function of the *HLA-A, -B* and *-D* gene products. As the understanding of the functions of these gene products increases, it should be possible to isolate these gene products and to study their function in artificial reconstituted systems. While this prospect is a long way off, it may well be necessary, before it is possible to understand how all of the gene products in the HLA system interact to regulate immune responsiveness, cell-mediated cytotoxicity, and such apparently unrelated parameters as hormone levels and intracellular cyclic-AMP levels. As the understanding of the genetic organization and function of the HLA system increases, it is almost certain to increase the understanding of the way in which this complex system contributes to susceptibility to such a wide variety of diseases.

References

1. Möller, G. (ed.) (1975) HLA and Disease *Transplant. Rev.* **22**, entire volume.
2. Dausset, J. & Svejgaard, A. (1976) *HLA and Disease* (entire volume). Munksgaard, Copenhagen.
3. Jersild, C., Fog, T., Hansen, G. S., Thomsen, M., Svejgaard, A. & Dupont,. B (1973) Histocompatibility determinants in multiple sclerosis with special reference to clinical course. *Lancet* **ii**, 1221–1225.
4. Shreffler, D. C. & David, C. S. (1975) The H-2 major histocompatibility complex and the I immune response region. Genetic variation, function, and organization. *Adv. Immunol.* **20**, 125–195.
5. McDevitt, H. O., Dead, B. D., Shreffler, D. C., Klein, J., Stimpfling, J. H. & Snell, G. D. (1972) Genetic control of the immune response: Mapping of the *Ir-1* locus. *J. exp. Med.* **135**, 1259–1278.
6. Debre, P., Kapp, J. A., Dorf, M. E. & Benacerraf, B. (1975) Genetic control of specific immune suppression. II. *H-2* linked dominant control of immune suppression by the random copolymer L-glutamic acid-L-tyrosine (GT). *J. exp. Med.* **142**, 1447.
7. Taussig, M. J., Munro, A. J. & Luzzati, A. L. (1976) *The Role of Products of the Histocompatibility Gene Complex in Immune Responses,* eds. Katz, D. H. & Benacerraf, B., pp. 541–552. Academic Press Inc., New York.
8. Tada, T. & Taniguchi, M. (1976) *The Role of Products of the Histocompatibility Gene Complex in Immune Responses,* eds. Katz D. H. & Benacerraf, B. pp. 506–512. Academic Press Inc., New York.
9. Dorf, M. E., Stimpfling, J. H. & Benacerraf, B. (1975) Requirement for two H-2 complex *Ir* genes for the immune response to the L-Glu, L-Lys, L-Phe terpolymer. *J. Exp. Med,* **141**, 1459.
10. Melchers, I. & Rajewsky, K. (1975) Specific control of responsiveness by two complementing *Ir* loci in the *H-2* complex. *Europ. J. Immunol.* **5**, 753.
11. Zaleski, M., Fuji, H. & Milgrom, F. (1973) Evidence for multigenic control of immune response to theta-AKR antigen in mice. *Transplant. Proc.* **5**, 201.
12. Rüde, E. & Günther, E. (1974) Genetic control of the immune response to synthetic polypeptides in rats and mice. *Prog. in Immunol. II* **2**, 223.
13. Debre, P., Waltenbaugh, C., Dorf, M. & Benacerraf, B. (1976) Genetic control of specific immune suppression III. Mapping of *H-2* complex complementing genes controlling immune suppression by random co-polymer L-glutamic acid[50]-L-tyrosine[50] (GT). *J. exp. Med.* **144**, 272.
14. Meruelo, D. & Edidin, M. (1975) Asso-

ciation of mouse liver adenosine 3':5'-cyclic monophosphate (cyclic AMP) levels with Histocompatibility-2 genotype. *Proc. nat. Acad. Sci. (Wash.)* **72**, 2644.

15. Ivanyi, P., Hampl, R.. Starka, L. & Mickova, M. (1972) Genetic association between *H-2* gene and testosterone metabolism in mice. *Nature (New. Biol.)* **283**, 280.

16. Murphy, D. B., Herzenberg, L. A., Okumura, K., Herzenberg, L. A. & McDevitt, H. O. (1976) A new *I* subregion *(I–J)* marked by a locus *(Ia-4)* controlling surface determinants on suppressor T lymphocytes. *J. exp. Med.* **144**, 699.

17. Okumura, K., Herzenberg, L. A., Murphy, D. B., McDevitt, H. O. & Herzenberg, L. A. (1976) Selective expression of *H-2 (I* region) loci controlling determinants on helper and suppressor T lymphocytes. *J. exp. Med.* **144**, 685.

18. Strominger, J. L., Chess, L., Humphreys, R. E., Mann, D., Parham, P., Robb, R., Schlossman, S., Springer, T. & Terhorst, C. (1976) *The Role of Products of the Histocompatibility Gene Complex in Immune Responses,* eds. Katz, D. H. & Benacerraf, B., pp. 621–643. Academic Press Inc., New York.